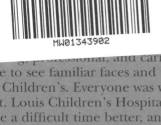

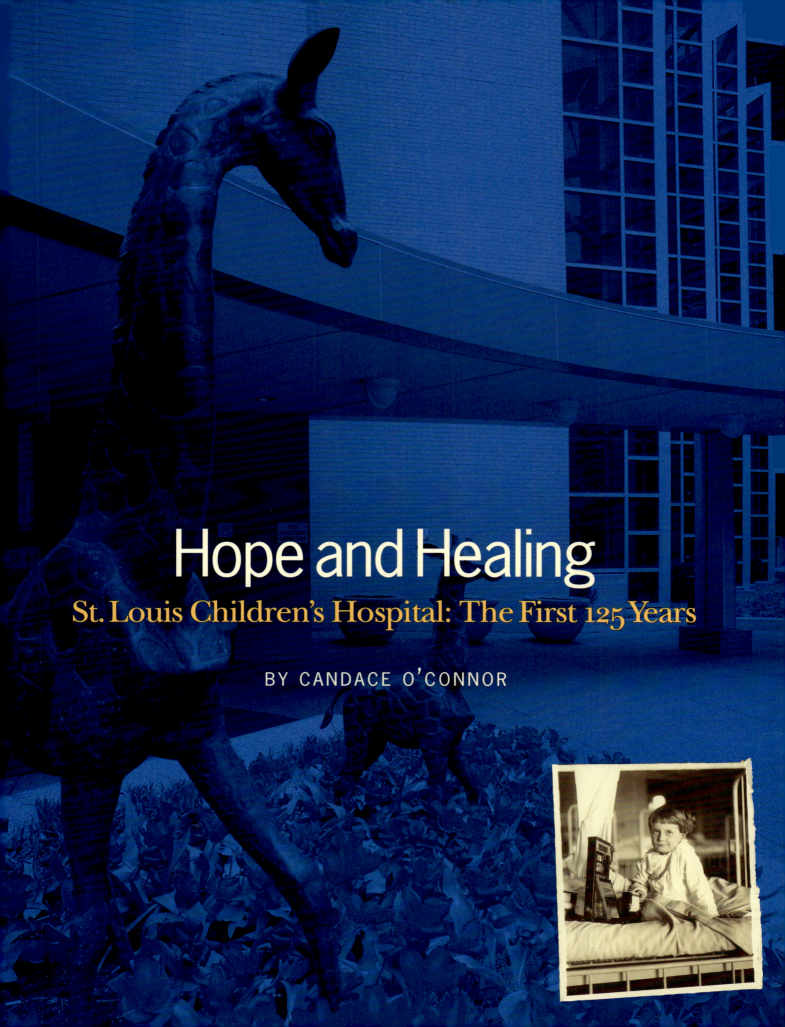

Copyright © 2006 by St. Louis Children's Hospital
All rights reserved
ISBN 0-9779339-0-3 (hardcover)
ISBN 0-9779339-1-1 (softcover)

No portion of this publication may be reproduced, stored in or introduced into a retrieval system, or transmitted, in any form or by any means (electronic, mechanical, photocopying, recording, or otherwise) without the prior written permission of St. Louis Children's Hospital.

PREVIOUS PAGE **Giraffe greeters.** These friendly animal sculptures welcome families, visitors and staff daily outside the ground level entrance to the hospital. Photo by John Twombly INSET **Young patient, ca. 1900s.** Becker Medical Library

NEXT PAGE **Exam time.** Toddler and care team, ca. 1940s. Becker Medical Library

TABLE OF CONTENTS

FOREWORD		by Lee F. Fetter and Charles W. Mueller	1
CHAPTER 1	1878-1884	"An Alluring Vision": Founding a Hospital for Children	2
		Homeopathic Medicine in St. Louis	14
CHAPTER 2	1884-1907	"A Sweeter Recompense": A Second Building for the Hospital	16
		Mrs. Jones and Mr. Brookings: Fellow Visionaries and Friends	32
CHAPTER 3	1907-1915	"Into the Promised Land": A New Beginning for the Hospital	34
		"The Magician": W. McKim Marriott	52
CHAPTER 4	1915-1936	"The Bold Experiment" Succeeds: W. McKim Marriott	54
		Marriott, Shaffer, Hartmann — and Insulin	76
CHAPTER 5	1936-1964	A Changing Pediatric World: The Alexis F. Hartmann Era	78
		Dr. David Goldring and the Gibbon-Mayo Heart-Lung Pump	100
CHAPTER 6	1964-1985	Personal Sacrifices: David Goldring and Philip R. Dodge	102
		Children's Hospital Nurses: "Devoted to the Care of Children"	128
CHAPTER 7	1985-1995	"Much Stronger National Force": A New Era of Leadership	136
		St. Louis Children's Hospital: Building "A Big Something"	156
CHAPTER 8	1995-2005	New Millennium: Synergy, Progress, and the Promise of Discovery	158
APPENDIX		Notable Faculty and Staff of St. Louis Children's Hospital and Washington University School of Medicine	182
ACKNOWLEDGMENTS			184
SELECTED BIBLIOGRAPHY			185
INDEX			186

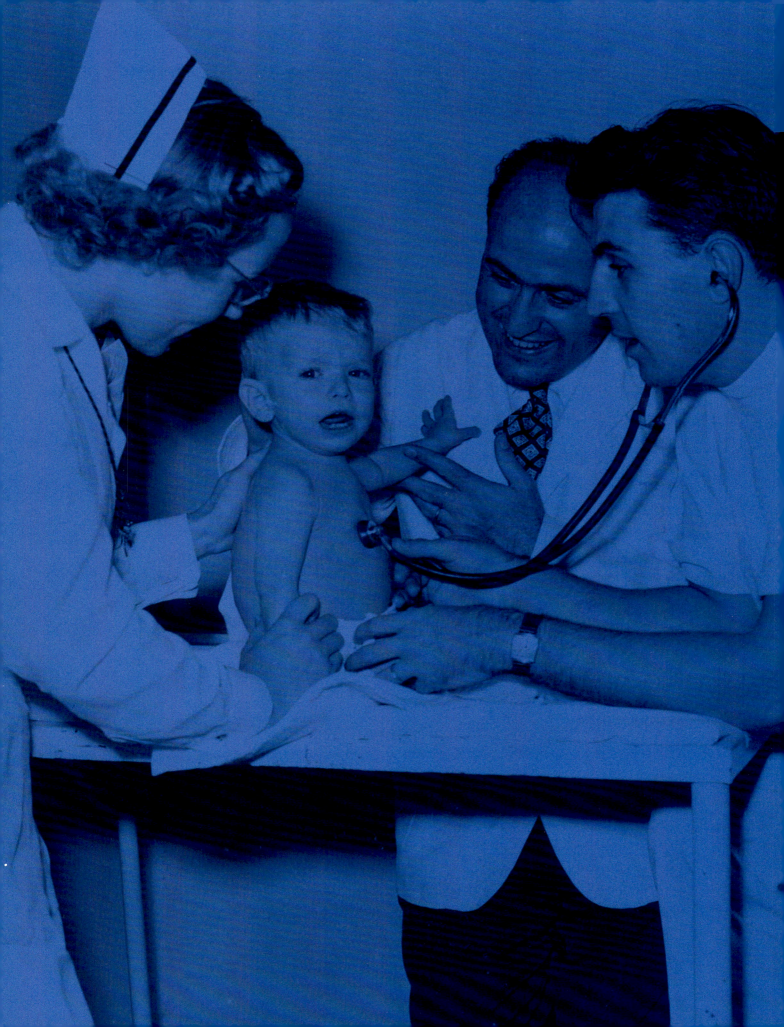

FOREWORD

This is a story of the people of St. Louis, and their love and dedication to children.

It is a story of how — over the past 125 years — our citizens, civic leaders, scientists, and caregivers have devoted their time, resources, and energy to providing a healthy life for kids.

The journey has not been easy. It has been filled with such deadly and debilitating roadblocks as typhoid, scarlet fever, diphtheria, tuberculosis, cholera, polio, encephalitis, diabetes, and cancer. In the early years of this journey, the statistics were grim: nearly 50 percent of children did not live to see their fifth birthday — a fact we can scarcely comprehend today. But medical discovery and technological advances, fueled by philanthropy and caring, have allowed more and more children to survive and prosper.

The history of St. Louis Children's Hospital is the story of pediatric medicine in St. Louis and in America. Over the last 13 decades and counting, individuals across our community have channeled abundant reserves of tenacity, vision, and compassion into making a difference for children.

It is this rich legacy of hope and healing that inspires us to continue the journey for the health of all children.

There are more young lives to save. Our work continues…

LEE F. FETTER
President
St. Louis Children's Hospital

CHARLES W. MUELLER
Chairman, Board of Trustees
St. Louis Children's Hospital

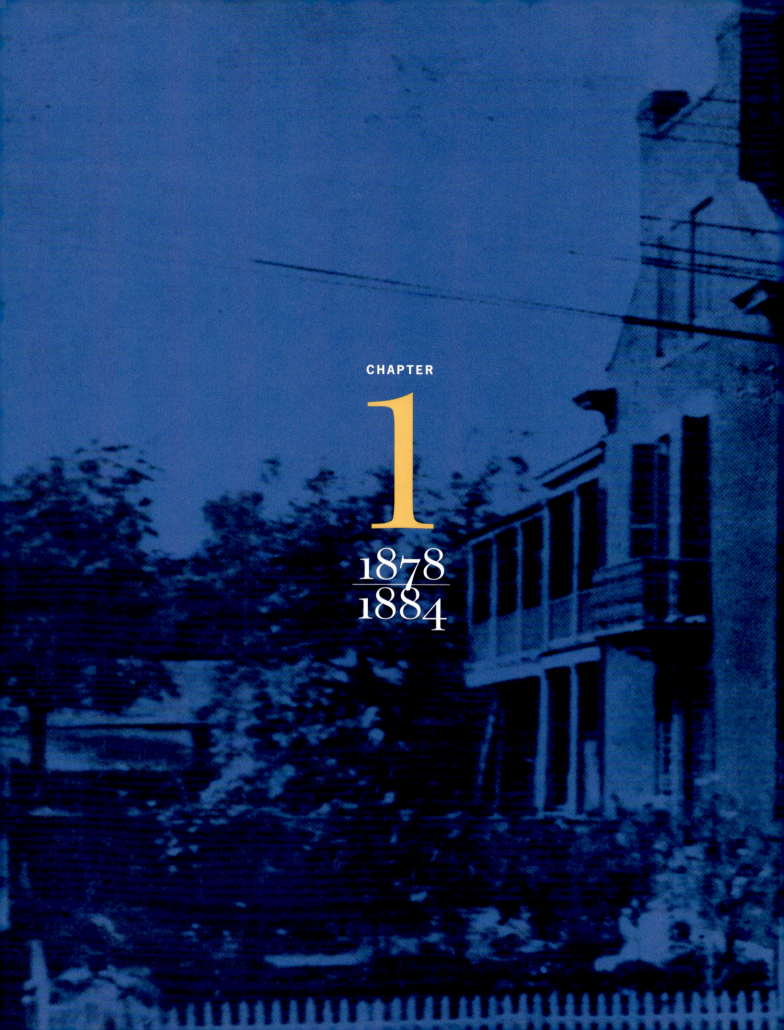

CHAPTER

1

1878
―――
1884

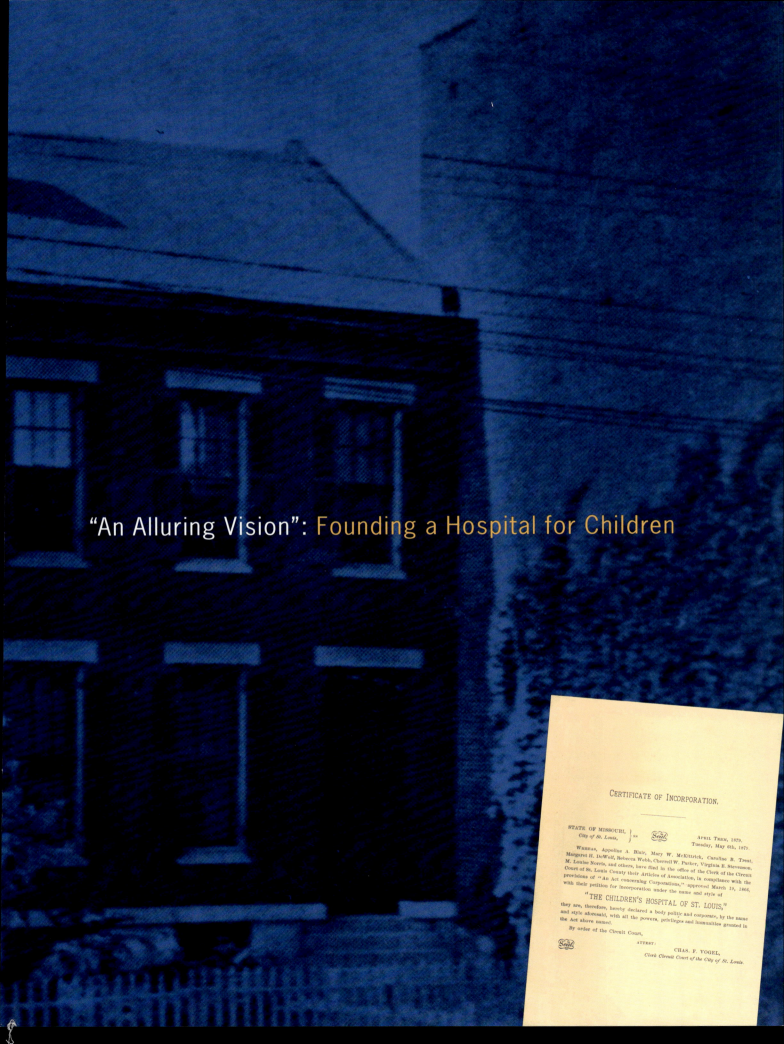

"An Alluring Vision": Founding a Hospital for Children

CERTIFICATE OF INCORPORATION.

STATE OF MISSOURI, } ss
City of St. Louis,

APRIL TERM, 1879.
Tuesday, May 6th, 1879.

WHEREAS, Appoline A. Blair, Mary W. McKittrick, Caroline B. Trest, Margaret H. DeWolf, Rebecca Webb, Cherrell W. Parker, Virginia E. Stevenson, M. Louise Norris, and others, have filed in the office of the Clerk of the Circuit Court of St. Louis County their Articles of Association, in compliance with the provisions of "An Act concerning Corporations," approved March 19, 1866, with their petition for incorporation under the name and style of

"THE CHILDREN'S HOSPITAL OF ST. LOUIS,"

they are, therefore, hereby declared a body politic and corporate, by the name and style aforesaid, with all the powers, privileges and immunities granted in the Act above named.

By order of the Circuit Court,

ATTEST:
CHAS. F. VOGEL,
Clerk Circuit Court of the City of St. Louis.

CHAPTER ONE "AN ALLURING VISION": FOUNDING A HOSPITAL FOR CHILDREN

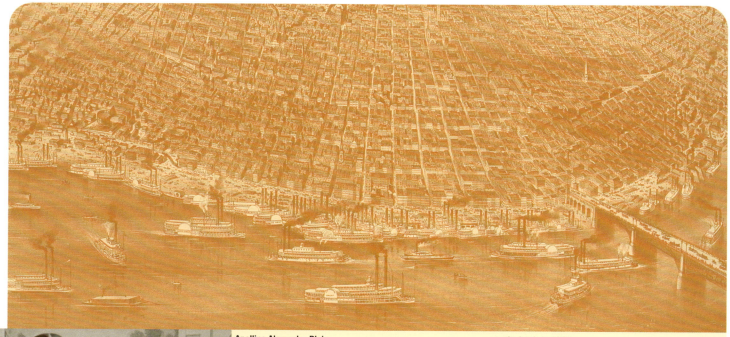

St. Louis in 1874.
Collection of A.G. Edwards & Sons, St. Louis

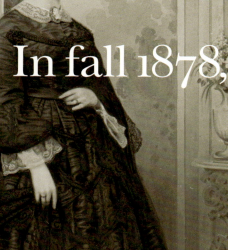

Apolline Alexander Blair (1828-1907). Widow of Frank Blair, a Civil War general and U.S. senator, Apolline Blair was president from the hospital's founding in 1879 until 1883, vice president to 1893, then "honorary president" until she died in 1907.
Becker Medical Library

In fall 1878, Apolline Alexander Blair received a visit from at least one — perhaps several — of the leading homeopathic physicians in St. Louis who had a proposal close to their hearts. They had often seen the suffering of children who were victims of injury or disease, compounded by poverty, malnutrition, and neglect. It was time, they said, to establish the first hospital in the city specially intended for such children. To bolster this effort, they would volunteer their help as attending physicians and consultants. Privately, they also planned to back the venture with a little money of their own; however, more financial help, and a board responsible for the hospital's day-to-day management, would certainly be needed.

PREVIOUS PAGE **First Hospital Building (1879-1884)** and **Certificate of Incorporation, 1879.** Becker Medical Library

1802
The first pediatric hospital is established in Paris: L'Hôpital des Enfants Malades.

1855
Children's Hospital of Philadelphia, the first pediatric hospital in the United States, is founded.

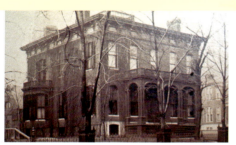

Blair home. The first meeting to discuss a hospital for children in St. Louis took place at the home of Francis and Apolline Blair at 2737 Chestnut Street. Becker Medical Library

RIGHT **Francis P. Blair, Jr. (1821-1875).** A St. Louis lawyer, Blair served terms as both a U.S. Congressman and a Senator and was appointed major general in the Union army. Courtesy of U.S. Senate Historical Office

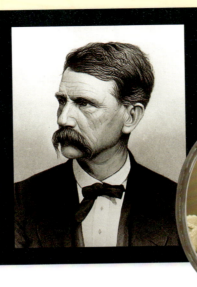

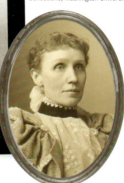

BELOW **Christine Biddle Blair Graham (1852-1915).** A board member of St. Louis Children's Hospital and a generous donor, Christine Graham was the only daughter of Apolline and Frank Blair who survived to adulthood. University Archives, Department of Special Collections, Washington University Libraries

The woman they were appealing to was well disposed to act upon their plea. The widow of Civil War general Francis P. Blair, Jr., she was an advocate of homeopathic medicine, a controversial form of treatment using tiny doses of drugs designed to stimulate the immune system by producing symptoms like those of the disease itself. Before his death in 1875, her husband had been treated by a prominent local homeopath, Edward C. Franklin, who became dean of the St. Louis-based Homeopathic Medical College of Missouri in 1876. That school had been founded in 1857 by homeopaths assisted by Frank Blair's older brother: attorney and state senator Montgomery Blair, who later served as postmaster general under Abraham Lincoln.

Like many women of her time, Apolline Blair had lost a child of her own to illness: six-year-old Eveline Martin Blair — seventh of her eight children and her second daughter — who died soon after her father in 1876. The painful memory of her death was still fresh in Mrs. Blair's mind when the physicians visited her two years later. And she was not the only one deeply affected by Eveline's death; her surviving daughter, Christine Blair Graham, widow of wealthy paper distributor Benjamin B. Graham, still remembered her young sister so acutely in 1915 that she supplied the funds for a new country hospital building for children, called the Eveline Blair Memorial.

Surely, Apolline Blair was also aware that well-to-do women across the United States — emboldened by their role in Civil War relief efforts — were actively taking part in a kind of humanitarian work that scholar Charles Rosenberg calls "pious activism," born both of *noblesse oblige* and religious responsibility. A particular focus of this movement was improving the welfare of children. Elizabeth Blair Lee, Apolline Blair's sister-in-law in the close-knit Blair family, was already manager of the Washington (D.C.) Orphan Asylum and would serve in this role for 57 years.

A MEETING OF PIONEERS
So on November 8, 1878, Apolline Blair followed up on the physicians' visit, inviting a group of friends to meet in the parlor of her home at 2737 Chestnut Street. The ten women in attendance, most of whom lived in the still-fashionable downtown district, seem to have been united mostly by proximity, social standing, and community spirit. One, Mary Foote Henderson — the wife of a former U.S. Senator, Gen. John B. Henderson — was described by a biographer as "a pioneer in the 'woman movement'" who "lent her active service to...new organizations designed to extend the sphere of woman's action and influence." Grace Allen, a young member of the gathering, was a daughter of the Blairs' next-door neighbor, Gerard B. Allen. The group was as diverse in religion as in age: among them were several Protestants and at least one Jew, Rose Harsh Fraley, wife of Moses Fraley, a founder of Temple Israel.

Four homeopathic physicians also attended, two of them named in later reminiscences as

1857

Homeopathic Medical College of Missouri is established in St. Louis.

1859

Good Samaritan Hospital in St. Louis opens its doors, staffed by homeopathic doctors.

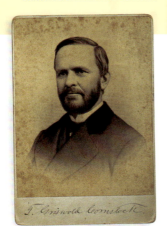

T. Griswold Comstock (1825-1909). One of the best educated and most successful of the local homeopaths, Comstock received a conventional medical degree, a homeopathic degree, and an advanced degree in obstetrics from the University of Vienna. At the Homeopathic Medical College of Missouri, he taught obstetrics; at Good Samaritan Hospital, he was a long-time senior attending physician. Becker Medical Library

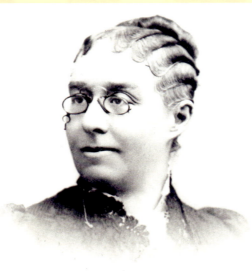

Mary W.C. McKittrick (1828-1908). Vice president under Apolline Blair, she served as board president from 1883 to 1907. A 1904 newspaper article said that "for twenty-five years (she) has been the gracious lady of the wards, not only cheering and helping the sick little ones with her personal attention, but exercising the wisest judgment and the most infinite tact in all that pertained to their welfare." Becker Medical Library

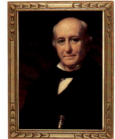

James Yeatman (1818-1901). A banker, railroad entrepreneur, and prominent Union supporter, he headed the Western Sanitary Commission during the Civil War and became a supporter of Children's Hospital. George Calder Eichbaum, Portrait of James G. Yeatman, 1890. Oil on canvas, 52-1/8" x 39-1/4". Mildred Lane Kemper Art Museum, Washington University in St. Louis. Gift of Joseph Gilbert Chapman.

> "...the word Hospital furnished an alluring vision of lines of white cots occupied

Mrs. Blair's initial visitors. One was Charles H. Goodman, a Yale graduate with an 1869 medical degree from Hahnemann Medical College in Philadelphia, who had "a large practice among the best people of the community," said one account; another was J.C. Cummings, only one year out of the nearby Homeopathic Medical College of Missouri. A professor from the college, William Collisson, was there, as was one of the city's best-respected homeopaths, T. Griswold Comstock. In 1849 Comstock had first received a conventional medical degree from St. Louis University before investigating homeopathy, "having observed while yet a student," said one source, "that in some diseases, at least, it was superior to the 'old school.'" With an added degree from Hahnemann, and advanced study abroad, he was "noted for his...liberal eclecticism, which gladly accepted all that seemed to be good in either school."

At this organizational meeting, a few key items of business were decided. First, as the board minutes noted, Comstock was appointed to chair the meeting, though Cummings quickly made clear that its object was "to appoint a board of lady managers, who should inaugurate and take charge of a Homeopathic Hospital for children." While the physicians present may have placed slight emphasis on the "homeopathic" aspect of their purpose, some of the women in the room were not parsing medical distinctions. Years later, early board member Virginia Stevenson recalled:

> "The color and size of the pills to be administered to the children did not particularly interest the younger members of the Hospital Board. To them the word Hospital furnished an alluring vision of lines of white cots occupied by rosy-cheeked, bright-eyed convalescents."

Next, three different boards were appointed, first the 16-member board of lady managers, with Mrs. Blair as president; Mary Webber Cutter McKittrick, wife of wealthy dry goods merchant Hugh McKittrick, as vice president; Mrs. Henderson as second vice president; and Miss Allen as secretary. "It was a most harmonious board," recalled Miss Stevenson, "we always voted 'aye.' Led by Mrs. Blair's vision and enthusiasm, and Mrs. Hugh McKittrick's profound common sense, we prospered greatly." An advisory committee of homeopaths was also named, including

1862
London Hospital for sick children opens.

1874
Joseph Lister develops use of carbolic acid as an antiseptic during surgery.

1876
Robert Koch discovers that a bacterium is the cause of anthrax, validating the germ theory of disease.

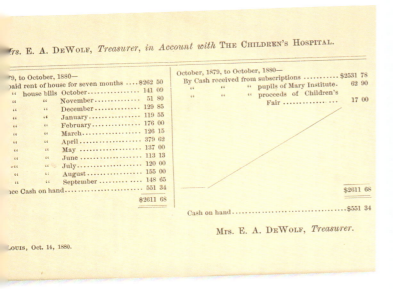

Treasurer's report. From the 1880 annual report.
Becker Medical Library

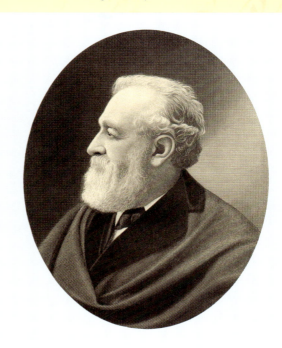

George S. Walker (1820-1895).
Becker Medical Library

-cheeked, bright-eyed convalescents."

Cummings, Collisson, Goodman, Charles H. Gundelach, William A. Edmonds, George S. Walker, and Diedrich R. Luyties.

The attendees also drew up an "advisory committee of gentlemen" that included some of the city's wealthier citizens: Samuel Cupples, head of the growing woodenware firm that bore his name; James E. Yeatman, a prominent banker who had headed a Civil War relief agency, the Western Sanitary Commission; Gerard Allen, an insurance company president; Col. George E. Leighton, an attorney; and Rt. Rev. C. F. Robertson, the Episcopal bishop of Missouri. Three were husbands of the lady managers themselves: McKittrick, Gen. Henderson, and Gen. J. W. Noble, well-known attorney and later secretary of the interior, whose wife Lizabeth Halsted Noble had earlier helped manage a Massachusetts sanitarium owned by her father, a physician. She and her husband lost their only two children, a son and daughter, in infancy.

Already, ties to prominent local institutions were becoming apparent. Virginia Stevenson was a long-time faculty member at Mary Institute; others, such as Mary McKittrick, had daughters there as students and sons at the affiliated Smith

George S. Walker, briefly a '49er in the California Gold Rush, graduated from the Jefferson Medical College in 1852, intending to become an allopathic physician. But in 1859, after moving to St. Louis and joining the St. Louis Medical Society, he began taking an interest in homeopathy. Later, the Society cited him to appear to defend his heretical practices.

"Pending the trial," said one biographical sketch, "controversies were carried on between Dr. Walker and members of the allopathic society, in which the latter used the bitterest invectives, hurled the fiercest denunciations, and showed the most malignant spirit of hatred and bigotry that the human mind can conceive. But all their arguments and senseless assertions were answered in a gentlemanly and dignified manner, in which the facts and truths... were presented." Still, he was expelled from the Society.

Walker, who became a surgeon in the Union Army during the Civil War, serving under Gen. William T. Sherman, later was professor of obstetrics at the Homeopathic Medical College of Missouri and co-edited two homeopathic journals published in St. Louis.

SEPTEMBER 1878

The *St. Louis Globe Democrat* prints a letter from James P. Kingsley, a local physician, pointing out the need for a children's hospital in St. Louis.

NOVEMBER 1878

Apolline Blair, prompted by a visit by several prominent physicians, holds a meeting with friends to discuss founding a pediatric hospital in St. Louis. During their second meeting, the Board of Managers expands to 20 women.

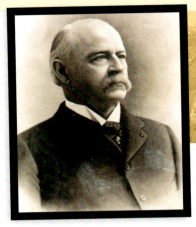

George Leighton (1835-1902). Leighton, general counsel of the Missouri Pacific Railway, served as long-time Washington University board member and its president from 1887-95. He was a member of the Hospital's "advisory committee of gentlemen." University Archives, Department of Special Collections, Washington University Libraries

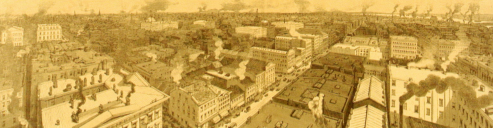

Pollution in the 1880s. Coal was an inexpensive and readily available fuel in the 1800s, but it created a tremendous amount of unhealthy smoke, especially in crowded urban areas such as St. Louis. Collection of A.G. Edwards & Sons, St. Louis

Academy. Washington University was also represented by lady manager Caroline Treat, whose husband Judge Samuel Treat was a charter board member. On the advisory committee were others with strong University links: Colonel Leighton, whose father-in-law, Hudson Bridge, was another charter board member and who would himself chair the board in 1887; Yeatman, board member and donor; and Allen, who was on the board of the O'Fallon Polytechnic School, which became part of the University.

Finally, the meeting gave shape to this new venture by giving the proposed hospital a title that seemed "sufficiently all-embracing and non-committal," recalled Stevenson. "On motion of Dr. Collisson," read the board minutes, "it was decided to name the institution 'The St. Louis Children's Hospital.'" Briefly, this name would later change to The Children's Hospital of St. Louis, but in 1885 it changed back again by action of the St. Louis Circuit Court — and remained so from that time forward.

THE BIRTH OF PEDIATRIC HOSPITALS

Other cities had stolen a march on St. Louis in founding a children's hospital. In Europe, where new views of the importance of childhood had been spawned by the Enlightenment, the first pediatric hospital — L'Hôpital des Enfants Malades — had been established in 1802 in Paris. In England, the London Hospital for Sick Children (Great Ormond Street) opened in 1852.

While Boston had failed in its attempt a few years earlier, the first successful effort in the United States to launch a pediatric hospital was the Children's Hospital of Philadelphia, founded in 1855. Five years later, German-born Abraham Jacobi founded the first children's clinic at New York Medical College and took a faculty chair in infantile pathology and therapeutics — thus signaling the birth of American pediatric instruction. A New York City colleague, Job Lewis Smith, was another giant in the young field, becoming clinical professor of the diseases of children at Bellevue Hospital Medical College in 1876. When the American Pediatric Society was founded in 1888, Jacobi became its first president and Smith its second.

Soon pediatric care would become more specialized. In 1889, L. Emmett Holt, Sr., took over the New York Babies Hospital, founded two years earlier — the first hospital in the United States focused solely on the care of infants and soon the most famous pediatric hospital of its period. He also wrote a seminal textbook — *The Diseases of Infancy and Childhood* — that went through some 20 editions.

CHILDHOOD MORTALITY IN THE LATE 19TH CENTURY

In the late 1800s, childhood was a minefield of potentially fatal diseases, such as measles, cerebrospinal meningitis, summer diarrhea, cholera, pneumonia, tuberculosis, influenza, and typhoid fever. Diphtheria outbreaks claimed thousands each year; in 1881, more than one percent of

NOVEMBER
1878

At their third meeting, Mrs. Blair and the Board of Managers create a pamphlet announcing the hospital to the community. Five-dollar subscriptions are welcomed.

JANUARY
1879

Subscriptions and donations for the new hospital are received.

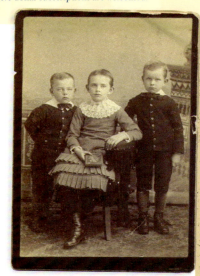

J.B. Gibson Collection

New York City children under ten died from this disease. Scarlet fever was another leading cause of death, with a mortality rate of 55 percent for children under two and 20 to 30 percent under five, while whooping cough killed at least one-fourth of all affected babies under one year old.

These grim statistics were only exacerbated by poverty. Joining the native-born poor in America's cities were waves of immigrants, many of them ill or malnourished. They crowded into tenements that were unheated, dirty and with a polluted water supply and terrible sanitation. Even the outside air was often unhealthy, infused with soot, sewer gas, or animal smells.

Still, middle-class or wealthy families were not exempt from loss. As homeopath T.C. Duncan said in his 1878 book on childhood diseases, "It is a justifiable opinion…that amongst those born with a normal constitution and under entirely favorable circumstances, the mortality during infancy and childhood ought to be less than at any other period of life. Yet it is a fact familiar to every one, that the reverse is the case in very many localities, most notably in large cities."

St. Louis was a prime example of urban growth and childhood loss. Between 1850 and 1890, the population soared from close to 78,000 to nearly 458,000, with immigrants from Germany, Ireland, and elsewhere. Increasingly, the downtown air was choked with coal smoke; drinking water, drawn unfiltered from the Mississippi River, was muddy. As Mark Twain noted in *Life on the Mississippi*, published in 1883,

"Hospitals for Children." Physician James P. Kingsley lamented the 50 percent mortality rate of children under the age of five in his 1878 letter to the *St. Louis Globe-Democrat*. Although they could afford the best medical care, middle- and upper-class families (above left) were not exempt from the dangers of illness such as diphtheria, measles, and influenza.

"If you will let your glass stand half an hour, you can separate the land from the water as easy as Genesis….The one appeases hunger; the other, thirst. But the natives do not take them separately, but together, as nature mixed them. When they find an inch of mud in the bottom of a glass, they stir it up, and then take the draught as they would gruel." This water was also tainted with sewage that flowed, untreated, into the river.

Amid such conditions, children easily became the victims of disease. In 1878, not long before Apolline Blair's meeting, the *St. Louis Globe-Democrat* printed letters from local physician James P. Kingsley, then traveling abroad, who wrote: "It is a well-known fact that the infant mortality in the City of St. Louis is something appalling, enormous. If you doubt it, take up the paper at the end of any week and see what the percent of

EARLY 1879

Hospital constitution, by-laws, and charter are drawn up; $650 in subscriptions have been collected.

MAY 1879

The St. Louis Children's Hospital is officially incorporated.

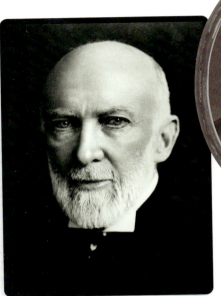

Samuel Cupples (1831-1925). President of the Cupples Woodenware Company and well-known philanthropist, he was a strong supporter and long-time advisory board member of Children's Hospital. He and his wife, Martha, had three children, but none survived to adulthood.
University Archives, Department of Special Collections, Washington University Libraries

Gerard Allen (1813-1887). Gerard B. Allen, a near neighbor of the Blair family on Chestnut Street, was a generous donor to the young hospital. His daughter, Grace Allen (later Dickson), was an active board member.
Becker Medical Library

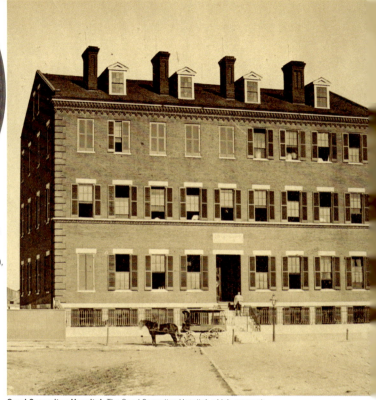

Good Samaritan Hospital. The Good Samaritan Hospital, which grew out of the older Protestant Hospital of St. Louis, was first occupied in 1861. It was used during the Civil War as a military hospital, then returned to civilian use. Staffed at first by homeopathic physicians, it became an allopathic hospital in 1902. Photograph by Emil Boehl, ca. 1870. Missouri Historical Society Photographs and Prints Collections

deaths among children are." His solution was a children's hospital — a cause that the *Globe-Democrat* took up editorially. With this support, Kingsley wrote again to promote his cause: "When one comes to consider that nearly one-half of all the children brought into existence die before they arrive at the age of five years, the necessity for children's hospitals, from a humanitarian point of view, is readily understood.... I presume it would be difficult to find anywhere this side of the water a city one-fourth the size of St. Louis without a children's hospital."

EXISTING MEDICAL ESTABLISHMENT

Every newspaper of the time ran ads for home remedies. In October 1879 the *Globe-Democrat* promoted "Vegetine for nervous debility," "Radway's Sarsaparillian Resolvent," and "Dr. C. McLane's Liver Pills." Even legitimate physicians had dispiritingly few remedies in their arsenal. Soon this picture would change with new medical breakthroughs, such as an antitoxin for diphtheria developed in the 1890s. At the same time, the germ theory of disease, promoted by Koch and Pasteur, was also gaining acceptance. But in the 1870s, those with traditional medical training — allopathic physicians — routinely used bloodletting or purging and such agents as quinine, calomel, opium, castor oil, and ipecac. In opposition to them were the homeopaths, who used a range of highly diluted natural products.

Whether they patronized allopaths or homeopaths, most well-to-do patients suffered through their illnesses — even surgeries — at home, not in the community's hospitals, which were places of last resort for the poor. By 1878, St. Louis had several hospitals already, including one owned by the city government and another by the Daughters of Charity. The Good Samaritan Hospital, funded by several Protestant churches and philanthropic citizens, was established in 1859, acquiring a new building at Jefferson and

OCTOBER 1879

The Hospital formally opens its doors at 2834 Franklin Street and welcomes the first two patients, Bennie and Mamie.

1880

Louis Pasteur develops method of weakening pathogen for immunization against cholera.

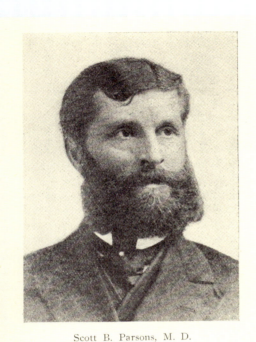

Scott B. Parsons. Becker Medical Library

In the 1883 annual report, surgeon Scott B. Parsons described several cases he had treated successfully that year:

"Hugh Shussler, aged 6 years, had been treated for two years for ulceration of the foot, and been subjected to two surgical operations...when he was immediately placed in the Children's Hospital, with his foot still painful and discharging.... Although it became necessary to remove all of the heel bone, there is but little deformity remaining."

"Margaret McMasters, 12 years old, had cerebrospinal meningitis, which produced curvature of the spine, for which she was treated for a long time by the Plaster Jacket and other methods, with only a small degree of benefit. She is now in perfect health, without the least trace of spinal distortion."

"Bessie Freesenmeyer, aged 7 years, was brought to the Hospital suffering most intensely from Hip Disease in its second stage, which, I am pleased to say, kindly yielded to the treatment adopted, without shortening of the limb, or deformity of any kind."

O'Fallon during the Civil War. While allopaths staffed other hospitals, local homeopaths staffed this one — among them, several of the same men urging formation of St. Louis Children's Hospital: Comstock, Luyties, Franklin, and Walker.

Nationally, these two communities — allopaths and homeopaths — were bitterly at odds with one another. In St. Louis, this antipathy had come to a crisis in 1860 with the case of George S. Walker, who began his career as an allopath and member of the St. Louis Medical Society, then switched to homeopathy. At this point, the Society charged him with heresy and expelled him, after a trial by his former colleagues. E.C. Franklin also sparred with St. Louis allopaths, notably M. L. Linton of the St. Louis Medical College (later part of Washington University), in a series of newspaper articles titled "Medical Science and Common Sense."

ST. LOUIS CHILDREN'S HOSPITAL IS BORN

Against this backdrop, Mrs. Blair and her friends were aiming to open a homeopathic hospital for children, funded by annual subscriptions solicited by the ladies themselves, who agreed to collect at least $200 each. Their first organizational meeting was quickly followed by a second, in which they decided to expand the board to 20 women "that an adequate amount of subscriptions might be secured." New members included Frances Pond Capen, wife of developer George D. Capen, creator of Portland and Westmoreland Places. Still in November came a third meeting during which they finished a circular announcing their new enterprise to the community.

In it, the women recognized their tardy start. "In almost every large city in the United States except St. Louis, there is a special hospital for children; and on account of the heat and malaria of our summers, there are few cities needing one so much as ours." The new hospital welcomed five-dollar subscriptions, they said; it would also accept contributions of food, clothing and furniture as

1882
Mary McKittrick takes Apolline Blair's place as president of the board of the hospital.

1883
Hospital board continues to report overcrowded conditions; 42 patients treated.

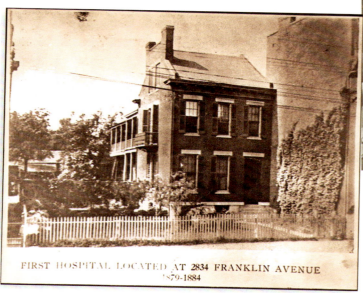

First hospital building (1879-1884). Located at 2834 Franklin Street, the first hospital building had room for 15 patients. Becker Medical Library

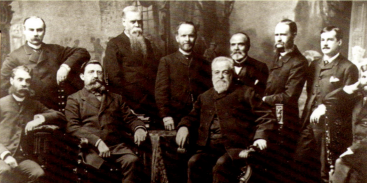

Children's Hospital medical staff, ca. 1879. Among the members of the first medical staff were surgeon Scott B. Parsons (far right) and specialist James Campbell (far left). T. Griswold Comstock is standing in the center. Becker Medical Library

soon as a building was secured. On no account would they incur any debt, but hoped "as soon as practicable, to provide a branch hospital in the country, where the little ones may be sent for pure and healthy air."

By the December meeting, subscriptions were coming in — $650 by mid-January 1879. Recalled Stevenson later: "It was a pleasure to me to visit my friends and acquaintances and ask them for the annual $5.00 subscription. One lady gave me $10 and thanked me for the opportunity to subscribe." One early supporter was noted educator Susan Blow, whose innovative ideas for kindergarten were taking hold locally and nationally; another was Virginia Kyle Campbell, wife of real estate tycoon Robert Campbell, who had lost 10 of her 13 children to illness before they reached age seven.

On May 6, the hospital was officially incorporated. Early in the year, the board also adopted a constitution, by-laws, and charter, drawn up by a committee that included Caroline Treat. The result was an institution that was "non-sectarian," said one account, "and the religious beliefs of patients are never questioned." Curiously, the hospital was not officially affiliated with the homeopathic college. Perhaps it was no coincidence that Treat's husband, Judge Samuel Treat, had earlier helped develop a constitution for Washington University that guaranteed the school would remain forever non-sectarian and non-partisan.

Although the board had money on hand, the problem was finding a suitable house at a reasonable rent. Finally, in September 1879, they had one: 2834 Franklin, "a modest two-story family residence," said one source, "capable of caring for only 15 patients." Still, said the first annual report, it "affords a sunny, cheerful home to its inmates." Now in-kind gifts began pouring in: bath towels, dolls, cradles, children's chairs, flannel nightgowns, brooms, apples and oranges, and "six pairs of drawers." Along with individuals, groups also donated, among them sewing circles and Mary Institute classes.

On October 29, 1879, the new hospital formally opened, with no fanfare in the newspapers of the day. "Many subscribers were present," said the minutes, and a local minister "made a few appropriate remarks." A matron was hired at a salary of $20 per month, and two children were admitted: a seven-year-old girl from the Presbyterian Home and a four-year-old boy from the Episcopal Orphanage. Years later, Stevenson remembered them: "a crippled boy named 'Bennie'" and "little Mamie, half blind and very frail," who "loved to sit in her rocking chair and sing in a clear sweet voice the old song 'Jesus Loves Me.'" Bennie (Benjamin Kelly) evidently improved, since in a later annual report he is listed as making a contribution to the young hospital.

1883

Edwin Klebs discovers microorganism responsible for diphtheria.

1883

To raise funds for a larger building, the Board of Managers stages a fair at the home of Bishop Robertson.

"Regulations Concerning Patients".
1880 annual report. Becker Medical Library

"Now wouldn't the community hearken to the 'Cry of the Children?'"

Over the following year, managers came and went — so did matrons, who sometimes did not measure up to board standards. New homeopaths volunteered for duty, among them surgeon Scott B. Parsons and "oculist and aurist" James Campbell, the only specialist among the physicians. Early on, the gentlemen's advisory board recommended buying the Franklin house, "as the possession of a building would give the institution a better position as a settled charity," said the annual report. So the women started a building fund, with Samuel Cupples and Gerard Allen heading the donor list at $500 each, Hugh McKittrick and Robert Barnes — later the benefactor for Barnes Hospital — at $250. In May 1880 the managers purchased the building for $4,500.

EARLY YEARS

In 1882, Apolline Blair stepped down as president and Mary McKittrick took her place, but the board continued much as it had done. A visiting committee, with a rotating membership of managers, closely monitored operations, though friends of patients could only visit from 2 to 5 p.m. on Thursdays. The patient load grew quickly. That year, said the annual report, "the house is now taxed to its utmost capacity. Having accommodation for only sixteen children, there are generally twenty under treatment at one time. Last week, admission was denied to seven applicants, because there was no room."

The 1883 report carried on the theme of overcrowding, declaring that "during this past summer, the applications were so pressing that two beds for convalescents were placed in the upper hall." Of the 42 patients treated over the past year, 22 had been discharged (16 "cured" and 6 "relieved"), and one child had died. Only those from two to 14 with acute diseases were admitted. Among them were cases of bronchitis, eczema, diphtheria, tonsillitis, malarial fever, epilepsy, paralysis, curvature of the spine, bone ulceration, disease of the knee joint, purulent otitis media with perforated ear drum, and catarrhal ophthalmia.

As board secretary Mary E. Bulkley later remembered: "Each child was personally known to 'The Board.' I'm sure all who were connected with the institution at that time remember the beautiful little 'Blossom,' and also poor little 'Fanny,' innocent victim, dying under our roof after many, many days in the only peace she had ever known….In those days the matron was to be found in tears when an operation was pending — and it was all very human, if entirely unscientific!"

With the hospital's stunning success, a new challenge was now on the horizon: the critical need for more space. To raise money for a larger building, the managers staged a fair at the home of Bishop Robertson and a successful parlor concert, held sales of their handiwork, and continued to solicit donors. For the first time, a new name appeared on their list: businessman Robert S. Brookings. With $4,000 from the sale of their old building, the Board of Managers bought a lot at Jefferson and Adams, though they still needed $6,000 more to construct a hospital, free from debt.

The board's executive committee issued a heartfelt appeal, begging the public to consider the hospital's pressing needs. "We have, in the past four years, proved our right to existence," wrote Bulkley, "we feel we have done good work in a quiet way." Indeed, the women's board *had* demonstrated "admirable management," agreed Charles Goodman, speaking on behalf of the homeopathic staff. Now wouldn't the community, asked Mary McKittick plaintively, "hearken to the 'Cry of the Children'?"

1884
Homeopathic Medicine in St. Louis

At the eighth annual session of the Missouri Institute of Homeopathy, held at the Lindell Hotel in March 1884, William R. Edmonds, A.M., M.D., physician at St. Louis Children's Hospital and president of the Institute, talked about the state of homeopathy. Although homeopathy was steadily losing its battle with allopathy, Edmonds expressed abundant confidence in its future:

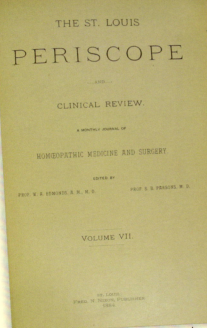

The St. Louis Periscope, 1884.
Becker Medical Library

ON THE NEED TO REMAIN TRUE TO HOMEOPATHY

"Loyalty to its great principle of cure, industry in work, with wisdom as to our surroundings, must ultimately place [homeopathy] high over all competition, as the great system of medical practice to take precedence of all others. In order to attain this honorable and most desirable end, let us as a band of co-workers quit ourselves as full-grown men and women, in a determined purpose to withstand enmity and opposition from without, while we toil and strive to correct mistakes within...."

ON HIS WISH FOR FEWER, BETTER-UNDERSTOOD DRUGS

"For twenty years my hobby, professionally, has been fewer remedies with a better knowledge of their toxic agency....We have too many remedies in use with no complete or sufficient acquaintance with their power in the cure of disease. Better infinitely to have fifty remedies in use, with a good knowledge of their powers over diseased conditions, than two or three hundred with the powers of which we have little or only guess-work knowledge....Let me feel that Corrosive Mercury is the surely indicated remedy for a given case of dysentery, and I shall feel or know no temptation to polypharmacy, crude quantities, alternation of remedies or short intervals between doses. These abuses are the forlorn resource of ignorance and incompetency.

"Then too, under a more exact acquaintance with our remedies, we shall have less of that unsightly and scandalous habit of routineism, so common, especially among older and busy practitioners in whose pocket cases of 50 or more remedies, we shall find 10 or 12 vials half empty, with soiled corks from too frequent use, whilst the remaining 30 or 40 vials remain untouched for months and years together. Let me not then be misunderstood; it is not the large list of remedies to which I object, but the long list, with no suitable exact acquaintance with their toxic action upon the healthy organism, as a key to their efficacy in the cure of disease."

ON THE RISKS OF AFFILIATING WITH ALLOPATHS

"We do not need and should not desire affiliations with other systems of medical practice. Such affiliations can only be held at the expense of a compromise of our leading principles. Compromise of principle we ought not, must not tolerate. Probably the best thing that ever transpired in the interest of homeopathy, after its birth and inception,

> "Better infinitely to have fifty remedies in use, with a good knowledge of their powers over diseased conditions, than two or three hundred with the powers of which we have little or only guess-work knowledge."

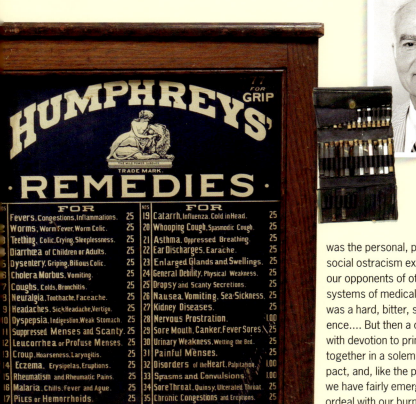

This drug kit was used in the late 19th century by homeopath James S. Read. His grandson, pediatrician **C. Read Boles (1920-2004)**, was a 1943 graduate of the Washington University School of Medicine and a long-time clinical faculty member, who retired in 1995. From the collections of the St. Louis Science Center and Becker Medical Library

Homeopathic drug cabinet and drugs, late 19th century.
"We have too many remedies in use with no complete or sufficient acquaintance with their power in the cure of disease," argued William Edmonds in 1884. From the collections of the St. Louis Science Center and St. Louis College of Pharmacy

was the personal, professional and social ostracism extended to us by our opponents of other schools and systems of medical practice. True, it was a hard, bitter, severe experience.... But then a common suffering, with devotion to principle, bound us together in a solemn league and compact, and, like the pure gold of truth, we have fairly emerged from the fiery ordeal with our burnished golden gems of truth all the brighter for the crucible of this early experience.

"Then perchance it might have been at times, in an emergency, very comfortable to have a little assistance from a neighboring allopath. But to-day it is far different, thanks to spread and increase in all that goes to make up professional success and co-operation among ourselves. We have our own colleges, a literature, societies, specialists and consultants equal to the best. Whose affiliations and recognitions do we need?"

ON HOMEOPATHY'S BRIGHT FUTURE

"The spectacle which we behold to-day is indeed a novel one. Less than a hundred years ago, we were the contemned of all contemners. Today, while our enemies all around us are openly or clandestinely using our remedies and views, others are clamoring to embrace us openly and formally by consultations and by admission into their societies. The bait, I confess, is a seductive one, but let us avoid its touch, and...treat it as a 'covenant with hell and a league with the devil.' The battle is fairly over, the victory and spoils are ours, and may the Lord have mercy upon our vanquished enemies."

– From *The St. Louis Periscope and Clinical Review, A Monthly Journal of Homeopathic Medicine and Surgery,* 1884, edited by Prof. W. A. Edmonds, A.M., M.D. and Prof. S. B. Parsons, M.D.

Foxglove. Originally used to treat ulcers in the lower abdomen, boils, headaches, abscesses, and paralysis, and externally for healing wounds.

HOPE AND HEALING — ST. LOUIS CHILDREN'S HOSPITAL: THE FIRST 125 YEARS

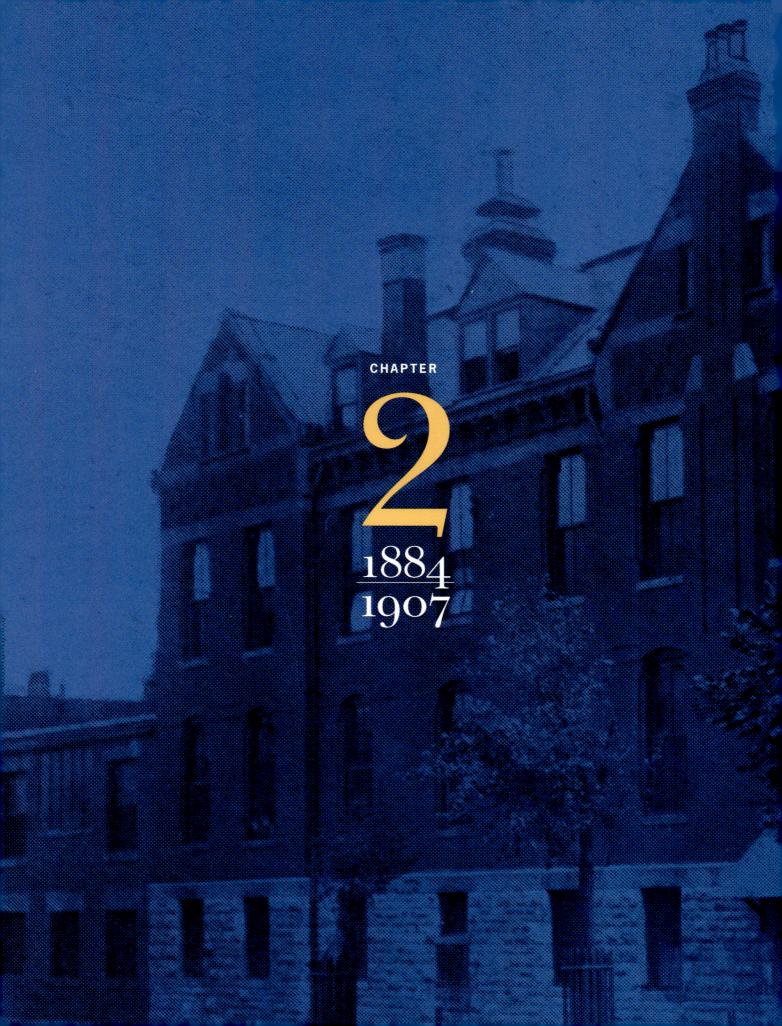

CHAPTER

2

1884
1907

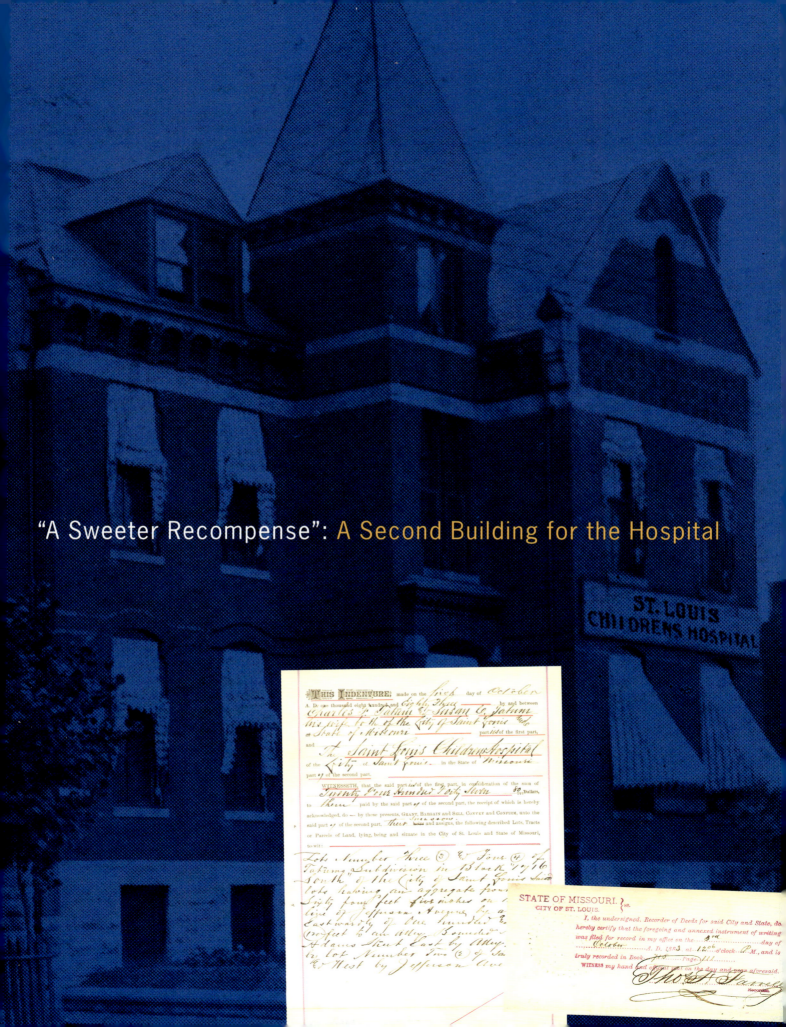

"A Sweeter Recompense": A Second Building for the Hospital

CHAPTER TWO "A SWEETER RECOMPENSE": A SECOND BUILDING FOR THE HOSPITAL

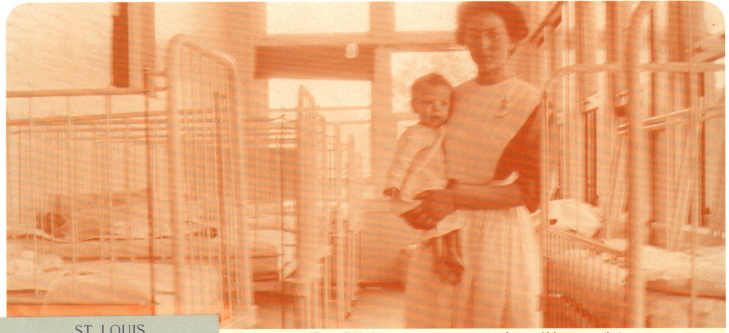

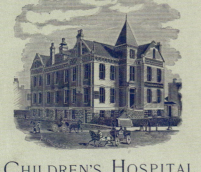

A lasting monument. The new Children's Hospital building at Jefferson and Adams, as depicted in the 1886 annual report. Becker Medical Library

A nurse with her young patient, ca. 1900s. Becker Medical Library

On the cloudy Sunday afternoon of June 15, 1884,

some 3,000 people gathered at Jefferson Avenue and Adams Street to celebrate a long-anticipated event: the cornerstone-laying of a second, much larger building for Children's Hospital. The hospital's entire homeopathic staff was there; so was a large contingent of women from its Board of Managers. Reporters from the major newspapers also were on hand to cover the ceremony, led by prominent Christian and Jewish clergy. Even the hospital's young patients were represented: "Little Blossom," one of the long-time residents, was chosen to spread mortar on the cornerstone of this "lasting monument to the benevolence of the ladies of St. Louis," said the next day's *Missouri Republican*.

PREVIOUS PAGE **Second Hospital Building (1884-1907) and Purchase Indenture.** Becker Medical Library

1880 — The U.S. Census shows that diarrheal diseases lead to the deaths of 20 percent of children two and younger.

1883 — The board locates a property for the new building, but negotiations fall through due to neighborhood objections.

CHILDREN'S HOSPITAL.

Laying of the Corner-Stone of the New Building on Jefferson Avenue and Adams Street.

Drs. Boyd, Betts, Snyder, Sonneschein and Rhodes Assist in the Exercises.

The laying of the corner-stone of the Children's hospital, on Jefferson avenue and Adams street, yesterday, was the external manifestation of an unostentatious charity that is present in our midst. The aims and objects of the movement are so unselfish, and the qualities of heart employed in its behalf are so elevated, that all who are engaged in the work honor themselves in no unenviable degree. To take care of the sick and helpless is always commendable, but when it is the pitiful voice of a child that moans, and when it is on a childish face that disease leaves its imprint, the care that changes the moan to the laugh of pleasure and restores the hues of health to the pallid cheek is doubly blessed.

In spite of the threatening weather 3,000

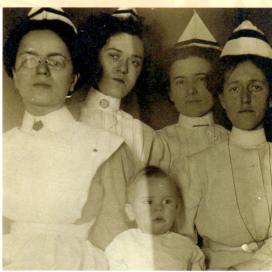

LEFT **Laying of the cornerstone.** From the *Missouri Republican*, June 16, 1884.

Nurses, ca. 1900s. In 1892, nurses' salaries were raised to $18 per month for those who had been working for more than a year. Becker Medical Library

Just as the program began, the skies opened and heavy rain began drenching the crowd. Still the exercises continued, "though in a somewhat abbreviated manner," added the newspaper. In his opening prayer, Rev. W.W. Boyd of Second Baptist Church adlibbed a reference to the inclement weather: "…as Thy rain falleth on the earth so may Thy grace and love fall on this institution." Rev. John Snyder — pastor of the Church of the Messiah since its founder, William G. Eliot, had left to become chancellor of Washington University — cleverly worked a bit of Shakespeare into his keynote address: "The quality of mercy is not strained. It droppeth as the gentle rain from heaven…."

Yet mere precipitation could not dampen the spirits of the managers who had struggled so hard to make this day a reality. They had met with obstacles at every turn, principally in marshalling enough money. Through heroic soliciting efforts — personal appeals and charity events, staffed by their own servants — they had raised nearly $21,000 for the land and hospital, which would accommodate as many as 60 patients and provide a dispensary for outpatient care. Many faithful friends had helped them: Hugh McKittrick, husband of board president Mary McKittrick, with $500; long-time donor Samuel Cupples for the same amount; Robert A. Barnes, soon-to-be-benefactor of Barnes Hospital for $250; Cupples' young business partner, Robert Brookings, for $125. The physicians all chipped in; even the architect, Thomas Furlong, gave $100. Leading everyone was a staunch new supporter: Jessie Wright Barr, wife of wealthy dry goods merchant William Barr, who donated $1,200.

Acquiring the new property had not been easy either. Briefly, the ladies thought they had secured a lot on Bell Street, but the neighbors "behaved in so excitable a manner that the negotiations had fallen through," reported the June 1883 board minutes. Finally, Grace Richards Jones, the board's energetic young treasurer, took charge of the building committee and the project moved more smoothly along.

There had been other bumps as well. Originally, James Yeatman, founding member of the male advisory board for the hospital, had promised the managers $500 from remaining funds of the Western Sanitary Commission, a

JUNE 15 1884

Some 3,000 people gather at Jefferson Avenue and Adams Street for the cornerstone-laying of the second building for the St. Louis Children's Hospital.

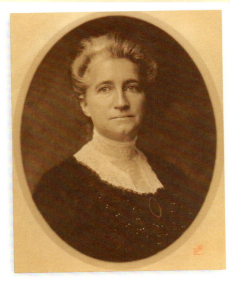

Mary E. ("Minnie") Bulkley (1856-1947). Minnie Bulkley, a skilled bookbinder, was also a social activist who participated in the settlement house movement and the suffrage movement. For Children's Hospital, she was a long-time manager, beginning in 1881. Photograph by T. Kajiwara, 1916. Missouri Historical Society Photographs and Prints Collections

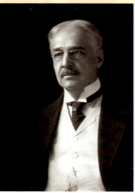

Charles H. Goodman (1844-1927). An 1867 Yale University graduate, who went on to finish Hahnemann Medical College in 1869, Goodman became a well-known St. Louis homeopath and member of the Children's Hospital staff. Photograph by Evans Studio, 1903. Missouri Historical Society Photographs and Prints Collections

Adoption letter. The first orphan in the care of the Hospital was adopted in 1885. The prospective parents had many recommendations as to their good character, as witnessed in this letter. Becker Medical Library

Civil War relief agency that he had headed, if the managers raised matching funds of $5,000. Once they had the $5,000 in hand, however, he tried to increase their target to $15,000 — a move that the women greeted with cries of indignation. One irately offered to pay the $500 herself, if someone would call on Yeatman "and communicate our entire rejection of this matter." In the end, Yeatman capitulated, and the $500 was theirs.

On this day of celebration, those battles were in the past. For today, the crowd was honoring the managers and staff as a group "of men and women who knew no limitation of creed or party," said Rev. Snyder, "but measured their mercy only by the needs of the sick and sorrowing." While their endeavor required "labor, faith, patience and untiring zeal," he said, in the end they would find a great reward:

> "To see the light of joy steal back into the shrunken eye; to see health plant once more in childhood's cheek the roses which disease had plucked away; to hear the...sound of the grateful voice that calls down childhood's blessings on your hearts — where can you find a sweeter recompense for all [your] self-sacrifice?"

Early one morning in August 1885, the hospital staff was shocked to find an 18-month-old child lying on their doorstep, "in an unconscious and apparently dying condition," said the annual report, adding: "taken in, careful nursing and medical treatment restored it to health." In October, the managers advertised in local papers for adoptive parents to come forward.

A couple passing through town on their way home to McPherson, Kansas, saw the notice and volunteered to take the child. For references, they provided letters from McPherson businessmen — jewelers, booksellers, attorneys, bankers, grocers — who attested to their status as "one of the best families in the city." "In October," said the report, "[the child] was placed in a good home, being adopted by kind and good people."

"...the coming year will be marked by a large increase in the number of patients, as well as more brilliant results in treatment..."

SUMMER 1884

Hospital patients and staff travel to Lake Minnetonka, Minnesota, to avoid the steamy St. Louis weather.

SEPTEMBER 18 1884

Patients and staff return to St. Louis from Minnesota and move to a temporary home, thanks to arrangements made by James Yeatman.

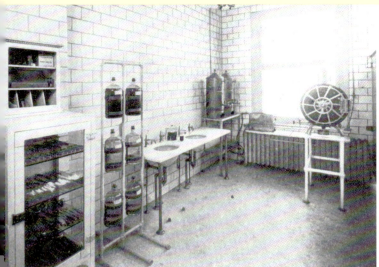

Sterilizing room, ca. 1890s. Hospital equipment and procedures were up to date and of the highest quality. Becker Medical Library

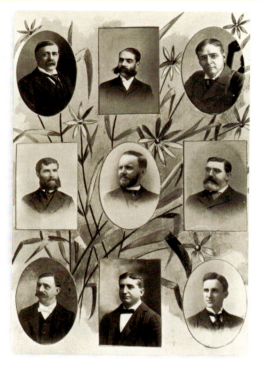

RIGHT **Medical staff, ca. 1890s.** Becker Medical Library

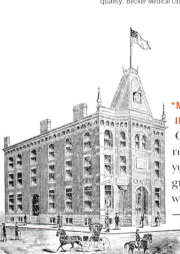

"MORE BRILLIANT RESULTS IN TREATMENT"

Once the festivities were over, recalled manager Minnie Bulkley years later, "the work grew and grew." The first challenge that year was what to do with their patients —15 or so on any given day — during the steamy summer? They had to vacate their old building by late June, and the new one would not be ready until November. Surgeon Scott Parsons proposed a solution: children and staff would travel at his expense to Lake Minnetonka, Minnesota, a watering hole for wealthy St. Louisans, where he and colleague George Walker both had summer homes. For $150, they could build a small cottage nearby and the patients could spend the season in comfort. "They returned Sept. 18th," said the board minutes, "all much improved by their stay but leaving one of their number, poor patient little George, to sleep in the quiet lake-side grave-yard." Perhaps to mend fences, James Yeatman then found them a temporary home in St. Louis until the new building was finished.

It was dedicated on November 12 and soon ready for occupancy, thanks to a host of well-wishers who contributed gifts: ranges, nightgowns, iron beds, books, dollhouses, blankets, a bird and cage, 50 window shades, 10 pounds of turnips, and three insurance policies. Several women, including Martha S. Cupples and Jessie Barr, sponsored the first memorial beds in the hospital; others, including Lizabeth H. Noble and staff homeopath Charles H. Goodman, fitted up rooms at their own expense.

The hospital remained closely tied to the homeopathic community, which in 1885 constructed a spacious new building for the Homeopathic College of Missouri not far away at Jefferson and Howard. With the expansion in their affiliated hospital and in their school, Children's Hospital homeopaths brimmed with confidence about the future. "With the present new and commodious quarters," reported Goodman for the attending staff, "it is believed the coming year will be marked by a large increase in the number of patients, as well as more brilliant results in treatment."

INSET **Homeopathic College of Missouri.** In 1885 the College constructed a new building at Jefferson and Howard described as containing "spacious and well-lighted clinical rooms, amphitheater, dissecting rooms and laboratories equipped with modern apparatus." It ceased operation in 1905. Becker Medical Library

NOVEMBER 12
1884

The new Children's Hospital building is dedicated and ready for occupancy soon thereafter.

AUGUST
1885

For the first time, an orphan is left on the doorstep of the hospital. "Kind and good people" from Kansas later adopted the child.

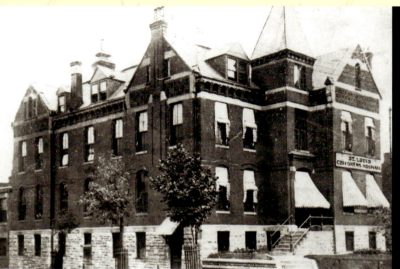

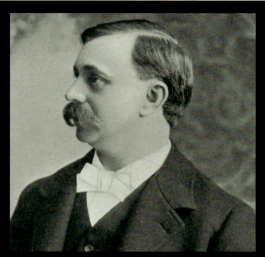

LEFT New hospital building.
The new buidling, located at Jefferson and Adams, was dedicated on November 12, 1884.
Becker Medical Library

Carl J. Luyties (1860-1916).
The hospital's first resident physician, Luyties was popular with patients, managers, and medical staff. An 1898 history of St. Louis called Luyties, who had also received a medical degree from Missouri Medical College, the city's best-known homeopath. From "A History of the City of St. Louis and Vicinity, 1898", p. 303. Missouri Historical Society Library.

Just before the new hospital opened, the medical staff met with the board and, on behalf of his colleagues, Goodman formally asked for three things: the appointment of a resident physician who could handle crises and dispensary care; a meeting with Grace Jones and her building committee to designate uses for the new rooms; and, most sweeping of all, full control of all medical matters. The board quickly voted to approve these requests; at their next meeting they appointed a "Medical Committee" — consisting of the two most senior managers, Apolline Blair and Mary McKittrick; a third woman; two homeopaths; and the resident physician — to work together on medical issues.

Clearly, the physicians were hoping to draw the lines of demarcation more sharply, claiming more authority for themselves. In coming years, the Medical Committee would make most of the significant decisions about medical care, with the managers intervening only occasionally as a group. The hospital by-laws soon reflected this change, giving the Committee medical supervision of the hospital and dispensary. More than ever, the board focused on fund-raising to keep the hospital solvent and on supervising its daily operations, especially the matron and nurses.

Indeed, the first resident physician, Carl J. Luyties — son of the late homeopath Diedrich R. Luyties, member of the hospital's first advisory board of physicians — was such a brilliant success that he left little room for dispute. His services "cannot be too highly commended, and are of the greatest benefit to our patients," wrote one manager in 1886. Luyties broadened the scope of the hospital's work by successfully building up the dispensary — which handled 497 patients during 1886 alone — and making house calls on sick children "when parents, in their ignorance and want of faith, have refused to leave them with us," wrote the board in 1887. Luyties was followed, however, by young homeopath Lucien C. McElwee, whose brief, unhappy tenure was tactfully overlooked in the annual reports, then by a long succession of others.

SURROUNDING HOSPITALS

No sooner was the new hospital well underway, with a growing number of inpatients — 41 in 1889, 55 in 1890, and a peak total of 56 in 1891 — than the medical staff begged the managers to undertake another improvement project: the addition of a ward for children with contagious diseases. Lacking such a facility, the hospital routinely turned these cases away; even so, patients sometimes developed surprising cases of diphtheria, measles, scarlet fever, or whooping cough that spread quickly among the other children,

1885
A new building for the Homeopathic College of Missouri is constructed at Jefferson and Howard.

1886
The hospital's dispensary treats 497 patients.

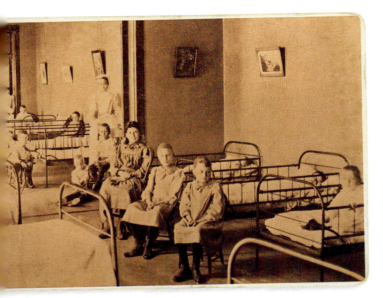

"A sweeter recompense". To see the light of joy steal back into the shrunken eye; to see health plant once more in childhood's cheek the roses which disease had plucked away."
From the address by Rev. John Snyder at the cornerstone-laying ceremony.
Becker Medical Library

already weakened by disease. "*Remember*," said the 1889 Annual Report, in a plea for donors to step forward, "that in all this great city…there is no place for a child with contagion."

St. Louis did have another children's hospital, however. In 1884, allopathic dermatologist W. A. Hardaway and his wife lost their small daughter Augusta to diphtheria and, in her memory, decided to fund a children's hospital: The Augusta Free Hospital for Children, located at Channing Avenue and School Street. Ready for occupancy in October 1886, said one reminiscence, "the hospital soon filled up, usually with a preponderance of crippled children, although all classes of ailments were treated." It was so successful that in 1890 it needed to expand; Charles Parsons, a banker and art collector, offered $15,000 if the hospital were re-named for his late wife, Martha Pettus Parsons. That change occurred in 1892, and the new building was soon completed, with beds for 40 children.

Why a second children's hospital? W. A. Hardaway was on the faculty of the Missouri Medical College, a bastion of allopathic medicine at odds with the homeopathic viewpoint. Another

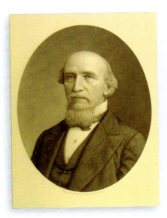

A 1952 reminiscence by Corinne Steele Hall recalled the founding of Martha Parsons Hospital: "In 1884, our close friends, Dr. and Mrs. W.A. Hardaway, lost a beloved child by diphtheria. Mrs. Hardaway was inconsolable, but my father [Missouri Medical College professor and orthopedist Aaron J. Steele] thought of a way to console her, and to fulfill his own dream at the same time.

"One Sunday morning, he took me by the hand and we walked together to the Hardaway home. I sat very still in little Augusta's rocking chair, and I remember how appealing Mrs. Hardaway looked with her light golden hair, pale face, and black dress. She was a Southern woman of great charm. Dr. Hardaway was an eminent dermatologist, and a man of means. My father spoke eloquently of the need for a children's hospital, suggesting in his ingratiating way that it might interest Mrs. Hardaway to establish such an institution in memory of her little girl. Before long the hospital on School Street and Channing Avenue, 'The Augusta Free Hospital for Children,' was well under way, and Mrs. Hardaway was a busy and happy board member."

In 1890, it was renamed the Martha Parsons Free Hospital after Charles Parsons (1824-1905), a prominent banker, philanthropist, and art collector, donated $15,000 in memory of his late wife, Martha Pettus Parsons. The hospital held 40 patients and was staffed by 21 prominent St. Louis allopaths.

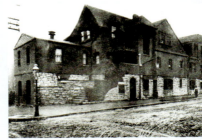

ABOVE **Charles Parsons (1824-1905).** A prominent banker, who served for several years as president of the American Bankers' Association, Parsons was also an avid art collector who left his valuable collection to Washington University. He endowed the **Martha Parsons Hospital** (right) in memory of his wife, Martha Pettus Parsons, who died in 1889.
Becker Medical Library

1886

Mary and Hugh McKittrick's son Alan dies at age 15, and the sorrowing parents donate a room at Children's Hospital in his memory.

OCTOBER 1886

The Augusta Free Hospital for Children, staffed by prominent St. Louis allopaths, opens its doors at Channing Avenue and School Street.

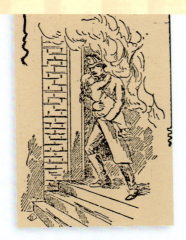

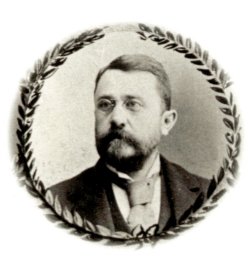

William A. Hardaway (1850-1923). A renowned dermatologist and the founder of the American Dermatological Foundation, Hardaway and his wife lost a daughter to diphtheria in 1884. They later established the Augusta Free Hospital for Children in her memory. Becker Medical Library

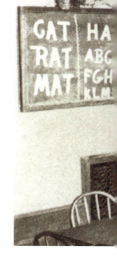

In 1889, the board minutes show that the resident physician suggested the need for fire extinguishers. Perhaps it was lucky that he spoke. Early on November 13, 1891, the basement laundry of Children's Hospital caught fire, probably because of a malfunctioning new dryer, sustaining considerable damage before the firefighters could douse the flames. "The paint upstairs was badly defaced by smoke," said the board minutes. "The children through the efficient exertions of the doctor, matron and servants, aided by kind neighbors, were all taken safely out of the building and kept in a neighboring saloon until the trouble was over." Altogether, 42 children were rescued, 20 of them bedridden and four having just undergone surgery. There were no casualties and only two serious injuries.

The insurance policies that had been donated by friends when the second Children's Hospital building went up then proved to be of key importance. In addition, the *St. Louis Post-Dispatch* offered to print a circular asking for help, the managers mobilized to solicit funds, and friends of the hospital also came through with special donations, thus carrying the hospital through this crisis.

Fire at the hospital. Pearl, an eight-year-old crippled boy, gave this account of the fire in the *St. Louis Post-Dispatch*: "I ran out myself. I can get along pretty fast on my crutches. I went down the stairs with all the well boys and they were crying and screaming, but I never cried once. The smoke was awful thick and I was afraid we were going right down into the fire. But we got out at last and ran over to the grocery where they kept us together until the fire was all out."

faculty member was pioneer orthopedic surgeon Aaron Steele, a founder of the St. Louis Polyclinic Hospital, which affiliated with the Missouri Medical College in 1885. When the Augusta Free Hospital wished to expand, Steele was the physician who approached Parsons for his major gift. Thus, Children's Hospital and Martha Parsons Free Hospital for Children represented very different, at times warring, approaches to medicine, and the two staffs did not in any way overlap.

Other local medical institutions were also changing. In 1891, the other major allopathic medical school in town — St. Louis Medical College, founded 50 years earlier — needed a new building, and the faculty approached young Washington University about an affiliation. Its faculty and staff had long-time ties to the College, and the University's chancellors, particularly Eliot, had for years dreamed of creating a medical department. Despite the school's precarious financial state, the board could not resist this appeal. Soon a new building went up at 1806-14 Locust Street, close to the University's downtown campus. At the same meeting that approved this department, the board appointed a new member:

1886

Caroline O'Fallon makes the first bequest to the hospital, amounting to $5,000.

1887

A small kindergarten is started for convalescents in the hospital. It is later given the name "The Laura Weil Kindergarten" in 1896 for a former manager who funds it.

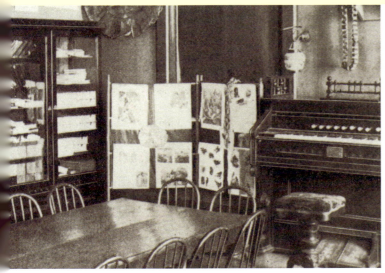

Laura Weil Kindergarten. Formed in 1887, this small kindergarten for convalescents had an average of 40 students daily by 1897. Becker Medical Library

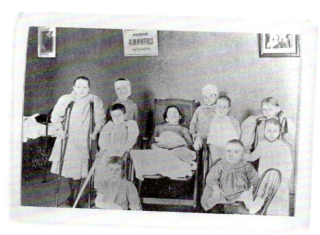

Surgical ward, ca. 1890s. Rooms were often dedicated to the memory of those who had passed away, such as this one given by Mary and Hugh McKittrick in the name of their son Alan. Becker Medical Library

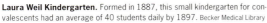

millionaire businessman Robert S. Brookings, who went on to become board president in 1895.

A NEW PROFESSIONALISM

By helping to specify uses for each space in the new Children's Hospital, the homeopathic physicians were squarely in line with the latest medical thinking. Since the early nineteenth century, when hospitals occupied former homes or other public buildings, the national attitude toward their design had shifted. As medical historian Charles E. Rosenberg explains, "by 1900 the hospital had assumed a characteristic physical form, its internal spaces defined by their functions and those functions understood in technical and bureaucratic terms."

This new hospital had a dispensary in its basement, with upper floors devoted to a surgical ward, convalescent ward, operating room, and wards for medical patients. In 1891, despairing of finding the money for a contagious disease annex, the managers remodeled the hospital's third floor for this purpose: "partitioned off, plastered, and windows cut in the roof, and now we have an isolated place, if contagious diseases break out in the hospital." Finally in 1899, as the annual report triumphantly reported, a heroic fund-raising effort had garnered nearly $14,600, and a three-story, fireproof addition at last went up: the first two levels for infant wards and the third for a self-contained contagious unit. In 1905, they managed to construct a two-story porch as well — open in the summer for a sleeping porch, then enclosed in the winter for tubercular patients thought to need some fresh air.

More rooms were furnished with new equipment in memory of St. Louisans who had passed away. Mary and Hugh McKittrick's son Alan died at age 15 in 1886, and the sorrowing McKittricks donated a room "sacred to the memory of a dearly loved little boy," said the annual report. In 1890, James W. Bell gave the hospital $2,500 to endow an entire ward as a memorial to his late wife, Jane Major Bell.

The homeopathic physicians, who still gave their time to the hospital free of charge, prided themselves on practicing in a thoroughly professional manner. "I would…draw your attention to the fact that there has been no hospital erysipelas, nor gangrene, nor any infectious disease developed in any of the cases operated upon," reported Parsons in 1887. "This result I attribute to the strict adherence in the treatment to antiseptic dressings, as well as the careful nursing, the perfect cleanliness of rooms, bedding and clothing, and proper dietary rules, that

INSET **Caroline Schutz O'Fallon (1804-1898).** Caroline O'Fallon made the first donation to the endowment of Children's Hospital. After her death, Julia Dent Grant, widow of President U.S. Grant, wrote to Mrs. O'Fallon's son: "Your mother…was the beautiful angel of my childhood; so many acts of kindness, so many kind words of hers fill my heart's memory." Becker Medical Library

1889

The hospital has 41 inpatients.

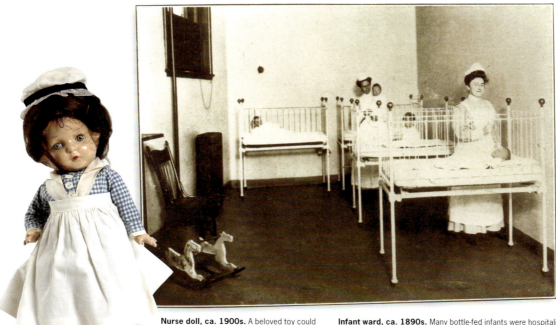

Nurse doll, ca. 1900s. A beloved toy could provide a great deal of comfort to young patients, whose parents were allowed to visit only a few hours each week. From the collections of the St. Louis Science Center

Infant ward, ca. 1890s. Many bottle-fed infants were hospitalized with diarrheal disease caused by contaminated milk. The Pure Milk Station began operating through the dispensary in 1904 and helped reduce the incidence of illness in these infants. Becker Medical Library

have been employed and are always adhered to in the management of this institution."

During these years, fund-raising took on a more professional cast. In the annual report, the list of donations now included a growing number from local companies, such as Ely & Walker Dry Goods. A civic group founded in 1893, the Saturday and Sunday Hospital Association Fund, was contributing nearly $1,500 a year by 1898. The managers even accumulated a small endowment, kicked off with a $2,500 gift from philanthropic widow Caroline Schutz O'Fallon, followed by a $2,500 bequest from long-time supporter Gerard Allen.

The patient population was also changing. Some came from the wave of German immigrants sweeping into St. Louis; in 1886, resident physician Carl J. Luyties asked that rules and regulations be printed both in German and English. Now African-American patients were treated in the dispensary, though not as inpatients. Over time, the age span of patients had expanded to include infants; while the upper end was still officially 14, the managers, moved by individual suffering, made exceptions. Said

the 1889 board minutes: "Dr. Boyce laid before the ladies the case of a girl of twenty who had been brought to the hospital for treatment of an abscess, which Dr. Parsons wished to open immediately. The ladies decided to keep the girl although she was over age."

In 1887, the hospital embarked on another new venture: a small kindergarten for convalescents, led by several young women, including Hattie Roth, who also taught a religious school on Sunday afternoons. By 1894, the school was thriving, with an average of 25 children daily, edging up to 40 by 1897. It had proved "a great blessing to the little sufferers," said one annual report, "…The Matron reports most favorably of the improvement in manners as well as mental quickening of the children." In 1896, the school got an official name: "The Laura Weil Kindergarten," in honor of one-time manager Laura Weil, now of New York City, who supported it.

Yet the original policy of no indebtedness was strained by these new initiatives. Managers still solicited money personally, but nearly all of them left town during the summer — which meant that fund-raising ground to a halt. In

1889
The annual report pleads for donors to fund a ward for contagious diseases.

1890
Emil von Behring discovers antitoxins and uses them to develop vaccines for tetanus and diphtheria.

To add to their nest egg, the women held events: fund-raisers, including an annual sale; private theatricals; a "Word Contest" in local papers; and a popular strawberries-and-cream party at Uhrig's Cave, "a beer garden on the corner of Washington and Jefferson avenues," said physician Robert Terry in a later reminiscence, which "...was a quiet, respectable, and delightful spot to go for supper, to meet friends and listen to light opera." At the May 1884 planning session for this event, said the minutes, "eight ladies volunteered to send men to wait on table and various ladies to send servants to attend to other matters."

In May 1888, the ladies considered one offer from a well-wisher: "Mrs. Allen's proposition to give an opera of her own composition at the Pickwick for the benefit of the hospital was discussed. The Managers felt obliged to decline the offer, with thanks."

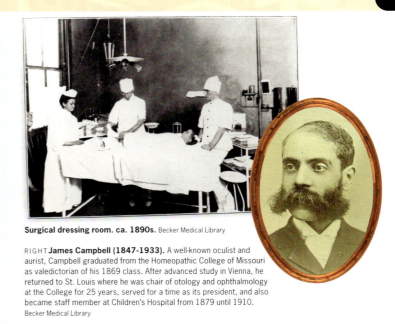

Surgical dressing room. ca. 1890s. Becker Medical Library

RIGHT **James Campbell (1847-1933).** A well-known oculist and aurist, Campbell graduated from the Homeopathic College of Missouri as valedictorian of his 1869 class. After advanced study in Vienna, he returned to St. Louis where he was chair of otology and ophthalmology at the College for 25 years, served for a time as its president, and also became staff member at Children's Hospital from 1879 until 1910. Becker Medical Library

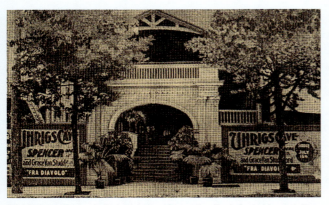

Uhrig's Cave. This popular St. Louis beer garden was the site of a fund-raising party for the hospital.

August 1889, for example, board secretary Minnie Bulkley recorded in her minutes that "she was the only Manager remaining in the city." In September 1890, board president Mary McKittrick chastised her board for their "thoughtlessness" in not raising enough during the previous spring to tide them over the summer months. "And as a consequence," she added, "this month found the Institution not only without any money but actually with a deficit." At the same time, the summer months always saw a dramatic upsurge in cases, especially in infants.

PURE MILK STATION

"Summer diarrhea," caused by contaminated milk, was common among children, particularly those who were bottle-fed. Amid the heat of summer, horse-drawn wagons carried fly-infested, five-gallon cans from one house to another, selling milk as they went. Not surprisingly, it became a potent bacterial brew. In an 1878 treatise on infant mortality, homeopath T.C. Duncan exclaimed: "Nothing in our mortuary statistics is more constant than the proportion between the number of deaths amongst young children and the excess of the daily temperatures above 95° Fahrenheit in the shade; indeed, we might safely say above 90°." Just as bad, milk sold in urban areas often came from cows kept in filthy conditions and enfeebled by disease. Altogether, the 1880 census showed that diarrheal diseases led to the deaths of some 20 percent of children two and younger — and that the poor or orphaned were most affected.

The country's leading pediatricians, among them Abraham Jacobi, Job Lewis Smith and L. Emmet Holt, Sr., strongly advocated breast-feeding, actively publicized the risks of bottle-feeding, and crusaded for milk sterilization. By the late 1890s, the young field of bacteriology gave

1891	1894	1899
NOVEMBER 13		
A fire breaks out in the hospital's laundry room and 42 children are rescued: two with serious injuries, but no casualties.	Apolline Blair suffers a debilitating stroke and is named "honorary president" of the Board of Managers.	Missouri Medical College affiliates with Washington University's medical department.

Allopathic physician John Zahorsky, later a member of the St. Louis Children's Hospital staff and a pediatric faculty member at the Washington University School of Medicine, wrote in issues of the 1904-05 *St. Louis Courier of Medicine* about the importance of pure milk in feeding premature infants, who became part of a popular incubator exhibit at the 1904 World's Fair:

"It is well known that the death-rate in foundling asylums ranges from 35 to 80 percent, enormously exceeding the mortality of infants in homes. The causes which lead to this are various but, as a rule, the high death-rate is principally attributable to the introduction of some pathogenic organism and its dissemination among the infants. Now, the same factors which cause this morbidity and mortality in foundling asylums are very prone to be operative in an incubator institute....

"In the first place no infant should be admitted that is several days old and shows some gastrointestinal or any other infection …. In the second place, only mother's milk should be fed to incubator babies, and even "graduates" must obtain a mixed feeding. At least mother's milk confers an immunity to infection on young babies which can not be supplied by any modification of cow's milk....

"The advantages are so many that it does not seem worth the while to make comparisons.... the comparative sterile nature, the easier digestibility and the immunity-conferring properties of human milk....We had five wet-nurses who, with their infants, slept in another part of the building. They furnished the milk but had nothing to do with the care of the incubator babies."

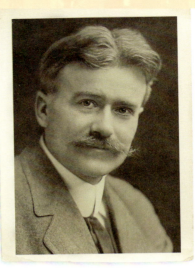

John Zahorsky (1871-1963). Allopathic pediatrician John Zahorsky joined the staff of Children's Hospital in 1910 as head of the Department of Infant Diseases. He was a strong proponent of feeding pure milk to premature infants in order to decrease the risk of illness. Becker Medical Library

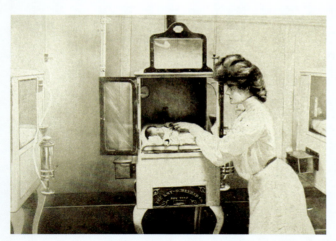

Early incubator. Incubators were a new technology in the early 1900's; an exhibit of infants in their incubators was a popular attraction at the 1904 World's Fair in St. Louis. Becker Medical Library

scientific underpinning to the health benefits of pasteurization, and in 1908, Chicago became the first American city to make it mandatory. Meanwhile, Thomas M. Rotch, a Harvard Medical School professor who received the nation's first chair of pediatrics in 1903, developed a revolutionary "percentage method" of mixing cow's milk with cream, water, lactose, and limewater to better suit an infant's digestion. During this same decade, iceboxes were becoming common in American homes, making possible the safe storage of milk.

At Children's Hospital, too, the patient population reflected the need for safe milk. Already in 1891, the managers considered and rejected the idea of raising their own cows to "improve the quality of the milk," said the board minutes. But in 1904, a Pure Milk Station did begin operating through the dispensary, which became a neighborhood center for milk distribution. "Although it has been installed only about two weeks," said the next annual report, "[it] has distributed 108 bottles of milk a day, part of that being the milk for some of the babies in the Hospital."

A CHANGING MEDICAL AND URBAN LANDSCAPE

By the early 1900s, either death or illness had stolen some of the hospital's earliest supporters. Among the managers, Apolline Blair suffered a debilitating stroke in 1894 and was named "honorary president," a position she held until her death in 1907. New managers — in some cases a second generation — were joining the board, replacing the pioneers. By 1904, Mary McKittrick's

1899

A much-needed three-story addition is added to the Children's Hospital building, with room for infant wards and a self-contained contagious unit.

1901

Overcrowding is a problem at the hospital, and patients sometimes must be turned away for lack of room, according to the annual report.

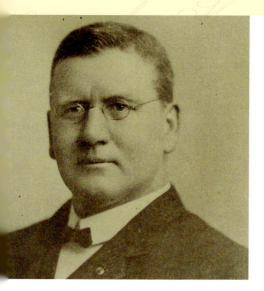

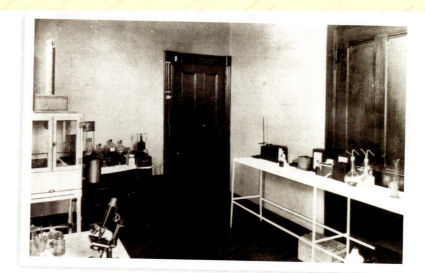

Laboratory, ca. 1900s. By 1905, the hospital had opened a department of pathology, which performed urinalyses, diphtheria cultures, and blood tests for malaria and typhoid. Becker Medical Library

LEFT **Lucien C. McElwee (1862-1921).** A Kentucky native, McElwee was an 1882 graduate of the St. Louis Medical College, then shifted to homeopathy. He received a degree from the Homeopathic Medical College of Missouri and, after serving as resident physician at Children's Hospital, became a faculty member of the College and finally dean in 1903. Becker Medical Library

daughter, Mary McKittrick Markham, was a member; Apolline Blair's daughter, Christine Graham, and daughter-in-law Apolline Blair, wife of James Blair, who was the hospital's attorney until 1902, also served for a time. After Graham's own death in 1915, a third generation would also get involved: her only daughter, Christine Graham Long.

The scope of health care was changing, too, both nationally and locally. By 1906, St. Louis had 32 major hospitals and as many as two dozen minor ones, with an average daily occupancy of around 2,700 patients. Missouri Medical College had decided in 1899 to affiliate with Washington University's medical department. Several smaller medical schools also existed, and along with the homeopathic and one "eclectic" college, these seven schools turned out some 600 graduates a year.

In contrast to earlier attitudes — that hospitals were exclusively places for the poor — patients from a much broader economic spectrum were choosing hospital treatment, in light of improved nursing practices, reduced institutional infection rates, and new procedures and equipment not available for home-based care. At Children's Hospital, the latest microscope, incubators, sterilizers, distillers, and X-ray equipment were now in use. By 1905, the hospital had opened a department of pathology, headed by homeopath L.S. Luton, which reported doing urinalyses, diphtheria cultures, and blood tests for malaria or typhoid.

Urban areas, too, were adopting stricter notions of cleanliness. In St. Louis, the 1904 Louisiana Purchase Exposition had focused civic attention on the city's shortcomings — its dirty streets, inadequate sewers, overcrowded hospitals, and particularly its muddy water supply, funneled straight from the Mississippi River. To prepare for the onslaught of visitors, the city's leaders paved streets, built hotels, and got engineers in the city's water department involved in cleaning up the water.

HOMEOPATHY — NO LONGER THE "GOLDEN MILESTONE"

Throughout these years, homeopathy was a field in transition. In 1905, the unsuccessful resident physician McElwee, by now dean of the Homeopathic Medical College, bemoaned the advantages offered in the east for the practice of homeopathy. "But we are equally convinced that with the same opportunities...the west will join hands with the east and they will sing in songs of exultation and triumph that will have as their refrain 'Homeopathy! The golden milestone of medical progress.'"

1902
The traditionally homeopathic Good Samaritan Hospital reconstitutes itself with an allopathic staff.

1903
The American Medical Association agrees to include homeopaths among its members.

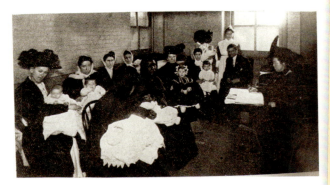

Dispensary, ca. 1890s. African-Americans were among the many patients treated in the dispensary after the new building opened. Becker Medical Library

RIGHT **Diseases report.** The number and types of diseases were carefully recorded in each annual report; this list is from 1904. Becker Medical Library

NAMES OF DISEASES.	Number of Cases.	Cured.	Improved.	Incurable.	Removed.	Died.	Still under Treatment.
Neurasthenia	1	1					
Nephritis	1	1					
Paralysis	2		1		1		
Pertussis	3		1		2		
Pneumonia	2	2					
Prolapsus ani	1	1					
Paraplegia	1			1			
Pleurisy	1	1					
Ptomaine poisoning	2	2					
Rhus poisoning	1	1					
Rheumatism	3	3					
Scabies	17	17					
Spasms	1						4
Stomatitis	3	1			1		1
Syphilis	2	1					1
Tonsilitis	6	6					
Tinea tonsur	1	1					
Tænia vermic	1	1					
Tubercular adenitis	2	2					
Tuberculosis	2					1	1
Tympanitis	1	1					
Tinea tryco	1	1					
Rhinitis	1	1					
Urethritis	2	2					
Vaginitis	3	3					
Vaginitis, gon	2	2					
Total	266	222	8	1	10	14	11

However, homeopathy as a discipline was already fading away. By the 1890s, homeopaths nationally were feuding among themselves, with the purists pitted against a growing number of eclectics, whose practices were drawing ever closer to those of the allopaths. At the same time, many allopaths were moderating their long-standing intolerance of homeopaths, and in 1903 the American Medical Association even agreed to accept "irregular practitioners" as members. As noted physician William Osler said two years later, extending an olive branch to the homeopaths: "A difference in drugs should no longer separate men with the same hope."

Meanwhile, some homeopathic colleges began closing or merging with allopathic medical schools, leading to a decline in numbers: from 22 nationwide in 1900 to only two by 1923. New state licensure laws favoring the allopaths were one reason; second-rate teaching and facilities were another. Financially, these chronically under-endowed schools could not keep up. Perhaps most important of all, research discoveries were advancing allopathic medicine — an antitoxin for diphtheria in 1896, an anti-meningococcal serum in 1908, among others — and giving it strong credibility, while homeopathy's fundamental tenets had changed little. In 1902, the traditionally homeopathic Good Samaritan Hospital of St. Louis reconstituted itself with an allopathic staff; by 1905, the graduating class at the Homeopathic Medical College of Missouri had dwindled to only seven students.

At Children's Hospital, old stalwarts of its medical staff were dying or retiring. William Collisson — whose "pleasant voice and face" had "won the hearts of the children," according to the annual report — had died in 1885; John C. Cummings had died in 1897; and Scott B. Parsons in 1899, succeeded by his son, Scott E. Parsons. George Walker retired to California in 1888 and died seven years later; and William A. Edmonds had left practice in 1899, retiring to his native Kentucky. Apolline Blair's family homeopath, E.C. Franklin, died in 1885, and by the time of her own final illness in 1907, she had switched allegiance to noted St. Louis allopath, Washington E. Fischel.

While the hospital was still thriving — a 1904 newspaper article called it "one of the most successful institutions in the west for the free treatment of children" — there were signs that its building needed serious overhaul. "Our expenses for the year have been very heavy," sighed one annual report writer, "owing to the fact that it became necessary to have the plumbing entirely done over." Again overcrowding became a problem. The 1901 report complained that "many

1904
Safe, sterilized milk is dispensed through the Pure Milk Station at the hospital, reducing the disease caused by contaminated milk.

1904
St. Louis hosts the Louisiana Purchase Exposition, a grand World's Fair that focuses civic attention on city improvements.

1905
A department of pathology is opened at the hospital.

BIG BENEFIT PLANNED FOR ILL AND MAIMED CHILDREN.

LADIES IN CHARGE OF GARDEN PARTY AT CARRSWOLD HOPE TO REALIZE LARGE SUM—HISTORY OF LITTLE FOLKS' HOSPITAL AND HOW MELANCHOLY LIVES ARE BRIGHTENED.

Last week there were sixty-five patients in the St. Louis children's hospital, and the most skeptical person in the world would look at life from a different point of view could he see the crippled, half-blind and the sick children who manage to look smilingly from their cots or chairs, helped, as they are, to endure pain by the splendid treatment supplied at the institution. Miss Ida Bisch, the competent matron, and her corps of nurses are in the closest sympathy with the little ones, and the ladies of the board of managers, who come to visit them, know most of the older children by name and

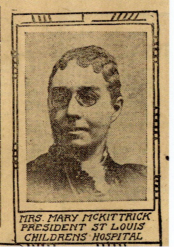

MRS. MARY MCKITTRICK PRESIDENT ST LOUIS CHILDRENS HOSPITAL

A **May 1905 newspaper article** touted a benefit garden party for the hospital given by E.C. Simmons, member of the original men's advisory board, and his wife, Carrie, at their country home, "Carrswold." The story also described the hospital on a typical day:

"Miss Ida Bisch, the competent matron, and her corps of nurses, are in the closest sympathy with the little ones, and the ladies of the board of managers, who come to visit them, know most of the older children by name and are fully acquainted with the nature of their illnesses....

"There is no hospital in which the patients are better cared for....A proper amount of study, amusement; good, nutritious food, the best of surgical and medical attendance — all these the child receives, and it is often the brightest spot in its existence when an accident or a troublesome disease sends it from its dark, crowded home in the slums to the light, well-ventilated ward, with its sweet, clean beds and kind attendants."

Fund-raising. Fund-raising events were often noted in the newpapers, giving much needed publicity to the campaign for new donors. Becker Medical Library

"...one of the most successful institutions in the west for the free treatment of children."

times the capacity of our building has been taxed to its limit, and we have been compelled to refuse patients for lack of room. This is especially true in contagious cases."

This report was written by President Mary McKittrick herself — an unusual gesture, since the board's secretary usually handled it. Increasingly, the annual reports were becoming more businesslike; the 1903-04 report, for example, rated St. Louis Children's Hospital against others across the country and its local rival, the Martha Parsons Free Hospital for Children, in terms of cure rates, mortality, percentage of improvements, and patients admitted overall. But McKittrick's message was more kindly, old-fashioned, thanking physicians for their "time and skill" given "with no remuneration...save the consciousness of doing good." In mentioning the new Scott Parsons, she insisted that he "has our unfailing dependence."

The day of the homeopath was ending, however, and so was McKittrick's era of leadership. In 1907, after nearly a quarter century of service, she stepped down from the job and died the following year. The hospital's third president was elected

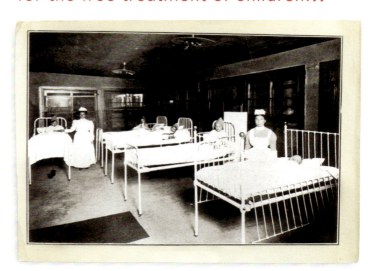

No shortage of patients. Twenty years after the second building was erected, it was nearly always filled to capacity and in need of repairs. Becker Medical Library

unanimously: board member since 1882 and long-time treasurer Grace Richards Jones, who would lead them into the uncharted future and, with her vision and personal connections, change the course of the hospital's history.

1907

Mrs. Jones and Mr. Brookings: Fellow Visionaries and Friends

Grace Richards Jones, named the board president of St. Louis Children's Hospital in 1907, took over an institution with an increasingly outdated building and the need for a new, non-homeopathic medical staff. Robert Somers Brookings, board president of Washington University since 1895, discovered in 1909 that he had to re-shape its medical school with a state-of-the-art campus and a brand-new faculty.

So these two leaders faced similar problems — did their respective solutions intersect? In resolving this question, it helped that they had much in common. They were long-time friends; in fact, Mrs. Jones's husband, Robert McKittrick Jones, was one of Brookings' closest confidants, served with him on the Washington University board as well as the Children's Hospital advisory board, and would soon play a role in the medical school's seismic change as a member of its reorganization committee. They were near Central West End neighbors — he at 5125 Lindell and she at 6 Westmoreland Place. Socially, they were both members of the wealthy, close-knit St. Louis elite.

Oddly enough, they even looked a little alike. "White-haired, tall, Mrs. Jones walks with a brisk step down the hospital halls," said one newspaper account from 1936, which commented on her singular "determination." Brookings' biographer, Hermann Hagedorn, described him as "a strikingly handsome man, tall and well-proportioned, with black hair and beard beginning to show the white later attained, and with a pair of dark eyes that one could feel piercing straight through to the back of one's head."

TWO VISIONARIES

They also shared a philanthropic sense that led them to devote decades of time and a great deal of money to their individual causes. Mrs. Jones was Children's Hospital board president until 1925, and her name regularly appeared on its list of donors. Brookings, who served as the University's board president until 1928, spent more than $5 million of his own on its rebuilding, and then urged his friends and future wife, Isabel Vallé January, to give as well. Later, G. Canby Robinson, dean of the revamped medical school from 1919-20, recalled that Mrs. Jones "combined unusual qualities of leadership with vision, energy, and charm comparable with those of Brookings."

Perhaps Brookings was a little in awe of Grace Jones. As a rule, he did not believe that women were the intellectual equals of men. However, Mrs. Jones — an 1877 graduate of Mary Institute — had a superior education to the one he had received in his native Maryland. At 16, he had quit school and followed his brother to St. Louis, where he

TOP **Grace Richards Jones (1860-1950).** At her death in 1950, after 69 years of service, Children's Hospital dedicated a floor to "a great lady and a great benefactress of children," said chairman Warren T. Chandler. She herself donated generously to the hospital, and made a gift of more than $2,000 to the hospital so that its soon-to-be-opened Ridge Farm country division would hold an annual celebration on March 1, her birthday, and May 8, her husband's birthday. University Archives, Department of Special Collections, Washington University Libraries

Robert S. Brookings (1850-1932). After Brookings' death, Washington University board president Charles Nagel said of him: "He stands out as a champion of education in the broader sense; for in realizing the chance for others, he achieved and enjoyed it for himself." University Archives, Department of Special Collections, Washington University Libraries

> **"We trust that in the future, as in the past, we may find that, whenever an ideal can be put into life, the material means for doing so will be at hand."**

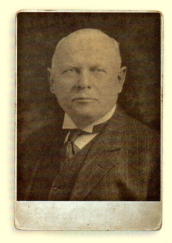

found a job at the same woodenware firm, then called Cupples & Marston. Eventually, he was promoted to partner and made a fortune, just as Robert McKittrick Jones had done in the cotton brokerage business after emigrating from his native Ireland. Brookings regarded Mrs. Jones, said Hagedorn, "as one of the ablest women of the city."

Their conversations about linking Children's Hospital and the Medical School were not formal meetings. Rather, said scholar Donna B. Munger, "this affiliation had been agreed to orally—over the tea table." Or as Helen Houston, wife of Washington University's then-chancellor David F. Houston, wrote to Isabel Brookings in 1934, two years after Brookings' death, "For years we went to Grace Jones's every Sunday evening and talked hospitals. Robert Jones and I frivolled occasionally but the others discussed every possible aspect of the question." During these discussions, Mrs. Jones was an eager visionary, "giving wings to the conception which filled Brookings' mind of a cluster of hospitals surrounding…a school of medicine," said Hagedorn.

"AN IDEAL…PUT INTO LIFE"

These sessions culminated in a formal agreement, with Brookings providing $75,000 for a new contagious disease pavilion. Still, a great deal of money had to be raised for the new Children's Hospital building, and Mrs. Jones committed herself to the task. On the dedication of the new hospital in 1915, she declared, with triumph likely tinged by relief: "We trust that in the future, as in the past, we may find that, whenever an ideal can be put into life, the material means for doing so will be at hand."

Brookings was impressed by her shining service. In 1921, he wrote to Abraham Flexner, whose critique had stimulated the re-founding of the medical school: "Mrs. Robert McKittrick Jones really is St. Louis Children's Hospital." Upon her retirement as board president, medical dean W. McKim Marriott offered another tribute: "In the early days of our country, the founder of the State of Maryland selected a motto: *Parole femina; fatti maschii* (words are feminine; deeds are masculine). Lord Baltimore had never dreamed of the existence of a person like Mrs. Jones."

Robert McKittrick Jones (1849-1940). A cotton goods commission merchant, he founded the firm of Robert McKittrick Jones & Company in 1883. He was a member of the Children's Hospital advisory board, along with Robert Brookings, and was active in other charitable work, including the Saturday and Sunday Hospital Association. In his will, he left $5,000 to Children's Hospital. University Archives, Department of Special Collections, Washington University Libraries

BELOW **6 Westmoreland Place.** The lovely home of Robert and Grace Jones was the setting for many discussions with Robert Brookings about the development of Children's Hospital.
Photo by Tim Mudrovic

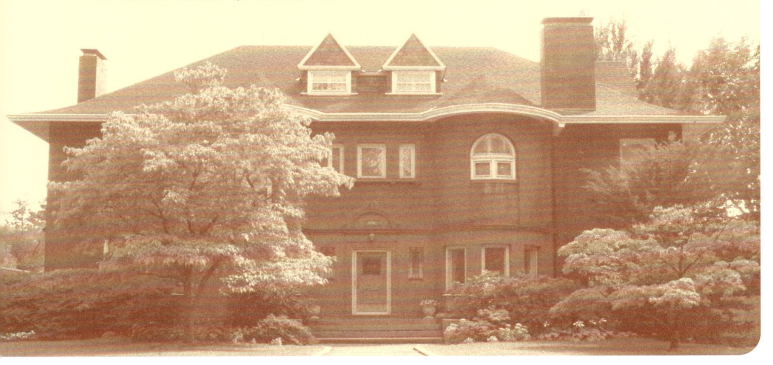

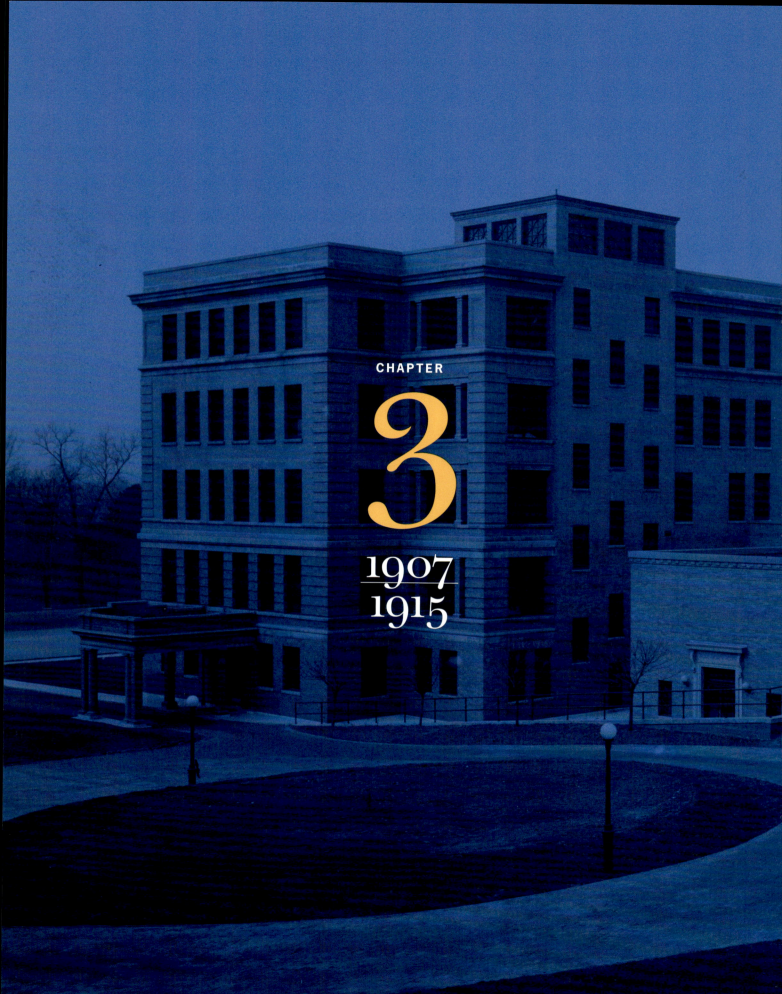

CHAPTER

3

1907
1915

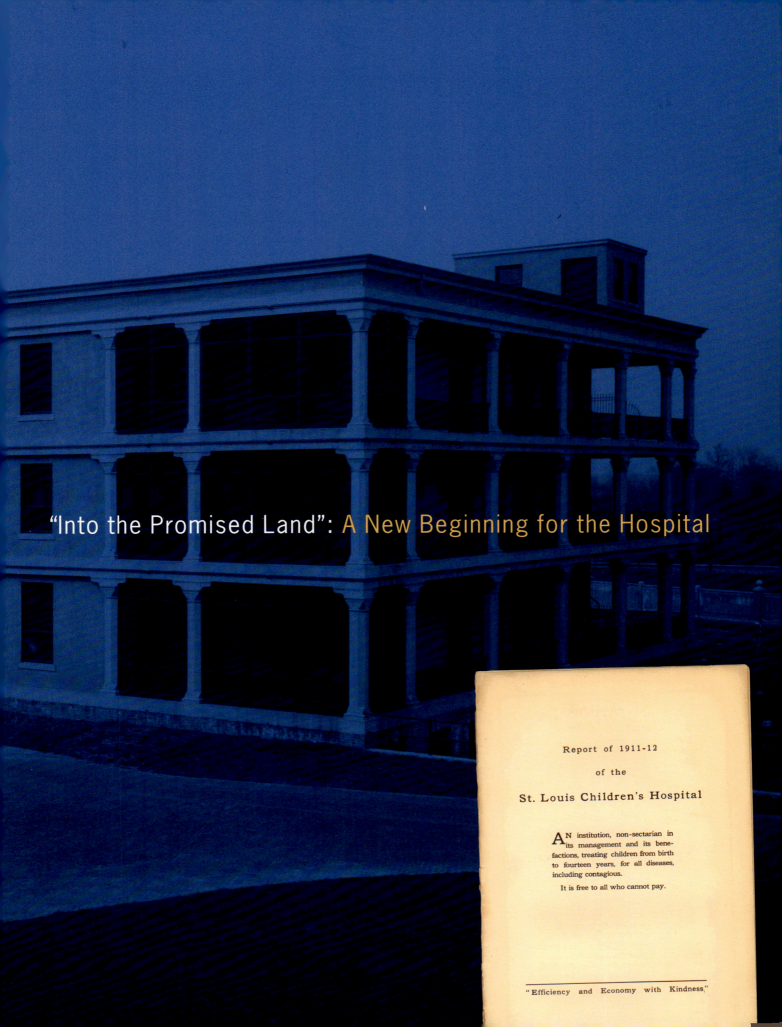

"Into the Promised Land": A New Beginning for the Hospital

Report of 1911-12

of the

St. Louis Children's Hospital

AN institution, non-sectarian in its management and its benefactions, treating children from birth to fourteen years, for all diseases, including contagious.

It is free to all who cannot pay.

"Efficiency and Economy with Kindness."

CHAPTER THREE "INTO THE PROMISED LAND": A NEW BEGINNING FOR THE HOSPITAL

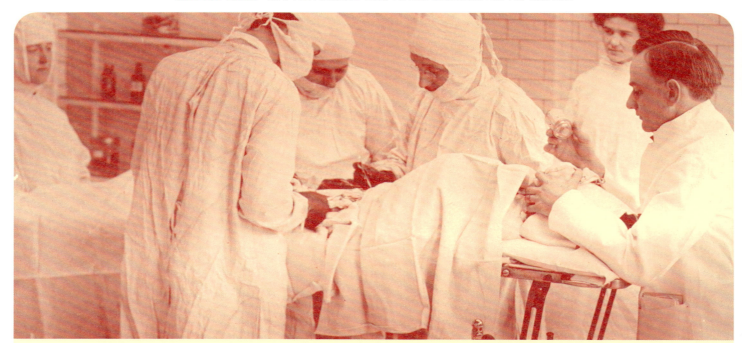

BELOW **Grace Richards Jones (1860-1950).** Borden Veeder remembered Jones, "a remarkable person of vision and courage." He said: "She ran that hospital the way a mother runs a big family. She knew everything that was going on, down to the last detail...." Becker Medical Library

Operating room, ca. 1911. Becker Medical Library

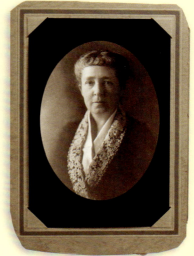

In 1907, Grace Richards Jones embarked on her job as board president with energy, fresh ideas, and an almost religious conviction that money would not be an obstacle when there was good work to be done. Years later, one board member recalled the kindness Mrs. Jones had shown her when she was a newcomer to St. Louis. "It may have been the pressure of a hand, a kindly light within the eye, a friendly smile — no matter — but the memory of it has sweetened my life," she said. Yet Jones, known privately as "Ma Jones" to the staff, was also a no-nonsense leader who soon told the board that she wanted Children's to "rank first in efficiency" among the hospitals of the Midwest.

PREVIOUS PAGE **Third Hospital Building, 1915.**
INSET **Title page from the 1911-12 annual report.**
Becker Medical Library

1905	1905	1906
Alexander Russell dies in Scotland, leaving a generous bequest to the hospital.	Robert Barnes' estate purchases a site on Kingshighway for a new hospital.	Frederick Hopkins suggests the existence of vitamins and proposes that a lack of vitamins causes scurvy and rickets.

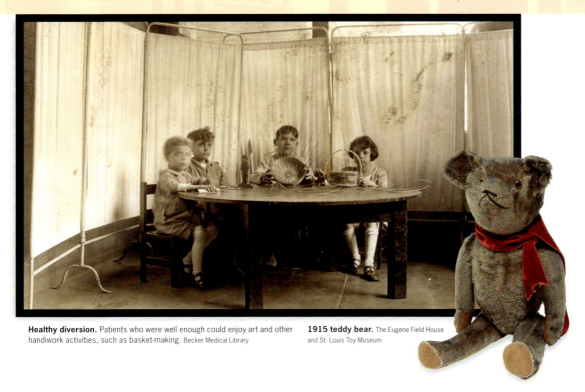

Healthy diversion. Patients who were well enough could enjoy art and other handiwork activities, such as basket-making. Becker Medical Library

1915 teddy bear. The Eugene Field House and St. Louis Toy Museum

Indeed, they *needed* efficiency to cope with a rapidly growing patient load in their increasingly outdated building. The first annual report after Jones became president noted 18,156 treatment days during fiscal 1906-07, up from 15,833 the year before. Pathologist L.S. Luton had attracted a record number of patients to the dispensary, and surgeon Scott E. Parsons had performed 103 operations, more "than in any year in the history of the Hospital," he said. Even the usually laconic C.H. Goodman, secretary of the homeopathic medical staff, wrote bluntly that the "present rooms are wholly inadequate for...increasing demands."

For the moment, the board's attention was distracted by a time-consuming new venture. In her last major act as president, Mary McKittrick had appeared before the St. Louis Circuit Court in May 1907 to request an amendment to the hospital's charter, allowing it to establish a new training school for nurses. For years the hospital had struggled to attract capable nurses, and then faced the problem of what to require of them. In October 1885, for example, the board minutes noted the decision to "enforce rule requiring nurses to wear uniforms."

This school would, they hoped, supply reliable staff to fill the hospital's burgeoning needs. As a profession, nursing had clearly acquired status in the managers' eyes. Now splitting it off from the Housekeeping Department, they hired a superintendent — Anna L. Wood, from Cortland, New York — to watch over seven trainees and six paid nurses. They also rented a four-room flat as a nurses' home and lined up physicians to provide lectures — all this, sighed board secretary Edith J. Davis, "in the face of many obstacles, both financial and otherwise. But it has added...enormously to the efficiency of the hospital, by putting it in the class of really up-to-date institutions."

What the board wasn't doing in the name of efficiency, it was doing in pursuit of money. The perennial need for funds to run this free hospital had not abated, though one year into Grace Jones's presidency, the board did manage to pay off its $6,000 deficit, with nearly $3,000 to spare. Quietly, they took prudent measures for the future: adding 11 members to the tiny all-male advisory board, previously composed only of Robert Brookings, Samuel Cupples, and Jones's

1907
The hospital's charter is amended to allow the establishment of a new training school for nurses.

1907
Grace Richards Jones becomes the new board president for the hospital.

William Barr (1827-1908). Barr, the dry goods merchant whose store was a predecessor of today's Famous-Barr, remembered the hospital with a bequest of $10,000. His wife, Jessie Wright Barr, was a loyal and generous member of the board. Becker Medical Library

husband, Robert McKittrick Jones. Now this group was awash in wealthy St. Louisans, most of them husbands of managers: dry goods tycoon John T. Davis, husband of Edith Davis; insurance executive George D. Markham, husband of current member Mary Markham and son-in-law of former president Mary McKittrick; and chemical manufacturer Edward Mallinckrodt, husband of member Jennie Mallinckrodt. Managers also formed a 50-member Auxiliary Board — Grace Jones's own daughter-in-law was among them — to stage entertainments that would raise money for the hospital.

Two bequests gave them, for once, a small cushion in a fledgling "reserve fund." Dry goods merchant William Barr, husband of long-time supporter Jessie Wright Barr, died in 1908, leaving $10,000 to the hospital. More mysteriously, a gift came from bachelor merchant Alexander Russell, who had lived for a time in St. Louis before his death in his native Scotland in 1905. He bequeathed a substantial parcel of real estate to the hospital, with more to come after his sister's death.

THE VISION OF "AN IDEAL MEDICAL SCHOOL"
To all appearances, the 1909 annual report heralded a future of modest struggles with the same familiar issues. "The attached report for the past year has followed along customary lines," wrote L.S. Luton comfortably that October. A couple of consulting physicians had been added to the staff; when long-time president T. Griswold Comstock died, C.H. Goodman had quickly taken his place. In the secretary's report, Edith Davis wrote blandly of the usual fund-raising events: a winter entertainment, a summer

On October 9, 1909, nursing head Anna Wood wrote a description of the Children's Hospital nursing school program. It was a two-year program in general nursing, she said, with special attention to the care of children and infants.

"Candidates must be between the ages of 18 and 35, have a fair English education, be of good physique, have sound teeth, good eyesight and hearing, be free from any constitutional disease and be of average weight and height."

From 30 applicants, they had chosen 16, though three of those dropped out during the year. Between October and May, they attended lectures in such areas as obstetrics and newborn disease, contagious diseases, anatomy, physiology, general surgery, and sanitary science, with special instruction in sterilizing and preparation of infant food. "All lectures are of an absolutely practical character," said Wood.

"Plans for the pleasure of the nurses: Tickets for entertainments, Christmas remembrances... Miss Bell donated a croquet set, also sent her carriage over several times in order that they might enjoy driving in the park. All served to break the routine of the year of hospital life."

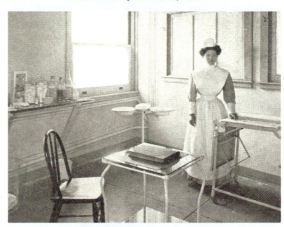

A member of the nursing staff.
Becker Medical Library

1908
Eleven new members are added to the advisory board, many of them husbands of the managers.

1908
William Barr, husband of long-time supporter Jessie Wright Barr, dies, leaving $10,000 to the hospital.

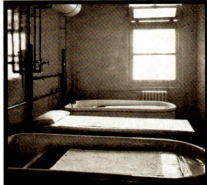

Infant baths. These state-of-the-art tubs for young children were installed in the new building on Kingshighway.
Becker Medical Library

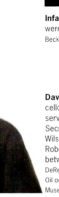

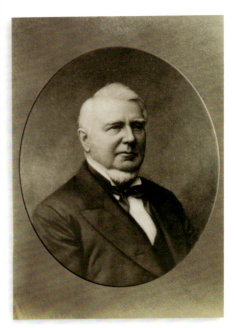

David F. Houston (1866-1940). Houston was chancellor of Washington University from 1908-13. He later served as U.S. Secretary of Agriculture, then U.S. Secretary of the Treasury under President Woodrow Wilson. He and his wife Helen were friends of Grace and Robert Jones and influential in achieving the affiliation between the University and Children's Hospital. J.W. DeRehling Quistgaard, Portrait of David Franklin Houston, 1923. Oil on canvas, 34-1/8" x 28-1/2". Mildred Lane Kemper Art Museum, Washington University in St. Louis. University acquisition.

Robert A. Barnes (1808-1892). A wealthy merchant and financier, Barnes left the bulk of his estate for the establishment of a hospital. Barnes Hospital opened its doors on December 7, 1914.
Becker Medical Library

operetta. But behind the scenes, events were brewing that would change the old order completely, sweeping away the medical staff and building, even reshaping the patient mix.

The first rumblings came in fall 1908, when Washington University's new chancellor, David F. Houston, gave a speech before the prominent Commercial Club. No doubt Houston — handpicked for his job by board president Robert S. Brookings, who was standing alongside him at this important event — was reflecting Brookings' wishes as well as his own when he described his dream of turning his largely local school into a "University for the Southwest." Part of that vision was an emphasis on research and laboratory science. "Most men overlook how practical pure science is and how powerfully it has served the world," he said. "Modern medicine is the creation of the laboratory scientist."

After he finished, Brookings — once a highly successful salesman — endorsed this lofty vision but proceeded to link it to money. On the medical side, he said, the University had acquired "the two oldest medical schools in the Mississippi Valley": the St. Louis Medical College in 1891 and Missouri Medical College in 1899. "Practically every physician and surgeon of any prominence in this city is a graduate of one or the other of these schools, and you will find their graduates in every state in the union." Likewise, the Washington University Hospital was providing "splendid service," including "considerable hospital charity...as many as fourteen thousand patients annually are treated at our clinics without charge."

This was all the praise he could muster, given his recent, disquieting visit to Baltimore. There he had met with Ira Remsen, president of The Johns Hopkins University, whose stellar medical school and affiliated hospital were well known as the finest in the nation. Brookings had been impressed; plainly, a new hospital would be necessary to help his school advance. "How long will it be," he hinted to this well-heeled crowd, "before some wise philanthropist gives to St. Louis and the Southwest a Johns Hopkins Hospital, by the erection and endowment of a hospital to be affiliated with our Medical School?"

Soon Brookings, still weary from his herculean efforts to establish the Hilltop campus, would

1908
Robert Brookings visits Johns Hopkins Hospital in Baltimore and develops his vision for expanding Washington University's medical school and hospital.

1909
Howard Ricketts shows that Rocky Mountain spotted fever is transmitted by ticks.

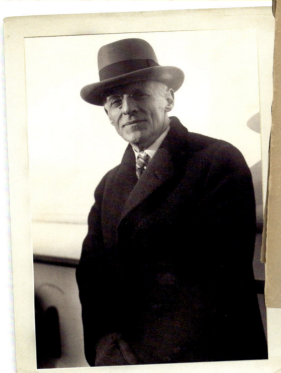

Abraham Flexner (1866-1959). A son of German immigrants, he grew up in Louisville, Kentucky, then attended Johns Hopkins. After teaching for a time, he wrote a book, *The American College*, a critique of higher education. These experiences qualified him to undertake his well-known survey of American medical schools. Later, he joined the General Education Board and raised millions to further medical education. Becker Medical Library

see that the need was still more desperate than he had feared. Just two months after Houston's seminal speech, the Carnegie Foundation for the Advancement of Teaching, a fund created by industrialist Andrew Carnegie, sent Hopkins graduate Abraham Flexner to survey 155 U.S. and Canadian medical schools, with the goal of assessing their quality. In April 1909, he made a two-day stop in St. Louis, inspecting the University's medical school and finding it, he wrote later, "a little better than the worst I had seen elsewhere, but absolutely inadequate in every essential respect."

Brookings was indignant, but he and Houston met with the medical faculty who confirmed that an overhaul was necessary. So Brookings named three of his closest friends — William K. Bixby, Robert McKittrick Jones, and Edward Mallinckrodt, Sr. — as a reorganization committee and, on a return trip to St. Louis, Flexner outlined for them the school's problems. "When I had finished, Mr. Brookings said: 'What shall we do?'" and, as Flexner later recalled, he replied bluntly: "'Form a new faculty, reorganize your clinical facilities from top to bottom, and raise an endowment which will enable you to repeat in St. Louis what…[Johns Hopkins] accomplished in Baltimore.'" The group voted on the spot to undertake this massive rebuilding effort.

To help fill in the details, Flexner recommended David L. Edsall, a brilliant young faculty member at the University of Pennsylvania — who eagerly devised plans for "an ideal medical school," with a faculty of "the best men available," practicing in a state-of-the-art hospital and laboratory buildings. A born dreamer himself, Brookings was star struck; he declared that he would supply $500,000 of the $850,000 needed for land and buildings, as well as one quarter of the revamped school's operating expenses. Then he and Houston began searching for the brightest young faculty they could find.

PLANS FOR A NEW BARNES HOSPITAL

Meanwhile, other forces were at work that would intersect with these plans. In 1892, St. Louis grocer Robert A. Barnes died, leaving $1 million to found a hospital "for sick and injured persons, without distinction of creed": $100,000 to build

1909
Abraham Flexner from the Carnegie Foundation surveys 155 medical schools and finds the University's medical school "absolutely inadequate in every essential respect."

1909
Brookings forms a reorganization committee to completely overhaul the University's medical complex; he vows to supply $500,000 of the funds needed for land and buildings.

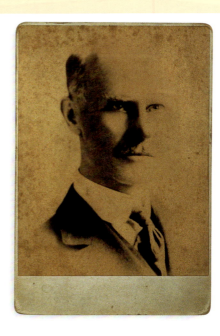

George M. Tuttle (1866-1926). George Tuttle, a Columbia University medical school graduate, remained at Children's from 1910 until his death. Not long before joining the hospital staff, he published a textbook on pediatrics that went through several editions; he was also instrumental in forming the St. Louis Pure Milk Commission. "A skilled clinician, a clear and stimulating teacher and above all a man of the highest ideals," said his obituary. Becker Medical Library

it and $900,000 to endow it. But in 1898, the trustees of his estate concluded, said one account, that it should be modeled after the Johns Hopkins Hospital, "the finest equipped and arranged in this country." Since the cost would be $200,000 — more than they could afford — they invested the money and waited for the fund to grow. In 1905, they bought a site on Kingshighway, and two years later hired architect Theodore Link to design the new building.

Well before Flexner made his scathing report, Brookings had become aware of the Barnes plans, and they tantalized him. Now he asked Houston to contact the Barnes trustees and discuss a formal affiliation agreement; he also secured a prime spot for the medical school by buying land adjacent to the Barnes plot. Likely, he felt confident in taking this step, since his business partner, fellow philanthropist and long-time friend Samuel Cupples was one of the three Barnes trustees.

A "MUNIFICENT GIFT"

Change was in the air, and during the winter of 1909, Grace and Robert McKittrick Jones met often on Sunday evenings with Brookings, David Houston, and his wife Helen, to talk over these heady possibilities. "The new Medical School and its affiliation with Barnes Hospital were the absorbing subjects," wrote Helen Houston later, but the possibility of another affiliation now entered their conversation as well. In November 1909, Cora Liggett Fowler — wife of bank director John Fowler and daughter of tobacco magnate John E. Liggett — wrote to the Children's board offering $125,000 for a new hospital building. It would honor her mother, Elizabeth J. Liggett, who had herself underwritten a dormitory on the Hilltop campus — Liggett Hall — in memory of her husband. Both Joneses must have felt ecstatic at this gift: Grace as the board's president and her husband, like Brookings, as a member of its male advisory board.

What led Cora Liggett Fowler to such munificence? Since 1898, she had been a member of the Children's board, though her previous donations — among them $25 in 1900-01 and $50 in 1905-06 — had been modest. In 1911, she would become the Joneses' neighbor, building a house at 35 Westmoreland designed by architects Mauran, Russell & Crowell. Yet even in 1909, she might already have been influenced, not only by the hospital's indisputable need, but also by Jones's compelling charm. Hinted G. Canby Robinson, later the medical school dean, in his reminiscence, "Mrs. Jones deserved a high place among those who helped to make the entire project a success…by stimulating the interest and backing of the leading people in St. Louis."

When Fowler made this gift, she knew nothing about the behind-the-scenes planning then in progress — and, apparently, neither did the joyful homeopaths on the Children's staff. "The very generous gift of Mrs. John Fowler…will

1909

David Houston, chancellor of Washington University, contacts the Barnes estate trustees to discuss a formal affiliation between their planned hospital and the University's; Brookings secures a site for the medical school adjacent to the Barnes hospital property on Kingshighway.

NOVEMBER 1909

Cora Liggett Fowler offers Children's Hospital $125,000 for a new building, to be named in memory of her mother.

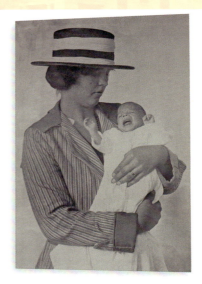

make possible efficient modern treatment in all departments," wrote pathologist L.S. Luton jubilantly in the 1909 annual report. Surgeon Scott Parsons expressed "a word of commendation for the noble and generous act of Mrs. John Fowler…it is hoped that the new St. Louis Children's Hospital, modern and replete, will rise to a greatness and prominence which has no equal in the West."

Just as one institution showed new promise, another — the Homeopathic Medical College of Missouri — finally closed its doors in 1909. For Children's Hospital, that meant no new graduates to fill its growing staff needs. Anyway, as Brookings and Jones both realized, the future lay elsewhere: in the new clinical discoveries and exciting research of conventional medicine. In coming years, Grace Jones would refer often, as she did in 1910, to the need for "doctors in active practice, who keep up to the advancing mark in medical science" and their co-workers whose "whole time is given to research into the causes of the diseases which all are endeavoring to cure, and who have the required laboratory facilities at their command."

A NEW REGIME

Sometime in the early spring of 1910, the entire homeopathic staff of Children's Hospital left except L.S. Luton, who remained as a general medicine "assistant." On April 1, 1910, a dazzling team of University recruits, chosen by internist George M. Tuttle, took over, with a host of talented

ABOVE First visit. This child visited the St. Louis Children's Hospital Infant Welfare Clinic for the first time at age 6 weeks, accompanied by his mother.
Becker Medical Library

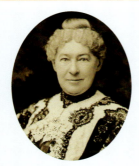

On November 19, 1909, Cora Liggett Fowler (1827-1928) addressed a letter to Grace Richards Jones and the board that must have been as exciting as it was unexpected.

"In view of the determination of the Board of Managers of the St. Louis Children's Hospital that the present building on Jefferson Avenue and Adams Street is no longer suitable or adequate for the needs of the institution…I will place at the disposal of the officers of the institution a sufficient sum of money not exceeding $125,000.00 to be used for the erection of a hospital building with modern equipment upon such ground as you may obtain suitable for the purpose."

In reply, the board passed a motion of thanks, adding: "A bylaw shall be duly adopted to be perpetually binding which shall assure the association of the phrase The Elizabeth J. Liggett Memorial with the name the St. Louis Children's Hospital on buildings, on stationery and in public print."

Letter from Cora Liggett Fowler to Grace Richards Jones, 1909.
Becker Medical Library

TOP Elizabeth J. Liggett (1827-1909).
University Archives, Department of Special Collections, Washington University Libraries

1909
Homeopathic Medical College of Missouri closes.

1910
Charles Henry Nicolle demonstrates that typhus fever is transmitted from person to person by body lice.

> Motto:— *Efficiency and Economy with Kindness.*
>
> **REPORT OF 1910-1911**
>
> OF THE
>
> **St. Louis Children's Hospital**
>
> Corner of Adams St. and Jefferson Ave.
>
> The City of St. Louis has no Hospital for sick children. Children admitted to the City Hospital are placed in wards equipped for and used by grown patients.
>
> The St. Louis Children's Hospital is the only hospital for children in the city, county or state, yet receives no appropriation out of the public funds. It provides the best possible treatment for the sick children of the city—even furnishing two nurses to one patient, when necessary. Since you are not taxed for this purpose, will you not aid in the support of this institution? It is non-sectarian, and free to all who can not pay.
>
> Children admitted from birth to 14 years. All diseases treated, including contagious.

"Efficiency and Economy with Kindness." This motto appeared in the 1910-11 annual report as the board's statement of the hospital's goal.
Becker Medical Library

department chiefs: Malvern Clopton, general surgery; Nathaniel Allison, orthopedic surgery; Selden Spencer, otology; John Zahorsky, "infant diseases"; Walter Baumgarten, pathology; and Greenfield Sluder, laryngology. Nominally, John Howland became head of pediatrics, though a leave to study in Berlin and Vienna took him away for his first year on staff.

Curiously, Grace Jones failed to mention this seismic shift in the 1910 annual report. Was the parting acrimonious? Did the homeopaths, who had served so long without pay, resent what was likely a rather abrupt dismissal? Tuttle alone referred to the change-over, and graciously said: "It seems only fitting that the reorganized medical staff should...acknowledge the excellent condition in which the hospital work was turned over to it by its predecessors. For a little more than thirty years the members of previous staffs have served the hospital faithfully and well, and we, their successors, have the advantage of building on their well-made foundations."

Within weeks, they were building on another foundation as well. The Martha Parsons Hospital, also burdened with an inadequate building in a deteriorating urban neighborhood, decided in April 1910 to unite with Children's Hospital. As Charles Parsons Pettus, heir to major donor Charles Parsons, later explained — in an echo of Grace Jones — the Martha Parsons board was eager "that the most efficient work might be accomplished at the least cost." In the next annual report, George Tuttle attributed the union to the fact that both hospitals were now "working for exactly the same end" — that is, they were both engaged in charitable work performed by an allopathic staff. With the homeopaths at Children's replaced by physicians committed to conventional medicine, the original distinction between the hospitals had disappeared. Perhaps it did not hurt that one member of the Martha Parsons board at the time of the affiliation also had a familiar name: Robert S. Brookings.

This move was welcome to the new Children's Hospital physicians, who now had plenty of patients: "The hospital bids fair to be crowded to its full capacity as long as it remains in its present quarters," said Tuttle. But these startling changes did not please one key person, Cora Fowler, who had envisioned a small, well-equipped hospital building, which her $125,000 could make possible. In May 1910, her attorney wrote a letter to Grace Jones that must have caused some consternation: "[Mrs. Fowler] is quite willing to put aside all questions touching the consolidation, etc., in deference to the opinions of her associates, but with respect to the size and cost of the

1910

The homeopathic staff of Children's Hospital, with one exception, is replaced by a team of talented allopathic physicians, including John Howland as head of pediatrics.

APRIL 1910

The Martha Parsons Hospital unites with Children's Hospital.

Borden Smith Veeder
spoke of the state of pediatrics in a 1910 address:

"I recently had a long discussion regarding medical education with one of the ablest educators in this country, and he told me most forcibly that an extended inspection of medical schools had convinced him that, considering its importance, pediatrics is more inadequately provided for in most medical schools than any other important subject; and he frankly said that, considering the importance inherent in this subject, the conditions surrounding it are, in most places, shameful....

"On the whole, I think we must agree with him in large part.... I would say that nowhere is the provision made for the subject as good, even relatively, as that which is made for general medicine, general surgery and obstetrics in a number of schools where these subjects are particularly well cared for....

"An extremely striking, and, I believe, direct result...is the fact that fewer able young men than might properly be expected to do so go into pediatrics as contrasted with the number of such men that go into general medicine, and the number is less even than of those who go into neurology for at the present day we may certainly say that there are in this country at least twice the number of men of recognized distinction in neurology than there are in pediatrics."

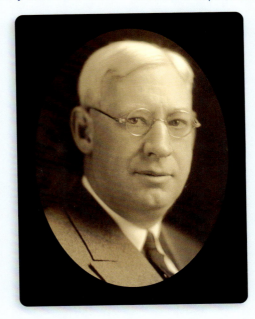

Borden S. Veeder (1883-1970). A graduate of Colgate College, with an M.D. from the University of Pennsylvania, Veeder came to St. Louis with John Howland in 1911 and served as professor of clinical pediatrics at the Washington University School of Medicine until 1951, when he was named emeritus professor. He served as co-editor or editor of *The Journal of Pediatrics*, 1932-58; founding member of the American Board of Pediatrics in 1933 and its president from 1933-41; founding member of the American Academy of Pediatrics; and president of the American Pediatric Society, 1934-35. Becker Medical Library

> **"The year just past has been the busiest and most effective in the history of the hospital."**

hospital, the proposed undertaking goes beyond what she feels she can provide...."

Somehow Cora Fowler was mollified and the planning went forward. Within months, the board had bought a parcel of land on Kingshighway adjoining the proposed medical school and Barnes Hospital. The purchase price — $26,142.20 — came from the hospital's reserve fund; it represented the entire bequest from William Barr and a like amount from the Russell fund. Thick and fast, other changes took place as well: the young nurses' school disbanded and was absorbed into Washington University's new program. The hospital's Auxiliary Board suddenly swelled by 50 percent with the addition of former Martha Parsons' members, and its board took on ten managers, though Grace Jones remained firmly in charge. "The year just past has been the busiest and most effective in the history of the hospital," said the 1910 annual report.

1911 ADVANCES:
SOCIAL SERVICE WORK AND RIDGE FARM

Yet 1911 did not lag far behind, since at least two landmark events occurred that would move the hospital forward. One was the successful launching of a new Social Service Department, an action taken by the board — rather brashly — while pediatric head John Howland was still away. Its goal, wrote Jones in the annual report, was "to better the home conditions of those poorest so that the child may not receive harm at home during its convalescence." Board secretary Emma U. LaBeaume, one of the Martha Parsons' transplants, bragged that this move was "in line with the most modern thought elsewhere, although this hospital is the first in the city to attempt it."

Heading this new department was a remarkable woman: one-time St. Louisan Julia Stimson, a 1901 Vassar College graduate who had trained

1910

Property adjoining the proposed medical school and Barnes Hospital is purchased for a new Children's Hospital building.

1910

The hospital's nursing school is disbanded and absorbed into Washington University's new program.

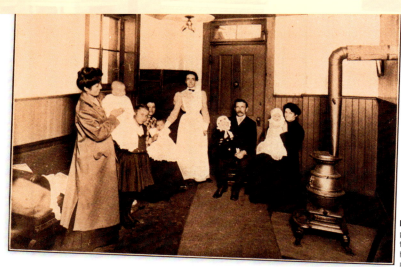

Dispensary. The hospital treated patients from infants to children up to age 14. In 1886 the dispensary handled 497 patients such as these.
Becker Medical Library

as a nurse at the New York Hospital Training School and would later receive a master's degree from Washington University. A born organizer, she was also energetic and politically savvy. Soon she had convinced the edgy medical faculty that she would only act "as the agent of the physicians and the executive management of the hospital," as she wrote to medical dean George Dock. She also built up the work of the department so that her one-person staff grew to eight, with some members funded by local church groups.

Stimson and her staff split their time between Children's and Washington University hospitals, and from October 1911 to September 1912, the number of visits they made was extraordinary: 1,535 to Children's Hospital families and 1,895 to University Hospital patients. Soon the hospital would award Stimson a substantial raise and a Ford runabout to make her home visits, bring children in for post-operative check-ups, and occasionally ferry emergency cases, as a kind of auxiliary ambulance. The car had "doubled the efficiency of the workers," wrote one board member approvingly.

In 1911, Children's received another boost for its mission when several long-time friends of the hospital — Christine Blair Graham, Anderson and Benjamin Gratz, Lorraine Jones, and John D. Filley — donated a 127-acre piece of woodland 25 miles south of St. Louis in Valley Park, overlooking the Meramec River. They also gave the hospital $4,000 to kick off a fund for a new "country branch" that would occupy the site. Orthopedic surgeon Nathaniel Allison was quick to praise this effort, contrasting the fresh air in this rural location with the hospital's current, smoky spot. "At the St. Louis Children's Hospital there are now under treatment approximately 100 children suffering from tuberculosis of the bones and joints. Surgically and medically all is being done for them that can now be done. They need fresh air, they need a life in the open as well as good food. The child from the city placed under proper care in the country where he can live out of doors, breathing clear air, will improve beyond belief."

Yet two simultaneous fund drives proved too much even for the tireless managers and their backers. When they sent out 5,000 fund-raising appeals with high hopes, "the response was small," wrote Mary McKittrick Markham, chair of the Ways and Means Committee. For the time being, they held the property and waited.

JOHN HOWLAND LEAVES THE UNIVERSITY

By mid-1911, the Children's Hospital plans seemed to be progressing. Perhaps to propitiate Cora Fowler, the board chose the same architectural firm she was using for her own house — Mauran, Russell & Crowell — and it designed a gray-brick building in three sections: a five-story, U-shaped, 120-bed general hospital, with space devoted to medicine, infants, surgery, and laboratories, plus residents' quarters; a three-story, 40-bed building for contagious diseases, with room for diphtheria, scarlet fever, and measles

1911	1911
A new Social Services Department, headed by Julia Stimson, is launched by the hospital "to better the home condition of those poorest."	Donors give a 127-acre piece of woodland in Valley Park, along with $4,000, to develop a "country branch" of the hospital.

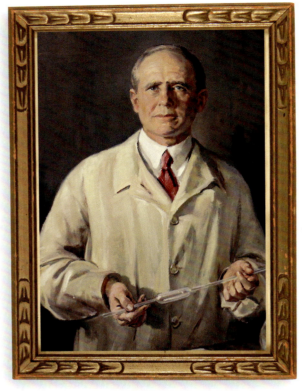

John Howland (1873-1926). A Yale graduate, with medical degrees both from New York University and Cornell Medical College, he had headed the children's clinic at Bellevue and worked with prominent pediatrician L. Emmett Holt, Sr. After leaving St. Louis, he became the first full-time professor of pediatrics at Johns Hopkins, modernizing the field by introducing quantitative research methods. An annual award, given by the American Pediatric Society for distinguished service to the field, honors him today.
The Alan Mason Chesney Medical Archives of The Johns Hopkins Medical Institutions

cases; and between these wings, an auditorium with private rooms above. The hospital would have no operating room, X-ray center, kitchen, laundry, or power plant; as efficiency dictated, it would share these facilities with adjoining Barnes Hospital.

Unfortunately, the Barnes project, which should have been well advanced, had run into a snag. In 1909, nephews of Robert Barnes challenged his hospital bequest, by now worth more than $2 million, and the case made its way through the courts until 1911, when the Missouri Supreme Court ruled in favor of the hospital. This delay had some advantages: It gave Robert Brookings more time to find money for constructing the new campus and convince Barnes to affiliate. But it also created ill will among the medical staff, who were promised gleaming new buildings as an inducement to come. Some left in disgust — among them, John Howland, who by the time of his departure on August 1, 1912, had spent less than a year on the job.

For Howland — one of the talented recruits known as "the Wise Men from the East" — this delay was only one of several reasons for dissatisfaction. Although he and an outside consultant, S.S. Goldwater of the Mount Sinai Hospital in New York, had given substantial help toward designing the new hospital, Howland now doubted that this building would happen at all. Since the board had no buyers for its current facility on Jefferson and Adams — which would languish until 1919, when it was finally sold to the Colored Methodist Episcopal Church — it did not have the cash it had expected. As his colleague David Edsall, another of the recruits who soon left, wrote to Abraham Flexner: "Poor Howland is in a pickle, with a wretched hospital, no *definite* prospect of a new one and not adequate funds to run it if built (no endowment at all)...."

In May 1912, a letter from Robert Brookings must have alleviated some of these concerns, since Brookings offered to pay the $75,000 cost of the proposed contagious pavilion himself. But at a meeting that same month, manager Katherine L. Guy moved "that the reception of colored children be discontinued in this hospital," and the board agreed. At the next meeting, member Mary McCall "voiced the feeling of many of the board in asking that this motion be not recorded without some expression of regret." Still, the result was a new policy of exclusion, and for Howland, this marked the breaking point; he wanted black children admitted, since he found them to be "among the most interesting cases of the clinic," according to a colleague.

This dispute was only one instance of a simmering feud between Howland and Grace Jones, who heartily disliked each other. During Howland's absence in Europe, when George Tuttle was acting head, peace had reigned. "It was [Tuttle's] interest, his good feeling and his faculty of smoothing out the rough places that secured the original staff and put the Hospital on its feet for better service to the public," recalled Jones in 1926, after his death. Howland possessed no such gift; in fact, said pediatrician

1912

Howland leaves the hospital in frustration over the delays in development of the new building; Borden Veeder assumes the position of pediatric head.

July 1912

Children's Hospital and Washington University sign their historic affiliation agreement.

The land in Valley Park was donated in 1911, and a 12-bed frame building at Ridge Farm opened in 1912 to patients who would recover more swiftly amid fresh air and a healthy country life. Local companies donated furnishings; Laura Weil's annual gift for a kindergarten at Children's Hospital now funded a teacher at Ridge Farm. At first, the daily cost per child was 86 cents but it rose to 96 cents in 1913. At a time of so many other expenses, Ridge Farm began to seem expensive to the jittery board.

But Ridge Farm was working, said a 1913 report: "One tiny four-year-old who has never walked, took his first steps, with the help of a brace and crutches, this week. One would scarcely recognize the pale, emaciated little sufferer of eight weeks ago in the apple-faced little lad who will soon be romping with the others." Added Borden Veeder: "It has been found that chronic and convalescent cases gain more in a week at the farm than they would during a month at the hospital in the city."

Late in 1913, Christine Blair Graham gave $25,000 for a new building and E.L. Opie, dean of the medical school, urged the board to continue this country department. With the help of an anonymous $51,500 gift, they did, building a 50-bed structure named for Graham's sister, Eveline Blair, who had died young. The managers also solicited people to perpetually support one day at Ridge Farm for a gift of $1,000.

Contract of sale of old Hospital. The second hospital building was not purchased until 1919, when it passed into the ownership of the Colored Methodist Episcopal Church for $12,500. Becker Medical Library

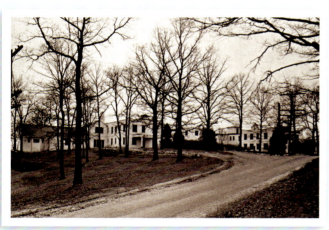

Ridge Farm. Becker Medical Library

Borden Veeder later, "his experience in St. Louis was unhappy for himself and for those who were associated with him." The board's independent attitude — establishing the Social Service Department and appointing Stimson in his absence — did not help either.

Only one curt line in the board minutes noted Howland's departure; another, that resident Kenneth Blackfan would leave with him. Until a new pediatric head could be found, Veeder took over, and his tact was a relief. "I never saw him lose his composure," wrote colleague Edwin H. Rohlfing. "[He was] always pretty sure of himself, but a good listener when he was trying to get the other fellow's exact position." As G. Canby Robinson put it: "He carried not only the charge of the entire department after Dr. Howland's departure, but reorganized the Children's Hospital."

1912

Work begins on the 220-bed Barnes Hospital and medical school buildings.

DECEMBER 1912

Ridge Farm opens on the donated property in Valley Park.

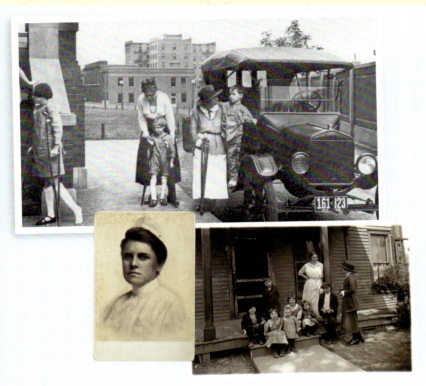

The 1911 annual report gave several examples of the kinds of cases that confronted Julia Stimson and her Social Service Department, which joined with the nursing department in 1913. In 1916, it would separate once again, and Stimson would become head of the Training School for Nurses:

"A doctor, in feeding a child at the feeding clinic, may see that he is making no headway, so he sends the Social Service worker into the home where, for example, she finds a history of syphilis in the family. She then takes the parents where they can be treated. It is this information which gives the doctors the means of making a correct diagnosis, and the child improves at once.

"A girl may be discharged from the hospital to a home where she is morally exposed through the absence of the mother. The worker tries to do preventive work by arranging to have the mother stay with her children.

"....Children who need braces and appliances are properly fitted and a loan is made to the family to cover the expense till it can be repaid, whenever that is possible."

Social Service Department's Ford. Provided by the hospital, this automobile allowed the members of the Social Service Department to make home visits and transport needy patients.
FAR LEFT **Julia Stimson (1881-1948).**
LEFT **Social Service.** The hospital established a Social Service division in 1910, with the aim of aiding in the treatment of patients by improving their social conditions. Social workers often paid home visits to see how former patients were progressing. Each of the seven children in the family pictured had been patients at Children's Hospital at one time.
Becker Medical Library (all)

CHILDREN'S HOSPITAL AFFILIATES WITH WASHINGTON UNIVERSITY

Ironically, just two weeks after Howland announced he would step down, the hospital and University signed their historic affiliation agreement on July 8, 1912. The document cited a key, but predictable, reason for the merger: the "efficiency" of a hospital associated with a research-oriented medical school. It also laid out the respective duties of both parties. While Children's Hospital would begin constructing "a first-class" building within six months and then operate it with the support of the medical faculty, the University would nominate the hospital's new administrative head, run a home for nurses, and build a dispensary along with its own medical school buildings.

The agreement also mentioned "pay patients." For the first time, the hospital was departing from its founding principle of providing all care free of charge and would now charge "reasonable fees" to those who could afford them. The Social Service Department began screening parents, finding some who wanted to pay when they couldn't and others who could but cried poverty. "Parents are expected...to recompense the Hospital up to the ward rate of $10.50 per week," wrote Jones, who had pressed for the change. In 1915, an additional $3 charge for tonsillectomies — proposed by physician Philip C. Jeans — drew fire from Fowler, who declared she did not approve.

In quick succession, the board approved a spate of other changes. A junior hospital auxiliary and sewing circles were formed. In December 1912, the board managed to open Ridge Farm, where they had renovated an old building on the property — a stopgap measure until they could finally put up a fine new 50-bed, fireproof facility, funded by Christine Blair Graham and an anonymous donor, in 1914. In May 1913, they attempted their most extraordinary fund-raising event yet, when they organized a "Cherry Carnival" at the Forest Park Highlands. The event made nearly $8,000, but it also convinced Grace Jones and her exhausted board that the future of fund-raising lay in individual and corporate giving.

MAY	JUNE
1913	1913
The largest fund-raising event yet for the hospital, the "Cherry Carnival," nets $8,000.	The cornerstone-laying ceremony is held for the Elizabeth J. Liggett Memorial Building.

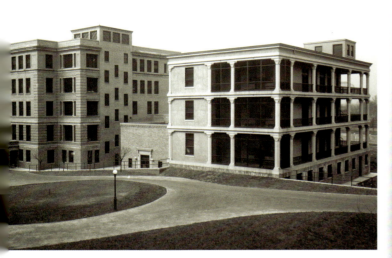

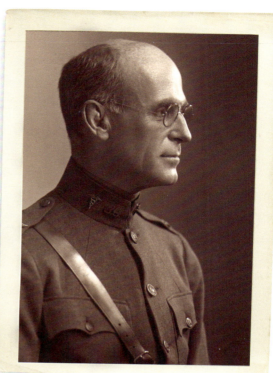

"AN IDEAL...PUT INTO LIFE"

Early in 1913, the board approved final plans for the new hospital and the construction contract was signed. Then on June 17 came the day they had all been longing for: the cornerstone-laying ceremony of the Elizabeth J. Liggett Memorial Building. Cora Fowler placed the stone and attorney Isaac Lionberger gave a brief, sentimental address. Paying tribute to Fowler ("herself denied the blessings of motherhood, she has gathered into her protecting arms unnumbered generations of little sufferers"), he also portrayed the future of this hospital: "There will be large and airy rooms and rows of little beds, each containing its small invalid. Neat and smiling nurses will tread softly its corridors, bearing balm for the afflicted. Doctors will come and go, watching and ministering, curing and alleviating. Mothers will steal in to see their children, and depart comforted."

During the months of construction that followed, recalled medical dean W. McKim Marriott in 1925, "Mrs. Jones was on the ground almost daily. She made herself familiar with every detail and added many improvements which before that time had not been present in children's hospitals. The result is a hospital building ideally adapted for its purposes." In fact, he said, "[Mrs. Jones] and her splendid Board have brought the Children's Hospital 'out of Egypt' as it were and 'into the promised land.'"

Some thought the board had made a mistake in settling so far west. "A lot of people thought we were crazy," recalled pediatrician Borden Veeder much later. "Kingshighway was very much in the country. We'd had a big outpatient clinic on Jefferson avenue, and there were many arguments that patients wouldn't go that far."

Meanwhile, work on the 220-bed Barnes Hospital and medical school buildings had already begun in 1912, but the wished-for endowment fund had not materialized. Still using Johns Hopkins as a model, Brookings applied in 1914 for a grant from the General Education Board (GEB), which now had Abraham Flexner on its staff. Quickly, they awarded the University $750,000, later increased to $1 million, provided the school produce a $500,000 match. With this money, the medical department would adopt a controversial new "full-time plan," in which faculty members agreed not to charge private patients within three departments: medicine, surgery, and pediatrics. Children's staunchly supported this bid to the GEB. "We pledge our every effort to afford the fullest facilities and support to a staff so constituted," said the board.

On January 9, 1915, the dedication of the

ABOVE **The third Children's Hospital.** "The St. Louis Children's Hospital is an institution that calls for all there is of cordial support and sustenance from the benevolent people in the city where it has done such a world of good work in child saving, and man and woman, making, in the course of one generation." — *Christine Blair Graham* Becker Medical Library

Fred T. Murphy (1872-1948). A Harvard graduate and faculty member of the School of Medicine, he became the head of surgery in 1915. Becker Medical Library

1914

Brookings applies for and receives a grant from the General Education Board, which awards the University $750,000 (later increased to $1 million).

DECEMBER 1914

Patients are treated for the first time at the new hospital building.

In May 1913, the board held a giant Cherry Carnival — such a stupendous effort that they never tried an entertainment on this scale again. Some 500 billboards and 300 streetcar signs announced the event, chaired by Grace Jones. The women volunteers wore white blouses and skirts with cherry-colored sashes, and white hats trimmed with cherries.

They had everything: dancing, merry-go-round rides, lemonade stands, a penny arcade, ice cream, cigars. There were contests for the best-dressed dolls and for the most beautiful baby; a Moon auto was raffled off "and a crippled child in charge of a pretty nurse" made "the drawing as the climax of the evening." A cherry tree offered cherries for sale, with "one lucky cherry bringing a Victor Talking machine."

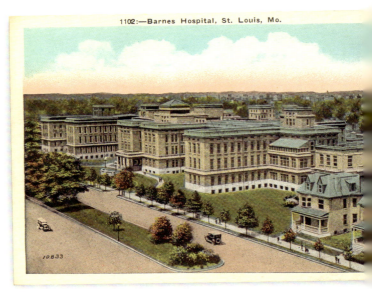

Barnes Hospital. The Barnes Hospital complex as it appeared after its completion in 1915. The two smaller buildings in the right foreground were first used as the "hospital for colored patients." Becker Medical Library

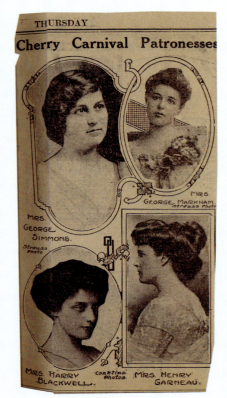

Cherry Carnival Patronesses This fund-raiser was organized by several society women and chaired by Mrs. Grace Jones. From Mary Margaret Mckittrick, Journal Vol II. Missouri Historical Society Archives.

completed Children's Hospital at last took place, though patients had already arrived in December. "Society men and women crowded the corridors all the afternoon," said a newspaper account. After George Tuttle gave the main address, he presented the keys of the hospital to Grace Jones, who in turn lauded generous donors. Borden Veeder spoke, mentioning a bronze tablet — "To the Sick Children of St. Louis" — mounted inside the hospital; he also described Children's efforts to help these patients, particularly through the new field of preventive medicine. "The one question we ask ourselves," he said, "is 'How can we be of service to the community?'"

Barnes Hospital, too, had opened on December 7, 1914; then Washington University Medical School was dedicated from April 28-30, 1915, in a lavish ceremony rich with high-flung rhetoric and distinguished visitors, among them William H. Welch, first dean of the Johns Hopkins School of Medicine. The occasion opened with prayer offered by Rt. Rev. Daniel S. Tuttle, Bishop of the Diocese of Missouri and father of George Tuttle; several speakers associated with Children's

DECEMBER	JANUARY		APRIL
1914	**1915**		**1915**
Barnes Hospital opens.	Dedication of the completed Children's Hospital is held.		Washington University Medical School is dedicated in a lavish ceremony.

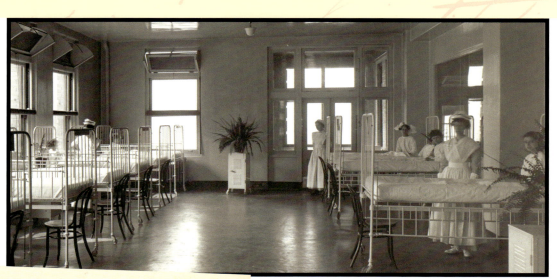

Spacious new wards. The new wards had plenty of space and ventilation, with fresh air provided through transoms and the large porches that flanked each room. Becker Medical Library

NATIONALITIES AND RELIGIONS OF PATIENTS TREATED IN WARDS

The 1636 children who were cared for in the wards of the hospital were of the following religions and nationalities:

American	1098	Baptist	116
Austrian	35	Christian	73
Bohemian	10	Congregational	11
Bulgarian	1	Episcopal	32
Danish	1	Greek Catholic	3
Dutch	4	Jewish	269
English	7	Lutheran	145
French	5	Methodist	196
German	124	Non-sectarian	102
Greek	4	Presbyterian	124
Hungarian	15	Roman Catholic	565
Irish	36		
Italian	42	Total	1636
Mexican	1		
Polish	28		
Roumanian	8		
Russian	203		
Spanish	2		
Swede	9		
Syrian	1		
Welsh	2		
Total	1636		

Nationalities and Religions chart. Along with other pertinent data, the nationality and religion of each patient was noted and recorded, as in this page from the 1914 annual report. Becker Medical Library

Hospital, including George Dock and surgeon-in-chief Fred Murphy, gave addresses. The star of the occasion was Robert Brookings, aptly described by Acting Chancellor Frederic A. Hall as "the one man, pre-eminently, whose dream is this day realized." Brookings described each new building in loving detail, including the Children's complex and a prospective "hospital for colored patients" that would accommodate pediatric and adult patients.

That year, one of the early Children's Hospital managers, Minnie Bulkley, reflected on how far the hospital had come in 36 years. "It seems as if ages of time and a continent of effort must separate the splendid new Children's Hospital, so efficient and so immaculate, from the old house…where the work began," she wrote. Christine Blair Graham and four other board members went farther in praise of the new facility: "In point of equipment, the hospital is unsurpassed and unsurpassable, and the organization of the service is as nearly perfect as anything human can well be."

With this building, which would require professional management, and its new ties to the academic medical world of Washington University, the board's long-time authority over hospital affairs would inevitably diminish. Although Grace Jones stayed on as board president until 1925, she had already made her major contribution to the hospital. It was a crucial one, however. As charter board member Virginia Stevenson said upon Jones's retirement: "How nobly she has done her work, with what energy and skill she has conducted the affairs of the St. Louis Children's Hospital, is shown in the present building on Kingshighway, in the lovely home out at Ridge Farm, in the loyal and enthusiastic Board that she has gathered around her, and, last but not least, in the gratitude and love which she has inspired in many hearts."

"The Magician": W. McKim Marriott

After John Howland's abrupt departure, Borden S. Veeder served as his temporary replacement, but Washington University School of Medicine still needed a permanent head of pediatrics. The job had become even more attractive since Howland had held it: The new head would also bear the title of pediatrician-in-chief at Children's Hospital. At the urging of Philip Shaffer, one of the University's 1910 recruits, the department turned in 1917 to Williams McKim Marriott, a talented researcher working at Johns Hopkins, who had little experience in clinical pediatrics and even less in administrative work.

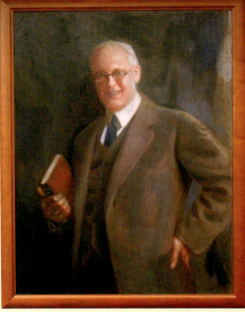

W. McKim Marriott (1885-1936).
As Chancellor George R. Throop said at Marriott's memorial service in 1937: "An inexhaustible store of vitality seemed to possess him. He was ready to assume any burden, to confront any situation, and to act under all occasions with an optimism and a cheerfulness that carried the strongest inspiration."
Unknown artist, Portrait of W. McKim Marriott, n.d. Oil on canvas, 47" x 36-1/2". St. Louis Children's Hospital.

Yet his choice proved one of the school's most fortuitous. For him, "everything was possible, simple, easy....He had a good deal of the magician in him," recalled a friend, Edwards Park, at Marriott's 1936 memorial service. "He worked with tremendous energy, and in a veritable and constant ebullition of enthusiasm." These qualities were apparent as he guided his department, his hospital — even his burgeoning field of pediatrics — to new heights of excellence. After his early death, *The Journal of Pediatrics* paid tribute to "the meteoric career of one of the most brilliant minds that has flashed across the field of pediatrics in America."

Marriott — "the Chief," as University faculty called him — was born in Baltimore in 1885; one grandfather was a minister and his father, James, was an inventor whose creations included a noiseless typewriter. "I have wondered," said Park, "if [Marriott's] combination of idealism and practicality was not a family contribution." A prodigy, he began at the University of North Carolina at age 15, graduating in 1904. He was first introduced to St. Louis during the 1904 World's Fair, where he worked in the U.S. Geological Survey exhibit.

"BEAR BITES" AND CHEMISTRY

During his last two years of college, he became intrigued by chemistry and, after graduation, followed a professor to New York City and acted as his assistant. There he met prominent chemist C.G.L. Wolf of Cornell University's medical school and transferred to Wolf's laboratory, where he learned biochemistry, taught medical students, and along the way — almost incidentally — picked up a medical degree in 1910. His only clinical experience came during a few summers at Yellowstone Park, where he served as hotel physician treating, as he put it, "bear bites and Geyser burns."

Late in 1910, biochemist Shaffer — a long-time friend — recruited him to Washington University as an instructor in biological chemistry. For four years, Marriott worked as part of the medical school's tiny chemical branch in its outdated building at

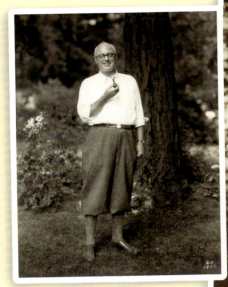
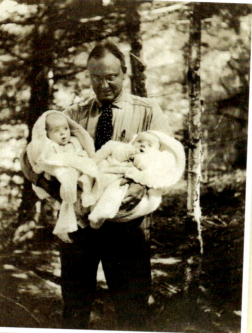
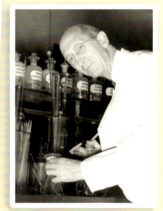

1806 Locust Street. Still, "there was a buoyant, youthful spirit among all of us in those days, felt by no one more keenly than by Marriott," wrote Shaffer later, adding that they wanted to build "a medical school in which…productive research would be recognized as an obligation of equal importance with teaching and practice."

By 1914, Marriott was restless and eager for more experience. After department head George Dock turned him down as a trainee in internal medicine, he accepted an offer to work in the chemistry lab of John Howland, by then at Johns Hopkins, in exchange for pediatric training.

"A BOLD PROPOSAL"

Over the next three years, the two produced work that was "perhaps the most important influence on pediatrics that took place in the United States, and one that extended far beyond this country," wrote Veeder later. Two research breakthroughs stood out: Marriott discovered that acidosis exists in the dreaded infant disease known as "alimentary intoxication" or cholera infantum, and that serum calcium concentration is low in the dangerous infantile tetany — a finding that led to an effective treatment.

With Veeder and other members of the Base Hospital No. 21 team away at war and with funding from the General Education Board to put the pediatrics department on a full-time basis, the medical school began searching for a pediatrics head — and in 1917 decided to take a chance on Marriott. "His selection was a bold proposal, and it is not surprising that it encountered criticism and even opposition…." recalled Shaffer. "But a number of the members of the faculty knew the sort of man he was…and had confidence that clinical skill and judgment would be quickly acquired." Despite Howland's disapproval, Marriott decided to accept.

"I remember well my own feeling of relief when his more experienced clinical associates first began to comment on his unusually keen insight into diagnostic difficulties and on his logical common sense in treatment," added Shaffer, "for I was then satisfied that the bold experiment would succeed."

> **"He worked with tremendous energy, and in a veritable and constant ebullition of enthusiasm."**
> —Edwards Park, 1936

LEFT As Philip Shaffer said of Marriott: "He believed in spending himself for ideals, in facing and accepting obligations without regard to personal cost. He focused his ideals on this medical school and gave himself without stint to it." W.M. Marriott Collection

MIDDLE Marriott and his wife had twin daughters, one of whom died in childhood, as well as a son, McKim. Wrote Edwards Park: Marriott "showed his lack of conventionality in his private life. When twins were expected in his family, Mrs. Park found him in great enthusiasm making the napkins [diapers] on the sewing machine." W.M. Marriott Collection

RIGHT Philip A. Shaffer (1881-1960). In 1910, Shaffer joined the medical staff as professor and head of biological chemistry at the age of 29. He recruited Marriott that same year, and later praised his nomination for the pediatrics head as a "bold experiment." Becker Medical Library

Marriott, who returned to Washington University during World War I, was an ardent pacifist, "and his views used to disturb Howland, who was an intense partisan," said his friend, Edwards Park. A St. Louis colleague, Park White, honored him at his 1936 memorial service with this poem:

> "He came and looked upon a stricken world
> And said, 'What these call sin is ignorance!
> We who love Truth must keep her flag unfurled,
> Must fight Destruction with invisible lance.
> Be ours the task to know what can't be known;
> Be ours to save while others blindly kill;
> Be ours the task to do what can't be done;
> Be ours not to destroy but to fulfill!'
> So patiently he set himself to learn
> The laws of health and sickness; his the prize
> To save young lives for those who gave them being-
> (No fault of his if fools should some time turn
> And rend them, raining havoc from the skies!)
> He learned – and taught.
> Blind followers left him seeing.

CHAPTER

4

1915
1936

"The Bold Experiment" Succeeds: W. McKim Marriott

INFANT NUTRITION

A TEXTBOOK OF INFANT FEEDING FOR STUDENTS
AND PRACTITIONERS OF MEDICINE

BY

WILLIAMS McKIM MARRIOTT, B.S., M.D.

PROFESSOR OF PEDIATRICS, WASHINGTON UNIVERSITY SCHOOL OF MEDICINE; PHYSICIAN
IN CHIEF, ST. LOUIS CHILDREN'S HOSPITAL, ST. LOUIS

ILLUSTRATED

ST. LOUIS
THE C. V. MOSBY COMPANY
1930

CHAPTER FOUR "THE BOLD EXPERIMENT" SUCCEEDS: W. McKIM MARRIOTT

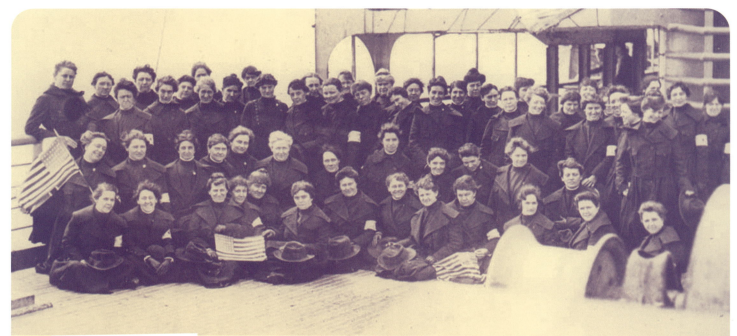

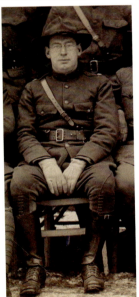

LEFT **Borden S. Veeder in WWI.** Veeder was quartermaster of the Base Hospital No. 21 group and served for a time as the group's commanding officer. He was awarded the Order of St. Michael and St. George for his service. Becker Medical Library

Red Cross Nurses. This contingent of 65 St. Louis nurses, headed by Julia Stimson, served at Base Hospital No. 21. Becker Medical Library

As the relocated Children's Hospital

began its new life on the Kingshighway campus, international events were occurring that would constrain its operation and shrink its staff for several years. World War I had broken out in Europe, and Americans were being drawn inexorably into the conflict as well. In the 1916 annual report, the president's letter couched the hospital's need for funds in the imagery of battle. "Continued support…will bring a preparedness for war on all that attacks the health and sanity of our children," wrote manager Grace Jones.

PREVIOUS PAGE **Hospital Medical Staff (1919).**
INSET **Infant Nutrition.** W. McKim Marriott developed a simple formula for modifying milk to meet the nutritional needs of infants. His popular textbook on the subject was published in 1930.
Becker Medical Library

| JUNE | APRIL 6 |
| 1916 | 1917 |

The hospital's Executive Faculty begins the search for a new head of pediatrics.

United States declares war on Germany; several Washington University medical school faculty, including Children's Hospital staff members, leave for France soon after as volunteers for Base Hospital No. 21, established by the American Red Cross.

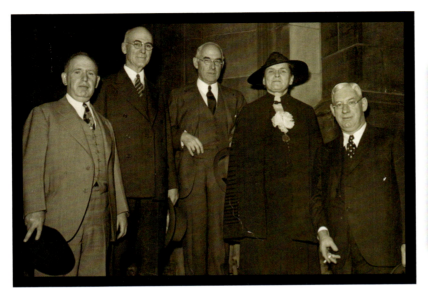

Key figures from Base Hospital No.21 at a reunion in 1943.
(from left: Walter Fischel, Fred T. Murphy, Malvern Clopton, Julia Stimson and Borden Veeder). Becker Medical Library

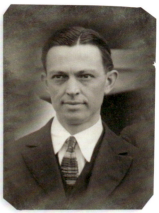

Philip C. Jeans (1883-1952).
A Johns Hopkins graduate, Jeans came to Children's Hospital as a resident in 1912. By 1917, he was chief of the pediatric clinic at the Dispensary, where he successfully built up attendance. His research focused on hereditary syphilis in children, later on fortifying foods with vitamin D. Becker Medical Library

On April 6, 1917, the United States declared war on Germany, and Washington University medical faculty soon left for France and Base Hospital No. 21, one of some 50 overseas hospitals established by the American Red Cross. Key hospital staff members were among those who volunteered for service: acting pediatric department head Borden S. Veeder, who turned that job over to Philip C. Jeans; surgeon-in-chief Fred T. Murphy; associate surgeons Nathaniel Allison and Malvern B. Clopton; pathologist Eugene Opie; assistant surgeon Vilray P. Blair and assistant physician Hugh McCulloch; neurologist Sidney Schwab; and residents John Murphy and Meredith Johnston. Just as important was the departure of nursing school head Julia Stimson, leader of the nursing contingent, who later rose to chief nurse of the American Expeditionary Forces and won a Royal Red Cross from the British government.

At Children's Hospital, everyone felt the pinch as more than half the medical team suddenly disappeared. Still, "the fine spirit manifested by those remaining, both doctors and nurses, made it possible for the work of the Hospital to continue," said the 1918 Annual Report. "The policy adhered to during this period was that of treating as many patients as possible in the Dispensary and admitting to the Hospital only seriously ill children....As barely enough nurses were available to care for patients in the partially filled wards, it was impossible to accommodate very many private patients, especially those requiring special nurses." The private pavilion closed for a time, and the hospital's country department, Ridge Farm, shut down for the duration.

Then a devastating new problem arose: the fall 1918 influenza epidemic, which sent nearly 100 young patients to the hospital and sidelined nurses — requiring the managers to volunteer as nurses' aides. "Whole families of children ill of influenza were brought to us," continued the annual report. "[I]n some instances both parents had died of the disease. The Hospital could not well refuse these patients if there were any possible means of caring for them. All floors of the contagious pavilion were opened and these, as well as the side rooms in the main Hospital, and a number of cubicles in the admitting ward, were filled with influenza patients."

1917 The hospital's country department, Ridge Farm, is closed for the duration of the war.

1917 W. McKim Marriott is appointed head of pediatrics and physician-in-chief.

For the most part, the underpaid nursing staff performed admirably, despite long hours and very hard work, especially during the training period. Infractions met with severe punishment. In 1918, a supervisor reported that "Miss Estes, a second-year nurse on night duty in the Infant ward in the Children's Hospital, had gone to sleep on the stretcher while on duty…It was recommended… that three months should be added to Miss Estes's training and public notice made of the same."

Also in 1918, committee minutes showed how some young nurses were treated. Nurse Flynn was "guilty of a callousness and lack of a proper spirit" toward her work as a nurse, since "it was reported (1) that Miss Flynn has refused to go to Dr. Sachs's home to take care of his children because she didn't wish to do 24 hr. duty (2) that she declined to go home with Mrs. Green, an obstetrical patient of Dr. Roysten's, for the same reason…."

Occasionally, there were genuine problems. In September 1916, Veeder reported that at Ridge Farm: "A nurse had put carbolic acid in the water pitcher on the medicine tray." She was temporarily suspended. In October 1917, another "allowed a baby to fall out of bed, causing a large hematoma on the right side of the head." Her case was referred to the nursing superintendent.

Gradually, the treatment of nurses improved, as the nursing school introduced a five-year B.S. degree in nursing in 1924. In 1926, Marriott wrote: "The time has passed when an educated girl will enter a hospital and spend several years in giving free service, often of a menial nature, unless she receives at the same time educational advantages."

What to do about nurses. This 1932 letter to the editor of the *St. Louis Post-Dispatch* highlights the difficulties of the nursing profession.

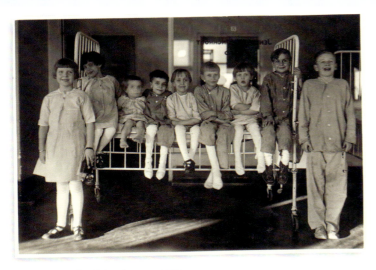

Cheerful young hospital patients, ca. 1920s. Becker Medical Library

> " …for the secret of the care of the patient is in caring for the patient."

"SOUGHT AFTER BY A NUMBER OF UNIVERSITIES…"

The leader who steered the hospital through the later crises and wrote these accounts of its success was the new full-time head of pediatrics and pediatrician-in-chief W. McKim Marriott. Appointed in 1917, he took a year's leave of absence and arrived in July 1918, quickly dispelling doubts among those who feared that this fine researcher would not function well as a clinical chief. Yet Marriott had not been the first choice of the Executive Faculty, the medical school's powerful decision-making group made up of the dean and key department heads. They had begun searching for a new pediatrics chief in June 1916, consulting some 20 medical giants around the country, including William H. Welch of Johns Hopkins, Washington University's former pediatrics head John Howland, and Abraham Flexner, whose damning report had precipitated Robert Brookings' reorganization of the medical school. The list that emerged from this name-gathering did not even mention Marriott, though it did include Borden Veeder, as well as Oscar Schloss of New York and Francis

1917	1918
Joint committee is formed for the operation of Barnes and Children's hospitals, supervised by Louis H. Burlingham.	A policy of admitting women interns on the same basis as men is adopted; Johns Hopkins graduate Katherine K. Merritt is the first to arrive in July.

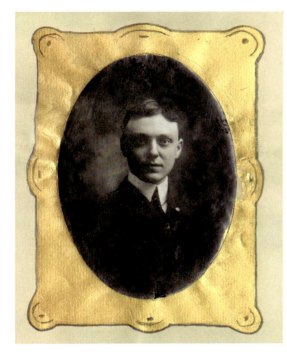

Weld Peabody of Boston. Unanimously, the Executive Faculty agreed to offer the pediatric chair to Peabody.

Peabody, a 1907 Harvard Medical School graduate with a stellar résumé, was an excellent, if optimistic, choice. Not only had he served as an assistant resident at Johns Hopkins and as a fellow under William Welch, but he had also been the first chief resident in medicine in 1913 at the new Peter Bent Brigham Hospital in Boston. A year later, he was named by the Rockefeller Institute to an advisory commission that traveled to China and helped shape the new Peking Union Medical College; by 1915, Harvard had named him associate professor of medicine. He was also an active researcher, making important strides in understanding typhoid, heart disease, and polio.

During his career, cut short by his early death in 1927, Peabody would earn an international reputation as director of Harvard's Thorndike Memorial Laboratory at Boston City Hospital, which became a model for rigorous scientific inquiry and humane patient care. Eventually, Columbia, Yale, and Stanford offered him professorships, while the University of Chicago invited him to become their dean. "He refused,

Williams McKim Marriott (1885-1936). Edwards Park, renowned Johns Hopkins physician, said of Marriott: "he suddenly appeared in pediatrics and for the space of a few years illuminated it, shedding light into some of its dark places, and then departed leaving behind him an influence and an accomplishment which few other pediatricians have equaled in a lifetime of endeavor." W.M. Marriott Collection

however, to leave his own university," said his obituary in *The Journal of Clinical Investigation*, "believing that here he could be of the greatest service."

Peabody also turned down the Children's Hospital offer. Reported the Executive Faculty minutes, ruefully: "While he felt the highest appreciation of the opportunities afforded, he preferred to adhere to his plan for a career in internal medicine rather than transfer his activities to Pediatrics." The board decided to defer any new decision until 1917 and listed seven likely candidates. Veeder was one, so was Schloss, and there was an addition: Williams McKim Marriott.

"A FAVORABLE IMPRESSION"

Behind the scenes, another party was quietly influencing this choice: the General Education Board (GEB) of the Rockefeller Institute, now staffed by the University's one-time critic, Abraham Flexner. The GEB had offered the university a $1 million grant to reorganize three clinical departments — pediatrics, medicine, and surgery — on a full-time basis, if the medical school could match it with $500,000 from private sources. This money would allow the medical school to adopt a new full-time plan, an idea pioneered at Johns Hopkins, in which faculty members would not take fees from private

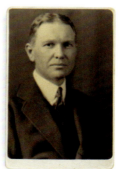

patients. At the urging of his old friend Robert Brookings, Edward Mallinckrodt, Sr. —whose late wife, Jennie, had served faithfully on the Children's Hospital board of lady managers — provided the one-third needed to fund pediatrics. With its grant, the GEB acquired the right to give advice on

Francis Weld Peabody (1881-1927). In a series of lectures to Harvard medical students in 1927, Peabody said: "One of the essential qualities of the physician is interest in humanity, for the secret of the care of the patient is in caring for the patient." Harvard Medical Library in the Francis A. Countway Library of Medicine

JULY 1918

Marriott arrives in St. Louis to begin his new position after a year's leave of absence in clinical work at the Boston Floating Hospital.

1918

Margaret L. Butler dies, leaving a bequest of $300,000 to the hospital as an addition to the James Gay Butler Endowment Fund, established at her husband's death in 1916.

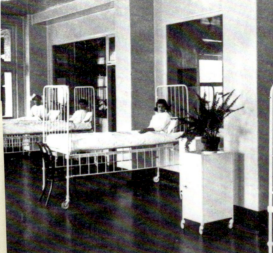

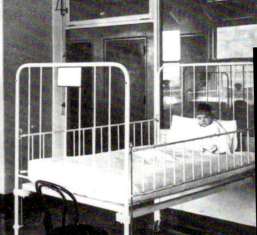

Jennie Mallinckrodt Ward, ca. 1920s. This ward was funded by Edward Mallinckrodt, Sr., and named in honor of his wife, Jennie, who was a long-time supporter of the hospital and served as the board's vice-president for the last 13 years of her life. Becker Medical Library

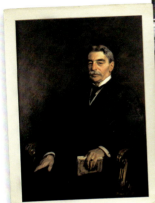

Edward Mallinckrodt, Sr. (1845-1928). In 1916, chemical company founder Mallinckrodt gave $166,666 to the Medical School to meet the General Education Board's required match for their $1 million gift. Similar gifts came from John T. Milliken for internal medicine and lady manager Mary Culver for surgery. Mallinckrodt Institute of Radiology

faculty additions and veto unwelcome choices. In July 1916, a disappointed Flexner exclaimed that, after Peabody's refusal, "it seems to me that there is no one now in sight who is clearly the ideal man for the chair or who is manifestly superior in qualifications to Dr. Veeder. And, while we appreciate Dr. Veeder's ability, we are not prepared to recommend him."

This lack of confidence did not please interim head Veeder, already feeling undervalued for this time-consuming work. In 1915, he complained to Dean Eugene Opie that "since I have been in charge…I have been unable to devote my time to anything outside of the clinical and executive work and I feel that this has very seriously hampered my own development." On a practical note, he added that "with the responsibilities and work I have had to assume, I have been very much underpaid, and that for the coming year my salary should be $3,000." Still, he chose to remain on the faculty for the rest of his career, though he was out of the running as a candidate.

By the November 1916 Executive Faculty meeting, the list of choices was narrowing. Surgery head Fred T. Murphy and physiology

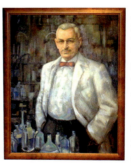

professor Joseph Erlanger were dispatched east to interview Marriott and Schloss and confer with Hopkins faculty. This time, Welch suggested "that individual fitness and laboratory achievement might outweigh clinical experience" — a vote for Marriott; Howland, unwilling to lose his prized collaborator, demurred, pointing to Marriott's limited clinical training. Altogether, said the committee's report, "Dr. Marriott has made a most favorable impression on the men at Hopkins…as a scientific investigator." They made less effort to assess Schloss's credentials: Murphy alone traveled to New York to meet with him, coming away with the positive yet non-committal view that Schloss "was an able investigator and clinician and would make an admirable head for a department of pediatrics."

Clearly, the Executive Faculty was intrigued by Marriott, but reluctant to overlook his lack of clinical background. After much debate, they

INSET **Jean Valjean Cooke (1883-1956).** Another Johns Hopkins alumnus, he was assistant physician at Children's starting in 1917, becoming a full professor in 1936 and emeritus in 1951. In 1949 he was president of the American Pediatric Society. His research focused on tetanus, diphtheria, scarlet fever, whooping cough, and later on leukemia. Viktor De Jeney, Portrait of Jean Valjean Cooke, 1963. Oil on canvas, 46" x 36". St. Louis Children's Hospital.

FALL 1918

Influenza epidemic breaks out in St. Louis.

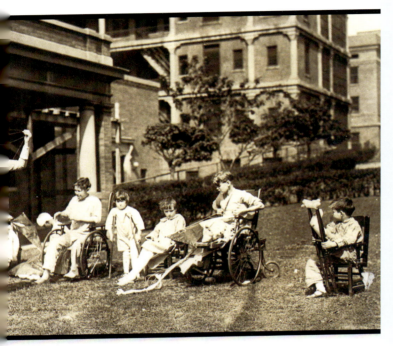

Fresh air and exercise. Children's Hospital physicians recognized and encouraged the therapeutic benefits of outdoor activity. *Becker Medical Library*

In a 1920 *Studies from the Department of Pediatrics* article, W. McKim Marriott described his collaboration with Joseph Erlanger in making ingenious use of prolonged artificial respiration to treat the paralysis of respiratory muscles in a child following her severe case of diphtheria:

"Rosie W., aged 10 years, was admitted to the St. Louis Children's Hospital, Jan. 3, 1920, six weeks after a severe attack of pharyngeal diphtheria....The patient was unable to move the legs or body or to hold up her head. She could swallow only with the greatest difficulty....The child's respiratory difficulties increased....Cyanosis deepened and [she] became semicomatose....It was evident that death from suffocation would result within a very short time.

"At Dr. Erlanger's suggestion, we made use of an apparatus described by Gesell and Erlanger ...designed to convert a continuous air current into an intermittent one of any desired rate and volume and has been used extensively in physiologic laboratories for administering artificial respiration to animals. A nitrous oxide mask connected to the apparatus was applied closely to the child's face.

"The effect was almost immediate; cyanosis disappeared, and the patient became sufficiently conscious to cooperate well.... The function of the respiratory muscles steadily improved, and at the end of a week it was possible to dispense entirely with the artificial respiration. The child was discharged from the hospital, January 31, in excellent condition. She is now (six months later) well and apparently normal in every way."

reached a compromise: hire the "productive and stimulating" Marriott, but grant him an immediate leave of absence for one year, so that he could gain hands-on experience in a large clinic, the Boston Floating Hospital. In the meantime, he would remain informed of all that happened and even suggest some changes himself, and then arrive in July 1918.

INHERITING A HOSPITAL

As soon as his appointment was official, Marriott began sending exuberant, hand-written letters to Philip Shaffer, his friend and the medical school dean, about plans for the future. In June 1917, he made a request, conveyed by Shaffer to the Executive Faculty, that acting head Jeans — who had also taken on the giant responsibility of directing the Dispensary's busy Pediatric Clinic — be promoted to associate professor. In July 1917, while on vacation in New York State, he wrote asking to hire a young bacteriologist, Jean Valjean Cooke, at the salary of $3,000 per year.

The hospital that Marriott inherited in summer 1918, amid the war and the incipient flu epidemic, was vastly different in size, sophistica-

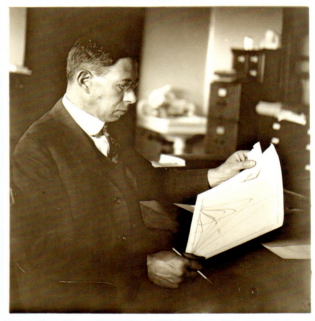

Joseph Erlanger (1874-1965). A Johns Hopkins graduate, Erlanger was recruited by Brookings and Houston and served as professor of physiology from 1910-65. In 1944 he and Herbert S. Gasser won the Nobel Prize for their work on the electrical properties of the nervous system. *Becker Medical Library*

MARCH 1919 — The first woman pediatric faculty member, Kirsten Utheim of Norway, is hired by Marriott.

1919 — Evarts A. Graham is appointed as the first full-time head of surgery, replacing Fred. T. Murphy.

> **WET NURSES**
> The Hospital will be glad to hear of women who would like to be employed as wet nurses either at the Hospital or in private homes. A certain number will be engaged by the Hospital; others after a physical examination and Wassermann test will be listed at the Hospital office. Physicians requiring wet nurses to go into private homes will be furnished names of available nurses registered at the Hospital. No charge is made by the Hospital for this service.
> The Hospital can best serve the community if there is the fullest co-operation between its medical staff and the medical profession outside of the Institution. In order to further this co-operation, the following notice is sent to physicians sending patients to the Hospital:

Filling a need. Marriott took note of the shortage of milk for infants in St. Louis and advertised for wet nurses to be employed at the hospital or in private homes, with no charge to the patients. Becker Medical Library

tion, and management from the outdated, downtown facility he had known as a young biochemist on the medical school staff. In 1917, Children's Hospital was operating on a reduced, wartime basis, but still had admitted 180 patients, 12 of them children under two who had died mainly of "nutritional disturbances." Although the managers worked hard as fund-raisers and hospital volunteers, most of the major decision-making had shifted elsewhere: to a joint committee, formed in 1917, for the operation of Barnes and Children's hospitals. The managers had a courteous, even cordial, relationship with this committee, which consulted them on important matters; still, no manager was a member. An experienced physician now supervised Children's as well as Barnes hospitals: Louis H. Burlingham, formerly of the Peter Bent Brigham Hospital in Boston, and member of the joint committee.

This wave of change had affected the faculty as well. Most core members were full-time, as stipulated by the GEB grant, but others were not — and they got a new title. Beginning in 1917-18, those who retained some private patients were known as "associate" (or assistant) "in clinical pediatrics." The full-time plan was also a boon to medical students, whose pediatric curriculum was progressive. "More time is devoted to the study of Pediatrics in the Washington University than in the average medical school," boasted a 1922 report. "Instruction is begun in the second year, which is a departure from the practice of most schools. This is done as it is felt that the student can best understand disease in the adult if he learns at the same time the manifestations of the same disease as they occur in childhood."

MARRIOTT'S VISION

As soon as the eager Marriott arrived on the scene, he continued to modernize the hospital and pediatrics department. In addition to Cooke, he appointed other talented young faculty, such as Maurice Lonsway, Sr., Samuel W. Clausen, Phelps G. Hurford, and Wayne A. Rupe, along with interns such as Harvey L. White. He even tried to attract his erstwhile competitor, Oscar Schloss — though he had to desist when Schloss

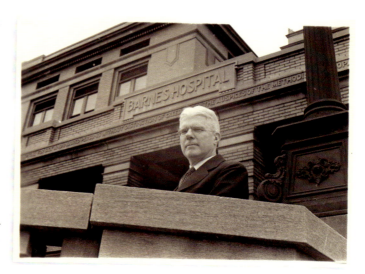

Louis Burlingham (1880-1946). Burlingham served as both the Children's Hospital Administrator and the Barnes Hospital Superintendent from 1918 to 1925. Philip Shaffer, dean of the medical school, had endorsed his hiring, saying that he wanted to ease the administrative load of physicians, "whose only concern should be with illness or the investigation of disease." Becker Medical Library

> **"More time is devoted to the study of Pediatrics in the Washington University than in the average medical school."**

1919
Ridge Farm re-opens and receives its first teacher from the Board of Education.

1920
Marriott establishes twice-yearly, post-graduate courses for out-of-town practicing physicians.

The new program in occupational therapy, said the 1919 annual report, was an instant success. "The happy, contented child is more receptive to treatment than the fretting, discontented one, and in cases of long periods of enforced rest in bed, as well as in the shorter, more acute cases, the provision of some form of directed activity for the hands and mind is essential."

Director Lois Keim went on to give examples of children helped by the program.

"One little girl, ten years old, whose leg was weighed down in a traction, begged that the weaving which had been given to her to do during the day be left over night, saying, 'I don't notice the pain in my leg when I have something to do.'

"Another child, scheduled for periodic return to the hospital, told her father that she would not come in again unless she was sure that she would have the same interesting things to make which she had had the last time.

"Two small boys have earned several dollars from the sale of bead chains and baskets. As one of these boys is permanently disabled, the practice of an interesting craft will relieve to some degree the tedium of his handicap.

"Still another boy, convalescent from pneumonia, became so interested in making baskets that he begged the doctor to keep him in the hospital for some time."

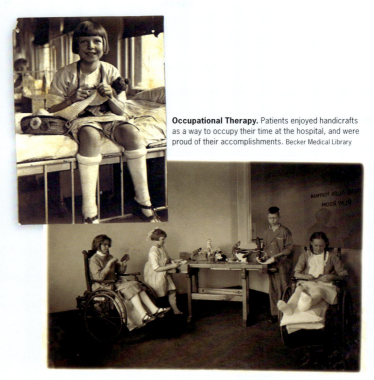

Occupational Therapy. Patients enjoyed handicrafts as a way to occupy their time at the hospital, and were proud of their accomplishments. Becker Medical Library

demanded at least $7,000 in salary. In other cases, he selected the cream of the interns to join his staff, and then sent them on to top pediatric posts. "Interns who graduated within the last three years are now instructors in Harvard, Yale and Washington University," he wrote in 1922. Among his own new faculty, he stressed the importance of engaging in laboratory research.

Marriott also reached out to the medical community. To reassure St. Louis doctors that the hospital was not trying to steal their patients, he sent them notices that patients "will in all instances be referred back…on discharge." For practicing physicians elsewhere, he established twice-yearly, post-graduate courses in 1920. Only two years later he wrote: "These courses were successful from the start. From 50 to 60 practitioners, coming from all parts of the country, have attended.…Several of these men have written us that they are now in charge of children's wards in hospitals in the towns from which they came."

At the same time, he took a new look at local needs and found that milk, especially for infants, was in acutely short supply. In response, he advertised in newspapers for wet nurses, to be employed at the hospital or sent out to homes; the hospital would provide this service free of charge. He inaugurated a series of lectures for the general public on disease prevention; they "have served to bring the community to realize the value of a modern Medical department," he wrote.

Quietly, he also worked to extend the hospital's scope. Two years before he arrived, the board of managers — thinking along the same lines — had arranged an affiliation with three St. Louis orphanages. Under Marriott, the hospital took on the care of newborns at Barnes Hospital in 1921. Then in the early 1920s, he began promoting an alliance with St. Louis Maternity Hospital — a step strongly supported by the GEB, which hinted that if a maternity hospital were built near the medical center, it would consider making a generous grant to endow a full-time Department of Obstetrics. The contract was signed in April 1923 — and Children's Hospital now had access to newborns for teaching and research. Soon construction of a new maternity hospital building was underway east of Barnes Hospital and completed in 1927; the GEB did come through with a large grant

1920
A nursing shortage is declared an "emergency" by Dean Allison; the census is cut to 70 on normal days, 75 in emergencies, due to lack of staff.

1920
The board of managers votes to set aside space on the first floor of the Pavilion building for black children, excluded from the hospital since 1912.

The first woman faculty member at the School of Medicine, physician Kirsten Utheim (1890-1949) impressed Marriott enough that he promoted her three times, took her on as a collaborator, and entrusted her with teaching, as well as the supervision of a hospital ward. In a 1923 letter of recommendation to the Director of the National Hospital in Oslo, where she was applying to become associate pediatrician-in-chief, Marriott testified to Utheim's ability: "In short, I may say that Dr. Utheim has shown herself to be a thoroughly competent clinician, investigator and teacher of Pediatrics."

After her marriage to Guttorm Toverud, a Norwegian dentist studying at Harvard, she returned to her native Norway and earned her PhD degree, based in part on her research at Children's Hospital. That same year she began at the National Hospital; later, she headed the medical staff of a residential treatment center for diabetic children. There, wrote her son, "she emphasized the need for children to have their insulin dose and diet adjusted while they attended school and participated in outdoor sports and play, a novel idea at that time."

During her subsequent career, she was a frequent lecturer throughout Europe on pediatrics. Her research interests centered on the prevention of rickets, anemia in pregnant and nursing mothers, vitamin B and C metabolism in pregnancy, and vitamin K usage for the prevention of neonatal bleeding.

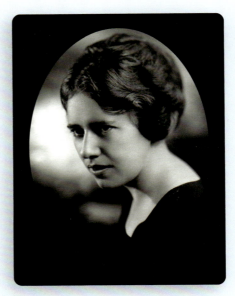

Kirsten Utheim (1890-1949). Courtesy of the Toverud family

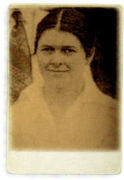

Martha May Eliot (1891-1978). After graduating from Radcliffe College in 1913 and Johns Hopkins School of Medicine five years later, Eliot wished to continue at Hopkins for her residency, but John Howland "flatly and promptly turned [her] down," she later said. Marriott accepted her for a residency at Children's Hospital in 1919.

Later, she became a medical pioneer, placing childhood disease within a social context and targeting public health, primarily as chief of the U.S. Children's Bureau, as a founder of UNICEF and the World Health Organization (WHO), and as a faculty member at Yale and at Harvard. Ironically, she won the American Pediatric Society's John Howland Medal in 1967. Becker Medical Library

aimed at newborn teaching and research. Another hospital, the 85-bed Shriners' Hospital for Crippled Children, was also going up around the corner, and its patients, too, would be available to University faculty for teaching purposes.

Still, Marriott faced disquieting problems, particularly a chronic shortage of nurses, which continued into the 1920s. At the beginning of that decade, the census of Children's Hospital had to be cut to 70 patients on normal days, 75 in emergencies, because there was not enough nursing staff to care for more. Dean Nathaniel Allison declared the situation an "emergency" in 1920 and attributed this shortfall to a need for "better education, better training, better living conditions" for nursing students.

"ON THE SAME BASIS AS MEN..."

Like most physicians of his time, Marriott routinely used the term "men" to describe house staff. "Interns on the pediatric service have been picked with considerable care," he wrote in 1922. "...Only those men of exceptional collegiate standing are accepted." In fact, he led Washington University in giving residency slots to talented women, most of them from Johns Hopkins. Almost as soon as he arrived, he announced this seismic shift with one terse sentence in the 1918 annual report: "The policy of appointing women interns on the same basis as men has been adopted."

The first two were Hopkins medical graduates Katherine K. Merritt, named intern, and Edith H. Maas, assistant resident, in February 1918; they were to take their places in July, just as Marriott arrived. Ironically, applicant Carol Skinner Cole was refused admission to the Washington University School of Medicine that same February, though she was finally admitted two months later when the school agreed — after Grace Jones and her board chided the faculty for its reluctance — to open to women "under the same conditions as men." However,

1920-25

Marriott develops a simplified formula for the artificial feeding of infants with evaporated milk, Karo Syrup, and lactic acid.

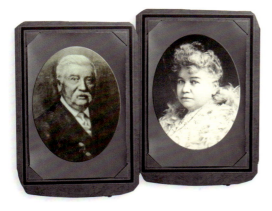

Colonel James G. Butler and Margaret Leggat Butler. The James Gay Butler Endowment Fund was established through generous gifts by Col. Butler and his wife Margaret; the first ward for "colored children" was later established in their names. Lindenwood University Archives

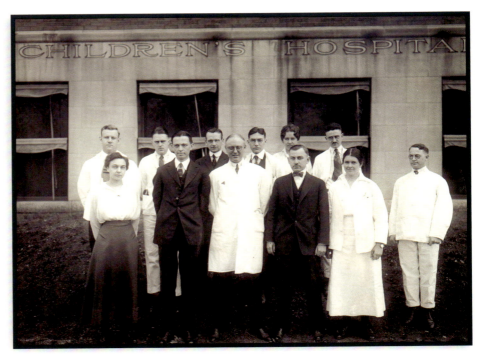

RIGHT **Staff of Children's Hospital ca. 1919.** Kirsten Utheim (top row, second from right), Mary Wright (bottom row, far left), and Martha May Eliot (bottom row, second from right) were among the first women appointed to the hospital's medical staff. Becker Medical Library

Maas never arrived in St. Louis; she resigned her place in April, married, and went on to make a distinguished career in New York City. Merritt came, and was followed in 1919 by two other Hopkins graduates: Mary Wright and Martha May Eliot, granddaughter of the co-founder and third chancellor of Washington University, William Greenleaf Eliot.

At the same time, Marriott hired the first woman faculty member on the pediatric faculty — indeed, in the entire medical school. Kirsten Utheim arrived in St. Louis in March 1919, having received her medical degree in Oslo, Norway. Letters from heads of Norwegian hospitals attest that "she had an inquisitive mind and a special interest in children." "Someone must have recommended Dr. McKim Marriott as an eminent mentor," wrote her son, Svein Utheim Toverud. At first, she worked as a volunteer assistant in the dispensary, then was promoted to assistant in pediatrics, in 1920 became instructor in pediatrics at a salary of $2,000, and in December 1922 was named "assistant physician for Children's Hospital." In addition to conducting research with Marriott on nutritional problems of infants and on dehydration, she served as a clinical supervisor and instructor for medical students before returning to Norway in 1923.

THE BUTLER WARD

More demographic changes were in the offing. In the same board minutes that announced Marriott's arrival was the notice of a new gift from the Butler estate. For years, tobacco producer and Civil War veteran Col. James Gay Butler and his wife Margaret had been generous to the hospital, beginning with a gift of 10 shares of stock worth $750. When Butler died in 1916, he left $25,000 to Children's Hospital, enough for the board to establish the "James Gay Butler Endowment Fund." After his wife's death in 1918, the fund ballooned with her bequest of nearly $300,000. The board began fretting about some "visible recognition" for the Butlers, as member Mary Markham put it — perhaps a tablet or room to honor them.

Soon an opportunity presented itself. Ever since they had made the decision to exclude black children from the new hospital, some of the managers had regretted it. In 1918, a

1921
Newborns at Barnes are taken into the care of Children's Hospital.

1921
At Marriott's instigation, Barnes' "Negro Wards" begin accepting patients 12 and under.

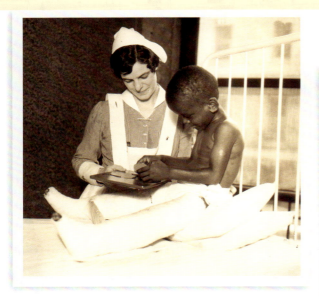

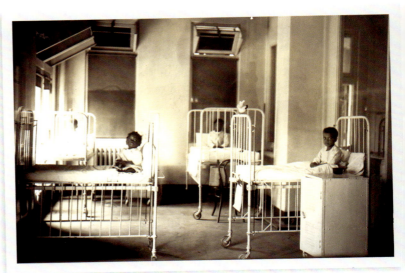

ABOVE AND RIGHT **Butler Ward.** In 1933 alone, the Butler Ward admitted 348 patients, with 3,491 total patient days and an average of 10 per day. Becker Medical Library

motion passed handily to reserve a bed in the Barnes Hospital "Colored Ward for the use of the St. Louis Children's Hospital, and for the length of time it shall be occupied the Barnes Hospital shall be paid at the regular ward rate of $14 per week with the regular charge of $5 for the use of the operating room if this is needed." By 1919, the board had extended its offer to more than one bed for "colored children."

Prodded by Marriott, they resolved in 1920 to find a place in their own building for this care. So the managers voted to set aside space on the first floor of the Pavilion, adding — perhaps for those offended by this move — that this area "has its separate kitchen, entrance, and stairway, so both its patients and their visitors will be entirely isolated from the wards of the hospital." By 1923, they had renovated an old orthopedic workshop and christened it the James G. and Margaret L. Butler Ward — a 17-bed area for "colored children." Also at Marriott's instigation, the "Negro wards" of Barnes Hospital had accepted patients 12 and under since 1921; treating them were pediatricians from the medical school, assisted by Children's Hospital house staff.

CLINICAL CHANGES
After the war, the original Executive Faculty began to disperse, including some who had played a role at Children's Hospital: pathologist Eugene Opie, who took a new job in Philadelphia, and surgeon-in-chief Fred T. Murphy, who retired from medicine. Opie was replaced by Leo Loeb, former head of comparative pathology, and Murphy by Bixby Professor of Surgery Evarts A. Graham, who would have a lasting impact on his field. Quickly, Graham became a member of the joint Barnes-Children's Hospital committee; he and Marriott, the only other regular attendee, made most hospital-related decisions between them with the help of Louis Burlingham.

During this era, others who would play a major role in the hospital first appeared: Park J. White was hired by Marriott in 1921 as assistant in clinical pediatrics and soon launched a class in medical ethics that stressed poverty and race as factors in childhood health; Glover Copher, an assistant resident, was asked to become a live-in staff member at Ridge Farm; William E. Shahan was named ophthalmologist-in-chief at

1921

The Sheppard-Towner Maternity and Infancy Act, the first federally funded social welfare bill in history, is enacted by Congress.

SEPTEMBER 1922

Treatment of the world's first diabetic infant with insulin is made in the Biochemistry Laboratories by Professor P.A. Shaffer.

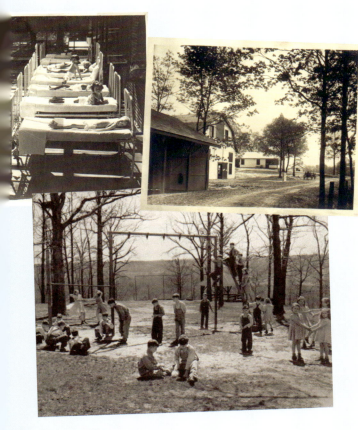

Ridge Farm, ca. 1930s. Becker Medical Library

In 1922, Marriott praised Ridge Farm — the hospital's country department located on 127 acres overlooking the Meramec River in Valley Park — as "an institution almost unique in America." By then, he said, it had moved beyond its original conception as a convalescent home for malnourished children to a place where "children with certain conditions, especially bone and joint tuberculosis, could be treated far more satisfactorily...than in the main hospital." Ads called it a "spacious and airy haven of health."

It specialized in open-air treatment and "heliotherapy" or sun bath, prescribing "fresh air, sunshine and pure food," as one headline put it. "The 70 children, suffering from bone and heart ailments, wear few clothes and spend virtually all their time outdoors, even sleeping in the open," continued the article. "They range from 2 to 15 years old and have regular school courses."

In 1929, Ridge Farm — which was actually a working farm — averaged 57 patients per day out of a total bed capacity of 60, an occupancy rate of 96 percent. The total number of patients admitted that year was 156, with an average stay of 134 days.

Children's Hospital, assisted by Meyer Weiner. Also in 1921, Marriott nominated a senior medical student — Alexis F. Hartmann — for the prestigious annual Gill Prize in Pediatrics. In recognition of the fact that dental disease and bodily illness were often linked, Virgil Loeb became "stomatologist," ensuring that every patient's mouth was examined and treated.

HIGHLIGHTS OF RESEARCH WORK

"Members of the Medical Staff have been engaged in numerous investigations of the cause and treatment of diseases of children and have made discoveries which have proved of distinct value in the saving of life and alleviation of suffering," said Marriott in 1919. To facilitate research, he had solicited a grant from the GEB toward construction of new research laboratories.

Many faculty put them to use. Borden Veeder, who studied mortality in pertussis and measles, had a clinical and research interest in hereditary syphilis, with 900 new cases in 1920 alone. Hereditary syphilis was also one focus of Philip C. Jeans, who in collaboration with Sidney Schwab and John Green demonstrated the involvement of the nervous system in such cases. Testing 80 young patients in his new Heart Station at Children's Hospital, Hugh McCulloch described the effect of diphtheria on the heart, as well as the cardiac impact of nutritional problems in infancy. T.C. Hempelmann studied juvenile tuberculosis and renal function in scarlet fever.

Marriott was the best known of all, primarily for his role in redefining infant feeding, previously "full of fads and fancies....In Boston and other

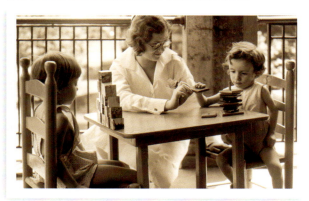

Play therapy. The hospital's spacious sun porches provided a refreshing place to learn and play. Becker Medical Library

1923
An alliance is formed between the Children's and St. Louis Maternity hospitals.

1923
James G. and Margaret L. Butler Ward — a 17-bed area for "colored children" — is completed.

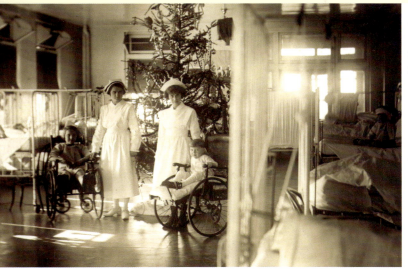

Christmas at Children's Hospital. The hospital's staff did everything they could to make the holidays cheerful for their young patients, including a beautifully decorated tree, lots of gifts, and even Santa Claus himself.
Becker Medical Library

cities, some physicians carried about cards containing mathematical calculations in order to facilitate the compounding of the proper milk formula," wrote Edwards Park of Johns Hopkins. "When Marriott taught that the artificial food mixture, as useful as any for the infant, was soured whole milk with 7 percent Karo syrup added to it, and this was found to be true, he reduced infant feeding to the simplest practice." With this formula, added C.V. Mosby, Marriott "threw out a life line to literally millions of mothers who could not afford expensive products for their babies." His popular textbook, *Infant Nutrition*, was published in 1930 and revised after his death by Philip C. Jeans, who would go on to convince the American Medical Association to endorse the addition of vitamin D in milk, effectively reducing the incidence of rickets — a practical application of Marriott's and Jeans' therapeutic nutritional vision.

Over the years, Marriott's work took other important directions. He devised one method for detecting acidity or alkalinity in the bloodstream and another for determining its lime and

Vilray Blair, a renowned plastic surgeon, became the leading U.S. surgeon in the new field of facial reconstruction. On the walls of his operating room were jungle scenes and cherubs, designed to make children feel more at home. In 1925, he hired one of his trainees, James Barrett Brown, a 1923 graduate of the School of Medicine, who succeeded him in 1940 as chief of plastic surgery.

Brown radically improved the treatment of serious burns with the innovative use of fine-mesh gauze for the dressing, and with the "split thickness-skin graft," in which he took larger, but thinner layers of skin from donor sites and grafted them on to burned areas. An even better solution came in 1927, when he and Blair pioneered the use of the homograft — skin from a person recently deceased — in children.

"Before this skin graft disintegrates," said a *Globe-Democrat* newspaper article, "it acts as a biological dressing, relieves pain, gets the victim out of shock, avoids handicaps and loss of function, shortens convalescence by weeks or even months. And it sets the stage for plastic surgery with the victim's own skin — the graft that 'takes' permanently."

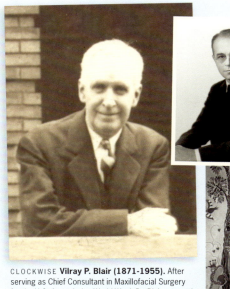
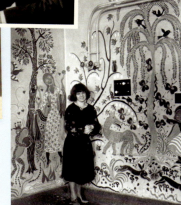

CLOCKWISE **Vilray P. Blair (1871-1955).** After serving as Chief Consultant in Maxillofacial Surgery for the U.S. Army during World War I, Dr. Blair returned to St. Louis and became a leading U.S. plastic surgeon. **James Barrett Brown (1899-1971).** Succeeding Blair was Brown, who treated conditions ranging from cleft lip and palate to burns to the reconstruction of injured hands and jaws.
Artist **Gisella Loeffler** painted elaborate murals in the operating room to soothe and distract young patients. Becker Medical Library (all)

1923
Claribel Wheeler is named superintendent of nurses at Children's Hospital.

1923
Marriott is named dean of Washington University School of Medicine after Allison steps down; Hugh McCulloch is appointed assistant dean.

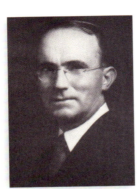

RIGHT **Hugh McCulloch (1888-1948).** Not only was McCulloch an administrator and physician-in-chief at Ridge Farm, he was also a talented pediatric cardiologist. A co-founder of the American Heart Association, he later became the first editor-in-chief of the journal *Pediatrics*, a publication of the American Academy of Pediatrics, and in 1952 president of the American Pediatric Society. Becker Medical Library

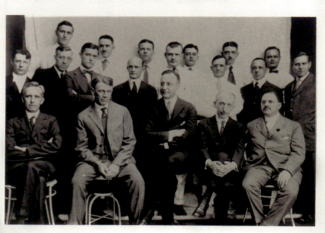

ABOVE **Surgical Staff, 1920.** Evarts A. Graham (front row, center) was appointed the first full-time head of surgery in 1919. Members of his staff included (front row, left to right): Vilray P. Blair, R. Walter Mills, Nathaniel Allison, and Ernest Sachs. Becker Medical Library

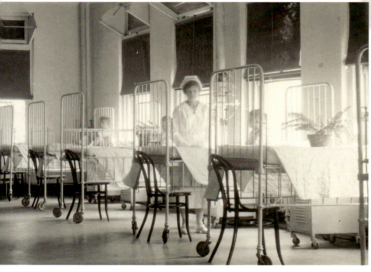

LEFT **Children's Hospital ward, ca. 1920s.** Becker Medical Library

magnesium content. He worked on the nature and treatment of Bright's disease in children, and developed new ways to treat hydrocephalus and convulsive disorders of infants. Newspapers began referring to him as "the most famous pediatrician in the world."

LADY BOARD OF MANAGERS

Meanwhile, the board of managers recast itself in response to this new regime of strong pediatric management. Not that their activity waned: they remained extremely active under Grace Jones's energetic leadership, while maintaining mutually respectful relations with Marriott throughout the changes. In 1922, Dean Allison praised the board's singular effectiveness. The Children's Hospital board of managers, he wrote, "is one of the most interesting and interested groups in the City of St. Louis."

Shortly after moving to the new hospital, board members formed six sub-committees — medical, infant, surgical, country, contagious, and social service — and each took pride in raising funds to meet its own budget. At one 1917 board meeting, the country and contagious units announced a surplus, while social service and surgical declared they would come out "even." When someone hinted that the infant and medical units might end in the red, those chairmen reported — with some asperity — "that they will see that there is no deficit in their Departments." For fund-raising, the board relied on advertising and direct-mail solicitation; as early as 1916, they reported a consultation with "Mr. D'Arcy" about daily ads in the *Globe-Democrat*, and sent 1,100 letters to lawyers asking them to mention Children's Hospital when clients were making wills.

The managers continued traditional activities, such as supplying the hospital's small needs out of their own pockets or through their own labor.

1924
A guidance service is established off-campus for children with behavioral problems.

1925
A sixth-floor addition for private patients is opened, funded by some 6,000 donors.

ST. LOUIS POST-DISPATCH
Only Place That Baby Should Be Kissed Is Top Of Head or on Feet, Says Medical School Dean
Mothers Told, in Public Lecture, How to Rear Healthy Infants — Warned on Peril From Unhealthy Persons.

During a series of public lectures at Washington University Medical School, W. McKim Marriott gave advice on the care and feeding of infants. The *St. Louis Post-Dispatch* reported, "Dr. Marriott, whose chair in the medical school is that of Pediatrics, or treatment of children, is not one of the grim and forbidding physicians who say that the baby never should be kissed. Under certain conditions, he is willing to permit a parent, or even a near relative, this privilege. The conditions were thus expressed:

"Before a person is allowed to kiss a baby, a thorough health examination should be made of the person, the hands and face should be carefully washed, coats and hats removed, and the infant should be kissed only on the top of its head or on its feet....

"The baby's daily schedule, Dr. Marriott said, should be about this: 'Sixteen hours sleep; three hours for bathing, feeding and dressing; one or two hours crying; one-half hour of exercise; the rest of the time, just being a baby.'

> **"...the very best work being done in the country is being done in our department of pediatrics."**

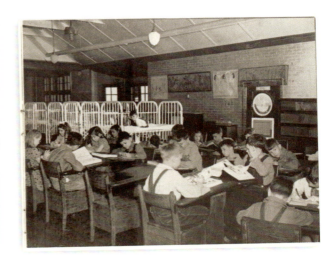

School at Ridge Farm. Prompted by an irate letter by Grace Jones, the Board of Education provided Ridge Farm with a teacher in 1920. Becker Medical Library

In 1916, they bought a victrola for the surgical ward, planned a privet hedge for the grounds, and sent a note of sympathy to Minnie Bulkley on the death of her mother, "who with failing eye sight hemmed over 160 dozen diapers."

But they also shifted firmly into an advocacy role, supporting causes that benefited children. In January 1919, Grace Jones noticed that patients were being sent to them from one children's home "in a most pitiable condition," said the minutes. They investigated this home, "and submitted the results to the people at a mass meeting." The next month, they lobbied the state government on behalf of a bill that would waive the inheritance tax on legacies left to hospitals, and later lobbied again "to further the passing of the law for better milk in Missouri." In 1920, Jones circulated an irate letter scolding the Board of Education for not providing vocational education to disabled children, such as those at Ridge Farm, which they had just succeeded in re-opening after its wartime hiatus. The board capitulated, and Ridge Farm had its teacher.

With fundraising in good order — the Butler bequest had erased the last of their indebtedness for the new hospital — the managers turned to enhancing hospital care. They hired a Montessori teacher to give lessons to patients, improved the chaotic food service, began a one-year training program for baby nurses, and established an occupational therapy program, headed by Lois Keim, in which children learned crafts. Social service got a boost when manager Adda B. Danforth, wife of William H. Danforth, underwrote a worker in the Orthopedic Clinic to supervise the long recuperation of children with bone tuberculosis. In fact, social service — which had separated from nursing in 1916 — was taking on new prominence, as managers joined others nationally in recognizing that "the mental and spiritual life of the people and its physical are inter-animated," wrote Jones. This

1925
Grace Jones steps down as board president; she is replaced by Mary Markham, daughter of Mary McKittrick.

1927
A new maternity hospital building is completed.

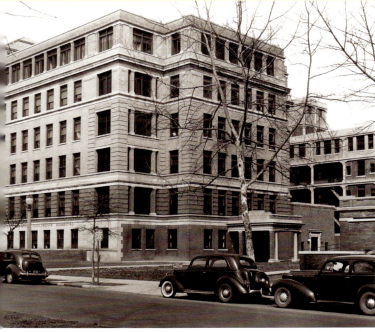

ABOVE **A new addition, ca. 1930s.** The whirlwind fund-raising drive of the board netted more than $300,000 in 10 days and allowed construction of a new sixth floor for the hospital. Becker Medical Library

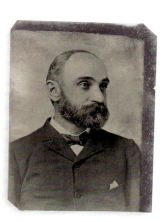

George F. Gill (1843-1892). The annual Gill Prize in Diseases of Children, still awarded annually to a medical student, was named for George F. Gill, faculty member at the St. Louis Medical College from 1887-1892 and a specialist in pediatrics. Becker Medical Library

understanding also led to the founding of a child guidance service in 1924 — located at first off-campus at 4746 McPherson — for children with behavioral problems.

Also in the early 1920s, the managers achieved a coup that surprised even them. They were planning to join the Community Fund, a forerunner of the United Way, but decided first to mount a giant drive to add to their endowment and raise funds for other purposes. Their goal of $300,000 would cover a sixth-floor addition to the hospital for much-needed private rooms to accommodate the swell of middle-class patients now embracing hospital care. With the help of some 6,000 donors, they exceeded their target in only 10 days, raising $320,000.

MARRIOTT BECOMES DEAN

By the early 1920s, despite the nagging shortage of nurses, Marriott — working in concert with the managers — had the hospital and his department running smoothly. In 1922, Dean Nathaniel Allison contrasted its success to the less-satisfactory operation of Barnes: "It is prosperous, it is about to enlarge its capacity, an excellent spirit of service exists throughout its organization, the very best work being done in the country is being done in our department of pediatrics. The development of the Children's Hospital is one of our most satisfactory achievements," he wrote.

Marriott himself was also sanguine. Over the past two years, he wrote in 1922, "the wards have been filled for a large portion of the year and there has been, at almost all times, a waiting list....The country department has been filled to capacity." At the hospital, he was adding to the personnel with the blessing of the managers who "had given him authority to increase the staff of the Hospital as he sees best." One of his appointments was Claribel Wheeler, already director of the School of Nursing, as superintendent of nurses in 1923.

A new appointment was in the offing for Marriott himself. When Allison suddenly stepped down as dean in 1923, the Executive Faculty elected Marriott — absent on vacation in Michigan — to take his place, at first calling it a temporary move "to see the school through the period of re-adjustment." Philip Shaffer got the job of telling him. "While walking along the lake shore late into the night, I persuaded him that he was the one best fitted to shoulder our administrative responsibilities," wrote Shaffer

1928
Alexander Fleming discovers penicillin in Oxford, England.

1929
On the 50th anniversary of the hospital, a "golden jubilee" tea is held.

memories *Helen Aff-Drum*

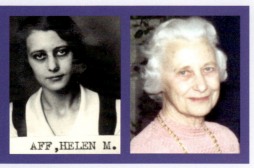

Helen Aff-Drum, as a student in 1934 at Washington University School of Medicine (above left), and today. Becker Medical Library

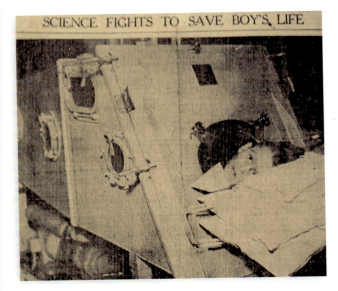

Children's Hospital in the news. Public interest was very high in the life-saving technologies and equipment used at the hospital, such as the "iron lung."

Helen Aff-Drum received her B.S. and M.D. from Washington University in 1934, with five other women in her class; she then interned at Children's Hospital. After doing her residency at Johns Hopkins and at Children's Hospital of Philadelphia, she returned to St. Louis in 1938 to join the clinical faculty at Children's Hospital. She retired as associate clinical professor emerita in 1977.

"What decided me to go into pediatrics? Well mainly, you couldn't do surgery – in those days they wouldn't let you. It was all right to do obstetrics, but you couldn't do gynecologic surgery. You could go into dermatology, psychiatry, or pediatrics, and you could go into eye, but you couldn't do eye surgery, not even a strabismus correction on the babies. It was so limited! It was a male thing....

"Dr. Marriott was very gracious and a wonderful lecturer. He was responsible for developing the standard formula for babies: 13, 17 and 2. 'Thirteen' was a can of evaporated milk, '17' was water, and '2' was Karo syrup. You would sterilize it and the babies would do well on it. For those babies who could not tolerate the formula, he invented the idea of adding so many drops of lactic acid and, as you poured it in, you had to beat the formula so it wouldn't curdle. Patients would come into the clinic and say: 'I need some more of that 'lassie' acid....'

"In those days, we had so many poor people, and they all brought their children to Children's Hospital because nobody was ever turned away. When they came in, one of the aides would bathe the child, give it a shampoo, and scrub the soles of its feet with Clorox before that baby came to the ward. If you had a baby with an acute illness, you wrote a special order: 'Please no admission bath.'"

later. "And I am ashamed to confess that I assured him he might do so without overburdening his departmental and research activities."

Marriott finally agreed, on condition that the Executive Faculty appoint an assistant dean to handle routine administrative tasks, and they immediately named Hugh McCulloch to that post. Somehow Marriott would also find time to remain as head of pediatrics, though his own research would suffer under the strain of the workload. "He tried to carry the full-sized load of two men on his shoulders," recalled Borden Veeder. "He worked day and night."

THE ROARING TWENTIES

In 1925, Marriott was pleased to note an addition to the hospital: the new private floor, funded by the managers' whirlwind campaign, which offered "home-like surroundings" and "convenient arrangements for mothers who desire to stay with their children." Increasingly, he noted, these patients were coming from out of town. Many of the hospital's ward patients were now "from families of the self-respecting middle-class... [who] in general are likely to be the most neglected

OCTOBER 1929	1930	1930
The Great Depression begins.	Marriott's popular textbook, *Infant Nutrition*, is published.	The American Academy of Pediatrics is founded with 304 charter members.

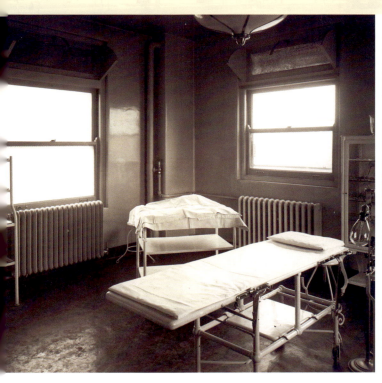

Operating room, ca. 1920s. Becker Medical Library

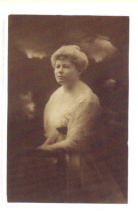

Mary McKittrick Markham (1875-1964). Wife of insurance broker George Markham, she served as fourth president of the board of managers from 1925 to 1945. Her mother, Mary McKittrick, had been second president from 1884 to 1907. Becker Medical Library

from a medical standpoint. The cost of medical attention in the case of minor illnesses can usually be borne, but when severe illness occurs, the family budget is likely to be insufficient." Since Children's Hospital used a sliding scale to calculate costs, he continued, it was "well equipped to render adequate medical care to [these] patients."

Changing hospital admissions also reflected another trend: the improving child welfare situation throughout St. Louis. Thanks to social service intervention, education, and earlier medical care, the number of children hospitalized with preventable diseases was decreasing, childhood neglect was down, and the infant mortality rate in St. Louis was reduced by more than half. At the dispensary, 17 pediatricians saw children daily — including visitors to the new well baby, nutrition, and speech defect clinics — for a total of 23,039 children seen as outpatients annually. On a national level, Congress passed the first federally funded social welfare bill in history: the 1921 Sheppard-Towner Maternity and Infancy Act, which helped reduce infant mortality by providing states with matching funds for maternity, child health, and welfare programs.

Generally, the '20s were a prosperous time for the hospital, with gains to the medical staff that included Daniel C. Darrow in 1925 and Harvey L. White a year later. Now women were appointed more frequently, with interns Dorothy Worthington in 1923, Caroline Whitney and Mary Pope in 1925, Katherine Bain — sister-in-law of Park White — in 1926; and staff pediatricians Edith Irvine-Jones, working with Hugh McCulloch on heart research, and Mary Spahr, relating infections to nutritional disturbances in infants. In 1927, Minnola Stallings became the first woman medical student to win the Gill Prize. Finally, the nursing staff was growing, thanks to better training, and a new hospital superintendent joined the staff: Estelle Claiborne, who would stay from 1925 until 1954.

Clinical work also advanced as Ernest Sachs developed new neurosurgical techniques in children; plastic surgeon Vilray P. Blair perfected methods for correcting cleft palate and lip, while James Barrett Brown performed the first homograft for burns in children; and Evarts Graham did several high-profile operations. By 1928, both otolaryngology and ophthalmology had re-organized on a full-time basis, with more time for Children's Hospital patients; the Mallinckrodt Institute of Radiology opened in 1931, offering state-of-the-art facilities for X-ray diagnosis; and a metabolism ward began with funding from manager Edith January Davis in memory of her mother, Julia January. In a key act of recognition, the GEB sent representatives

1931 Mallinckrodt Institute of Radiology opens, offering state-of-the-art facilities for X-ray diagnosis.

1932 An epidemic of encephalitis sweeps across St. Louis and continues into 1933.

JULY 1936 Marriott leaves Children's Hospital to take a position at the University of California.

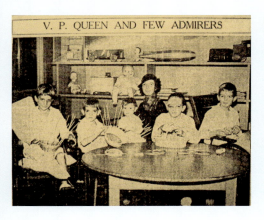

In 1934, Jane Wells visited Children's Hospital and wrote an account of her experience for the *Globe-Democrat*. It read in part:

"Today, I made some new friends. At the St. Louis Children's Hospital I met 3-year-old Danny whose happy blue eyes and chubby body belie the fact that he has recently had a serious throat operation, and Maria, the little Italian girl who made me understand that she likes spaghetti. There were Dorothy, who plays happily in her crib while recovering from a major stomach operation, and Bob, whose big wheelchair carries him over the floor of the hospital since his right leg has been in a cast, and Johnny who accepts philosophically the fact that the various bone operations the doctor found necessary to make on his hip keep him out of school and away from play....

"I saw one little boy who is 1 year old but he weighted only 10 pounds. His family had not had the funds to buy milk for five children, and this little one never seemed hungry. A 2-year-old girl, weighing 14 pounds, was brought in last week, the nurse told me, from a home in which the grandparent couldn't even tell the name of the baby. Undernourishment had caused such a weakened condition that the nurses had to inject food under the tiny patient's skin for immediate relief."

from leading medical schools to observe the work at the hospital, while its own staff lectured at medical society meetings. Meanwhile, resident exchanges began with Johns Hopkins, Harvard, Duke, Michigan, the Princess Elizabeth of York Hospital in London, and the Hospital for Sick Children in Toronto.

Within the area of research, Theron Catlin and his wife memorialized their young son by endowing a fellowship in infectious diseases, held in 1928 by Dorothy Wilkes Weiss, who investigated causes of influenza and meningitis. Alexis Hartmann developed the "Lactate-Ringer's Solution," also known as "Hartmann's Solution," for infants with severe diarrhea and dehydration; Jean V. Cooke worked on scarlet fever, discovering "an important new original idea of the disease which... would refute the general opinion as to its great similarity to diphtheria," said Marriott; F. Scott Smyth and Katherine Bain, now a staff physician, researched asthma, hay fever, and eczema; Marriott himself, able to do little research because of his administrative load, was still able to make an important link between mastoid and other infections to nutritional disturbances in infants.

Some losses also occurred in 1925: After 18 years, Grace Jones stepped down as board president, replaced by Mary Markham, member since 1904 and daughter of second president Mary McKittrick. Marriott paid tribute to Jones for not contenting herself "with cutting coupons and viewing the hospital from a distance" but taking "an active and personal interest in every part" of its work. That year, the University's chancellor and former classics professor, Frederic Aldin Hall, died; he was a favorite of the medical school and especially of Children's, since he had helped win crucial GEB grants. "We perceived in him...one interested in every detail of the School and tireless in working for its welfare," said Marriott's eulogy.

The 50th anniversary "golden jubilee" tea in 1929 was a festive affair, attended by current managers, long-ago staff member and homeopath James Campbell, and original board members Virginia Stevenson and Rose H. Fraley. St. Louis newspapers tallied up the hospital's successes: 57,756 patients cared for through the years, with an annual inpatient average of 2,800 — up to 77 percent of them for free. The *Globe-Democrat* called this record "glowing in character," while the *St. Louis Star* said the hospital was "a monument to the fine spirit of humanity that prevails in this metropolis of the Mississippi Valley."

THE DEPRESSION STRIKES

Just as malnutrition seemed on the decrease and childhood medical care was improving, the Depression began in October 1929. Soon Marriott was speaking bravely of "a decreased

The Community Fund Campaign. As one of the United Charities agencies, Children's Hospital received an allotment of funds from the Community Fund. Campaigns were essential for raising the funds necessary to continue the work of the hospital.

NOVEMBER 1936

Marriott dies of an infection after abdominal surgery.

1936

Philip C. Jeans persuades the AMA Committee on Foods to recommend fortifying milk with vitamin D, thus reducing the rate of rickets in the U.S.

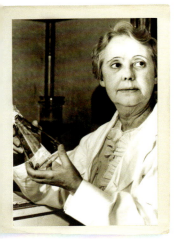

income and necessary retrenchments," but still hoping to "accomplish the greatest good with the limited funds available." The number of free patients soared to the highest percentage in the hospital's history, babies were coming in severely malnourished, and the Social Service Department was swamped. Early in 1932, Ridge Farm closed until the Community Fund found money the next year to re-open it, the January Metabolism Ward shut down until 1935, and one floor of the Contagious Pavilion emptied for most of that year. "Fortunately there was relatively little infectious disease," said Marriott, speaking too soon.

In 1932 and particularly 1933, an epidemic of encephalitis, or sleeping sickness, struck St. Louis. The sudden influx of patients as young as three months old meant that the contagious pavilion was pressed into service. At the same time, pediatric researchers — especially pathologist Margaret Smith — worked to find the cause. With the waning of encephalitis came an outbreak of polio; a new mechanical respirator or "iron lung," donated by manager Edith Davis and local schoolteachers, saved many lives. "This is the first year since I became connected with Children's Hospital that we have received no bequests at all," said Mary Markham in 1936.

Despite redoubled efforts to cut back, Marriott could not resist noting in 1935 the needs that still existed: air-conditioning in the hospital, particularly in the infants' ward; a ward exclusively for premature infants since "the mortality among premature infants is high"; the relocation to the hospital of the successful Child Guidance Clinic, still off campus and under the leadership of Paul Kubitschek; a new fluoroscope for diagnosis. Soon there would be another need: a new head of pediatrics. Marriott, weakened by a bout with viral encephalitis in 1933 and by years of overwork, accepted a job offer in July 1936 to become dean and professor of research medicine at the University of California.

Tragically, he died that same November of a streptococcal infection after abdominal surgery.

ABOVE **Margaret G. Smith (1896-1970).** A pediatric pathologist, Smith helped find the cause of the 1933 encephalitis outbreak in St. Louis by discovering the presence of a non-filterable virus in the kidneys. In 1956, she also first isolated the human cytamegalo virus in culture. Becker Medical Library

Former student, resident, assistant physician, and now associate physician Alexis F. Hartmann took over the Washington University pediatrics department. In his eulogy to Marriott, offered at a January 1937 memorial service, Hartmann spoke of Marriott's influence on the many residents who vied to come to Children's Hospital, with the result that "there are now many well trained and successful pediatricians who owe much of their skill to him." Perhaps he was also speaking of himself: for nearly three decades, he would use this training to shape the future of pediatrics at Children's Hospital.

It would be impossible to replace Marriott, however. The eulogy in *The Journal of Pediatrics* called him "the most important individual influence that developed in American pediatrics in the first half of the present century." And Chancellor George R. Throop said at the 1937 service, "The life of Williams McKim Marriott marks the greatest epoch of development and progress in the School of Medicine," but added, "Though we are greatly the losers by his going, the inspiration of his work and the breadth of his view will not soon fade from us."

Excerpt from Park White's letter to Dr. Marriott's widow, November 11, 1936:
"I heard the news from Dr. Shaffer in the cafeteria today. None of us could think or talk of anything else. The school and hospitals seem to be under a pall of real grief. I saw Dave Barr and Alex Hartmann during the afternoon and it seems as though each had lost a near relative. As I got off the elevator on the fifth floor of Children's, I could hear the 'Hello, Park, come in!' — to which I had grown so accustomed. But the 'Big Chief' who was mostly responsible for my coming to St. Louis wasn't there."
W.M. Marriott Collection

1928
Marriott, Shaffer, Hartmann — and Insulin

In the early 1920s, research groups in the United States and abroad were actively working on the development of insulin, among them a team led by biochemist Philip Shaffer of the Washington University School of Medicine. With the assistance of Alexis Hartmann, then a medical student, Shaffer and his two faculty colleagues — Edward A. Doisy, who would win the 1943 Nobel Prize for his work on vitamin K, and biochemist Michael Somogyi — developed a new technique in 1920 for finding sugar in the patient's blood. This method proved to be of key importance to Frederick G. Banting and Charles H. Best, the Toronto-based scientists credited with isolating insulin; Banting received the 1923 Nobel Prize in Medicine for his work.

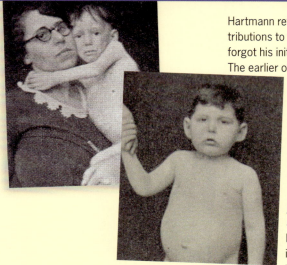

A drastic difference. Photographs were taken of one of the first children treated with insulin at Children's Hospital, a three-year-old named Billy, who was "literally skin and bones" and weighing only 16 pounds, according to Hartmann. Three months after his treatment with insulin, he was "fat and rosy" and weighed 32 pounds.
Becker Medical Library

Hartmann retained his interest in sugar metabolism and went on to make critical contributions to the understanding of pediatric diabetes and hypoglycemia, but he never forgot his initial experience of saving two diabetic children through the use of insulin. The earlier of these cases was also significant since the child was the first treated with insulin in the United States. Hartmann described these incidents in his eulogy for Marriott at a memorial service held in St. Louis on January 3, 1937:

"In September 1922, a diabetic infant of 18 months was brought to the hospital in a state of coma. Although he was temporarily helped by palliative procedures, it was not expected that death could be long postponed. Dr. Marriott had, however, just returned from a medical meeting in Toronto, where he had heard reports on the use of insulin, which had just been discovered. Dr. Marriott brought no insulin with him, nor was any available from the laboratories of Toronto, or elsewhere. He did bring back with him, however, a very brief description of the method of its preparation and the knowledge that here in Washington University there was a man who could and would rise to the occasion.

"Consequently he went to Dr. Shaffer, talked to him enthusiastically about this diabetic infant of ours, and the results obtained by the Toronto workers. Both to his surprise and satisfaction he found that Dr. Shaffer had already become interested in the extraction of insulin and very quickly persuaded him to make some for our infant. The result was not only the miraculous saving of a life (the infant of 1922 is now a strapping boy of sixteen) but possibly also proved an incentive which led to the discovery, by Dr. Shaffer and his co-workers, of an important principle in the extraction of such substances from tissues — the so-called iso-electric precipitation of proteins." Although he did not mention it, Hartmann had helped Shaffer prepare the batch of insulin and administered the injections himself.

Hartman then described the second child helped from the same formulation. As he continued, "A month or so later, another diabetic patient was admitted, a boy of

"…there has not been a day in which some children with diabetes have not been under treatment by the hospital and the lives of all of these have been saved."

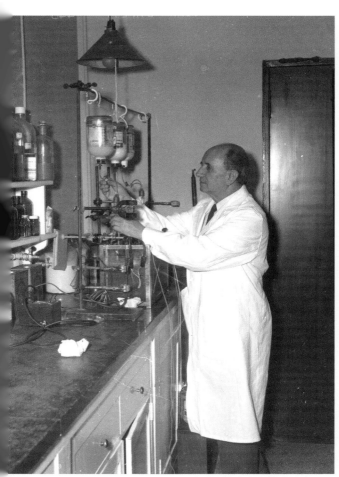

LEFT **Michael Somogyi (1883-1971).** Hungary-born Somogyi graduated in chemistry from the University of Budapest in 1905 and then moved to America. He became assistant in biochemistry at the Cornell University Medical College, where he worked with Philip Shaffer. In 1922, Shaffer persuaded him to teach biochemistry at Washington University medical school, and in 1926 he became the first chemist at the Jewish Hospital. The first insulin treatment of a child with diabetes in the U.S. took place in October 1922 with a preparation of insulin produced by Somogyi, Hartmann, and Shaffer. Becker Medical Library

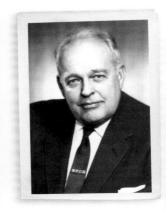

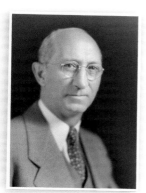

ABOVE LEFT **Alexis F. Hartmann, Sr. (1898-1964).** Hartmann was head of pediatrics at the medical school from 1936-64. He is known for his research showing the differences in serum electrolyte patterns in dehydration and designing a new method of fluid replacement. Becker Medical Library

ABOVE RIGHT **Philip A. Shaffer (1881-1960).** Shaffer came to the University in 1910 as professor and head of biochemistry and stayed on the faculty for 50 years, serving as dean from 1915-19 and 1937-46. He extracted the needed insulin from beef pancreas. Becker Medical Library

almost four, in the most pitiable condition imaginable. He was literally skin and bones, too weak even to raise arm or leg; his ankles and eyelids swollen as a result of prolonged and severe malnutrition, his skin covered with hemorrhages and xanthomata,— his weight being but 16 pounds. In three months, again as a result of insulin made in Dr. Shaffer's laboratory, this boy was fat and rosy, weighing 32 pounds."

DOISY'S MEMORIES

In his autobiography, written in 1975, Doisy also recalled these life-saving incidents. The two children were admitted, he remembered, "shortly after the startling announcement by Banting and Best of their success in the treatment of diabetes with an extract of pancreas. Because of the limited supply produced in the Connaught Laboratories and by Eli Lilly Company, insulin could not be obtained for them. So the Chief of the Children's Hospital, Dr. McKim Marriott, asked Dr. Shaffer for help. He enlisted me and Dr. Michael Somogyi, who had worked with Dr. Shaffer before the First World War, had returned to Hungary and was food administrator for Budapest during the war, and subsequently returned to work with Dr. Shaffer. The first product which was prepared was active and the diabetes was treated successfully; according to a report received about 15 years ago, both men were alive, married, and had children."

This work also contributed to promoting the survival of infants suffering from malnutrition. Hartmann continued in his eulogy, "Dr. Marriott asked, 'If insulin fattens diabetic babies so quickly, I wonder what it would do for other athreptic [malnourished] infants?' The question thus raised was soon put to the test and answered by Dr. Marriott himself, with the result that a new treatment for malnutrition was begun — the repeated intravenous administration of dextrose and insulin to infants unable to digest and assimilate sufficient food to satisfy their nutritional requirements."

At Children's and around the world, the rescue of this first diabetic child was followed by many other such victories. As Marriott put it only a few months afterwards, "since that time there has not been a day in which some children with diabetes have not been under treatment by the hospital and the lives of all of these have been saved."

CHAPTER

5

1936
1964

A Changing Pediatric World: The Alexis F. Hartmann Era

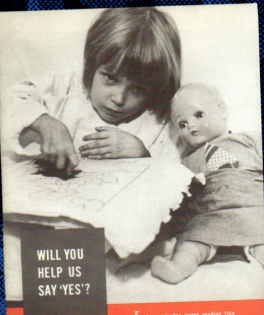

CHAPTER FIVE A CHANGING PEDIATRIC WORLD: THE ALEXIS F. HARTMANN ERA

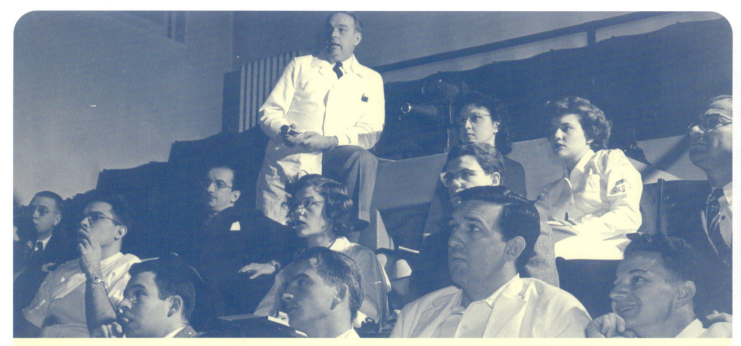

Alexis F. Hartmann, Sr. (1898-1964). Hartmann earned his B.S. degree from Washington University in 1919, followed by his M.S. and M.D. in 1921 when he was not quite 23. He was awarded the medical school's prestigious Gill Prize in 1921. First a resident at Children's, then instructor, assistant professor, and associate professor, he became head of pediatrics and physician-in-chief in 1936, serving until 1964. An avid tennis player (below) he was a regular at the courts outside the hospital. Becker Medical Library

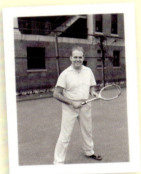

Apparently there were no other serious candidates to succeed pediatric head W. McKim Marriott. Alexis F. Hartmann, Sr., was his undisputed heir, recommended by a special committee approved by the chancellor. Still, the transition was not an easy one. The Depression was abating but it had not yet ended, and Children's Hospital continued to feel the pinch. What's more, the dynamic, forward-looking Marriott had left a void that would be nearly impossible to fill. As surgeon-in-chief Evarts A. Graham wrote in 1937, "The guiding hand of Dr. Marriott has been greatly missed during the past year." Still, he added hopefully, "all of us feel that under the able direction of Dr. Hartmann the hospital will go on to achieve even more fame than it has now."

PREVIOUS PAGE **Ground-breaking, 1952.** Becker Medical Library
INSET **Cover, fund-raising brochure, 1950.** Becker Medical Library

1936
Alexis F. Hartmann, Sr. becomes head of pediatrics and physician-in-chief.

1936
Sulfa drugs are first used in medical practice with an astonishingly successful impact on patients with bacterial infections.

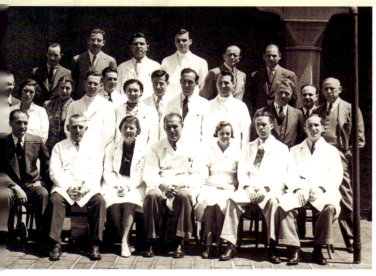

Department of Pediatrics staff, 1939. Becker Medical Library

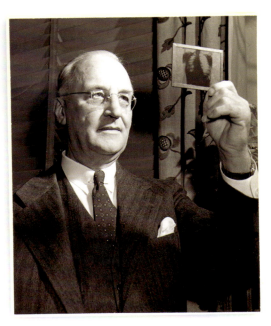

Evarts A. Graham (1883-1957). Appointed the first full-time head of surgery in 1919, Graham served in that capacity for 32 years. At the time of his death, he was considered to be the leading surgeon of his day. Becker Medical Library

There was good reason to hope for a bright future under Hartmann, whose entire academic life had been, and would be, spent at Washington University. Already a successful researcher, he would go on to produce some 90 publications during his career, including a seminal paper describing the Shaffer-Hartmann method for true blood glucose, written as a master's thesis. Pediatric cardiologist David Goldring later called these articles — covering such topics as diabetic acidosis, dehydration and anhydremia, salicylate intoxication and hypoglycemia — "pediatric classics." His work also inspired others, including Carl and Gerty Cori who undertook, at his instigation, their revolutionary studies of glucose-6-phosphatase in glycogen storage disease.

At the same time, he was a superb clinician. "He brought the laboratory to the bedside," wrote Gilbert B. Forbes, a former resident and instructor, in 1964. "The twinkle in his eye when he perceived some hint of metabolic aberration in a patient who had baffled the rest of us bespoke his primary interest in biochemical phenomena." Most of all, Hartmann — known to his residents as "the Chief" — was an inspiring teacher, training some 30 students who went on to hold key academic posts around the country. In the lecture hall, he spoke without notes but with contagious enthusiasm, added Forbes, "standing erect at the podium, hands thrust deeply into his coat pockets, a gleam in his eye....The quality of freshness (one felt that he had made the observation in the laboratory that very morning) was invigorating." The same quality was evident in the postgraduate courses he offered: "You seem to have one of the finest medical schools in the country as well as one of the best professors of pediatrics," said one physician attendee.

Hartmann also excelled on Wednesday morning ward rounds. "We all marveled at his keen observation, his brilliant analysis of the patient's history and his intuitive, almost uncanny, diagnostic ability," wrote White. But his residents knew that these rounds inevitably meant more work. "Provocative suggestions for further research were the order of the day: The laboratory staff learned to be ready late Wednesday morning for the parade of residents bearing samples for analysis!" said Forbes. To unwind from his own hectic schedule, Hartmann turned

1937
A nine-year-old Children's Hospital patient with pneumococcal meningitis is the first to recuperate under the treatment of sulfa drugs.

1938
With a grant from the Rockefeller Foundation, the School of Medicine opens a Department of Neuropsychiatry.

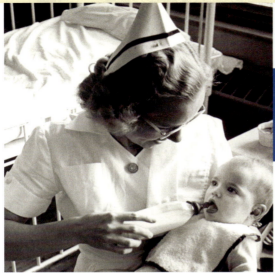

Dorothy Glahn Herweg. A long-time member of the nursing staff, she served as head nurse in charge of the infant ward. Becker Medical Library

memories *John Herweg*

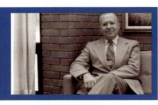

A 1945 School of Medicine graduate, Herweg did a nine-month internship before leaving for military service. He was appointed assistant resident in 1949 at a salary of $300 per year, and subsequently was chief resident and then instructor in 1951. In 1962, he was asked to head the junior pediatric clerkship and clinical research unit; in 1965, he became associate dean for student affairs.

"When I was chief resident, the Wednesday morning rounds at 9:00 often lasted two, two-and-a-half hours, sometimes almost until lunchtime. The chief resident was responsible, literally, for knowing everything about every patient in the hospital, because you would have to give Dr. Hartmann, at the bedside, a brief 30 or 45-second summary. That meant the salient features of the case: history, physical findings, clinical course, lab data, and so on. So Tuesday night was usually an all-nighter, especially if there were a lot of admissions that night, since by Wednesday morning you had to know who came in overnight — and the ones who came in were often the sickest ones.

"It was a great learning experience for the resident, but it was stressful. You were on call every other night. The nights you were off call, you usually finished about 7 or 8 o'clock. We lived in the hospital; I was single then. I had a bed on the fifth floor that actually had a straw-tick mattress. It was not luxurious, I can tell you — but we didn't have much time to sleep anyway."

to his beloved game of tennis, played faithfully at noontime on the courts outside the hospital.

Now only 38, he was head of the pediatrics department, which Marriott had described just before his departure, in a candid letter to Chancellor George R. Throop, as "very short-handed....There has been barely sufficient personnel to carry the routine work required, and investigative activities have been at a minimum." Further, Hartmann was an inexperienced, untried administrator, who would have the complex job of keeping the department and hospital moving ahead on many fronts: with cutting-edge research, strong clinical care, up-to-date building space, and able young recruits. During the coming decade, the world of pediatrics was about to undergo a seismic shift with the introduction of sulfa drugs and penicillin. Increasingly, too, the hospital's very personal, small-scale style of management — and the Board of Managers itself — would prove obsolete, and Hartmann would face a daunting challenge: the need to find a new approach.

THE FIRST FIVE YEARS

In the first few years after Hartmann took over, a crop of new pediatric staff members joined the department, including assistant physicians Dorothy J. Jones, Joseph C. Jaudon, Paul Zentay, and Sol Londe; and assistant surgeons Louis T. Byars, Robert Elman, and Peter Heinbecker. New pediatric residents included Alfred Schwartz, Merl J. Carson, and in 1941 David Goldring, Gilbert Forbes, and Mary McFayden Bishop; and in surgery Eugene Bricker, Samuel Harbison, and Vilray P. Blair, Jr., in 1940. Residents from other specialties also came on board, such as ophthamologist Ben H. Senturia. The exchange program with the Princess Elizabeth of York Hospital for Children in London continued, with Russell Blattner taking part in 1937, while Theron Catlin fellowships still supported able young doctors, such as Charles R. Anderson in 1939-40. Howard Murdock was appointed pathologist to succeed the legendary Leo Loeb.

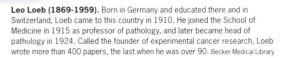

Leo Loeb (1869-1959). Born in Germany and educated there and in Switzerland, Loeb came to this country in 1910. He joined the School of Medicine in 1915 as professor of pathology, and later became head of pathology in 1924. Called the founder of experimental cancer research, Loeb wrote more than 400 papers, the last when he was over 90. Becker Medical Library

1939
The Child Guidance Clinic moves to the hospital's second floor.

1939
The hospital treats 679 paying patients, up from 631 in 1937.

RESIDENT PHYSICIAN

Woman Heads Hospital Staff

Precedent Is Set at St. Louis Institution

August 14, 1938.

The house staff of St. Louis' Children's Hospital is under the direction of a woman resident physician for the first time in its history.

Dr. Eleanor Johnson Rector, M.D., a graduate of Washington University's School of Medicine in the class of 1936, has had under her direction two assistant resident physicians and seven junior resident physicians, one of whom also is a woman.

Starting out as Miss Johnson, Dr. Rector took a nursing course at the University of Washington in Seattle, Wash., her home, exercised a woman's privilege, changed her mind, took a premedical course instead and obtained both B. S. and M. S. degrees. While obtaining the latter she met Lewis E. Rector, who also had hopes of being a doctor, and they both came east to Washington University.

Dr. Rector was married to Dr. Rector before their first year of medical school. Later she was graduated with honors. He is a resident pathologist at the Boston's Children's Hospital. They see each other about three times a year.

Dr. Eleanor Rector plans to join her husband some day in the future when and where he obtains an appointment as a pathologist. She will enter private practice then, specialising in pediatrics. Now she is too busy to think in any terms save those of a resident physician, which she will be until July, 1939.

Dr. Eleanor Johnson Rector, St. Louis Children's Hospital's first woman resident physician. Dr. Rector was graduated cum laude from Washington University's School of Medicine in 1936. She is the wife of Dr. Lewis E. Rector, also a Washington University graduate, who is a resident pathologist at a Boston hospital.

—Staff Photo

Becker Medical Library

1936-37 Budget. Hartmann inherited a tight budget in 1937: pediatrician Lawrence Goldman would later help found the Children's Research Foundation to increase the annual budget.
Becker Medical Library

In the late 1930s, pediatric residents still had opportunities for clinical work beyond Children's Hospital. Under the supervision of Joseph Jaudon, whose specialty was endocrinology and the problems of infants, they staffed the newborn service at St. Louis Maternity Hospital. The pediatric department, like the rest of the medical school, also became consultants to the St. Louis City Hospital and Homer G. Phillips Hospital, under the direction of Wayne A. Rupe.

Women were playing an ever-larger role in the hospital, occupying four out of 28 physician slots in 1939. This record paralleled their increasing representation at the medical school, which in 1938 admitted 22 women out of 348 students. Katherine Bain was still on staff, a fine pediatrician who developed clinical tricks that really worked, recalled Helen Aff-Drum, an assistant physician at Children's in 1939: "She said that if babies looked as if they were going to cry, just whistle," and they would forget what they had intended to cry about. Anne Perley was a dedicated biochemist who ran tests for the medical staff; Margaret Smith became assistant pathologist for Children's. "Woman Heads Hospital Staff," announced headlines in a August 1938 newspaper article, when Eleanor Johnson Rector, a 1936 School of Medicine graduate, became the first woman chief resident, supervising two assistant and seven junior residents.

Not only did residents have long, grueling hours, but they also felt perpetually hungry. In 1940, they and the graduate nurses were given food vouchers of only $25 per month to spend on their meals, and by September this lean amount was causing vocal comment. One resident protested to Estelle Claiborne "that food prices had been increased in the Barnes Hospital cafeteria, and the House Staff members were unable to get enough food with the $25.00 per month allowance."

During this period, the unpaid faculty in clinical pediatrics included some well-known names, among them Park J. White, Adrien Bleyer, Lawrence Goldman, and Maurice J. Lonsway, Sr. A few years later, Goldman, a

1939

World War II breaks out in Europe.

EARLY 1940s

Penicillin becomes widely available for use as an antibiotic.

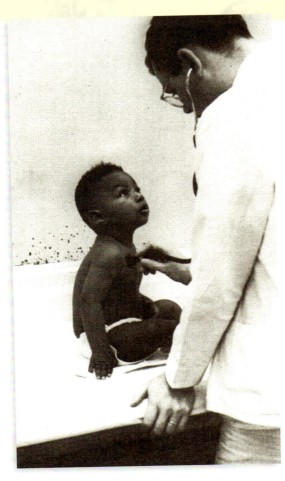

Doctor with young patient in outpatient department, ca. 1949.
Becker Medical Library

NEW EFFORTS

Beginning in 1938, one of Hartmann's major goals was to revamp Children's outpatient department, then part of the nearby Washington University clinics. "The diminishing attendance of the Pediatric Out-Patient Department during the past several years has reached the point that now there is no longer sufficient material for teaching purposes," he wrote, pleading for change. One problem was the limited afternoon hours of the clinic; another was its policy of charging for treatment. As a result, patients were beginning to shift to competing clinics: St. Mary's, DePaul, Jewish, Desloge, and the St. Louis City Hospital. Hartmann proposed to relocate the clinic to the current Admitting Ward — thus necessitating the move of Admitting patients to the Butler Ward and Butler patients to the unused contagious floor.

After years of effort — even including a $1,000 donation to the cause from his own pocket — Hartmann's efforts finally succeeded in 1945, with the Children's Research Foundation helping to fund an expansion of the outpatient department's hours to seven days a week. Even so, the clinic "packs them in daily," said a newspaper article. "Drop in at the clinic any morning, and you will see the drama, sorrow, and comedy attending a sick youngster in the family. A child as white as her many bandages is wheeled into the elevator while her anxious parents go slowly through the exit door. A very little girl screams at the approach of the needle...while her older brother disgustedly holds his fingers to his ears."

Hartmann was also eager to upgrade the care of premature infants. "Because of lack of available space it is necessary to care for these infants...in a special room which is not very satisfactory for the purpose and by the same nurses who are responsible for sick infants," he wrote. "A study has just been started to determine whether it will be possible to sterilize the air in this room by ultra violet irradiation. Even if this proves possible, there should also be available

beloved local pediatrician, inspired local business leaders — dress manufacturers, lawyers, insurance men, department store heads — to found the Children's Research Foundation. Within five years, the Foundation had contributed some $50,000 to the hospital for new equipment, a larger nursing staff, and, most of all, research. In one encephalitis experiment, supported by the Foundation, "a Foundation member even helped to the extent of recreating swamp conditions by means of an air-conditioner in reverse," said a *Post-Dispatch* article.

> **"Drop in at the clinic any morning, and you will see the drama, sorrow, and comedy attending a sick youngster in the family..."**

1941
David Goldring joins the hospital as a pediatric resident.

1944
Many members of the hospital staff join the armed forces, placing a heavy burden on those remaining behind; Ridge Farm closes for lack of personnel.

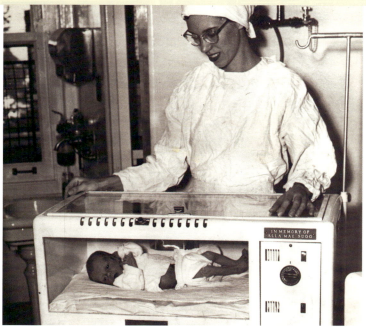

Premature infant ward. Said Jean O'Rear, head nurse: "The first thing we have to do is keep them warm. 'Preemies' are unable to maintain heat because they don't have the fatty tissues under the skin....Secondly, you must maintain nutrition....Third, we have to maintain respiration. Some of them are too lazy to breathe, so we have suction machines between every two incubators ready at all times. And fourth, just as important as anything else is prevention of infection." Becker Medical Library

premature incubators." His dream of a premature baby center would not be realized until 1949, however, when a 10-bed unit opened.

Further, he hoped to meld the Child Guidance Clinic more closely into the hospital's work, so that pediatricians could be trained in the psychiatric problems of children. Instead, the clinic continued on the fringes of pediatric work, functioning, said Hartmann in a 1937 memo to Dean Philip A. Shaffer, as "an outpatient department where particularly social agency children with behavior problems could be examined and treated." Thanks to a grant from the Rockefeller Foundation, the School of Medicine opened a Department of Neuropsychiatry in 1938, with new faculty David Rioch, John Whitehorn, and Carlyle Jacobsen, who received joint appointments at Children's.

The next year, the Child Guidance Clinic finally moved from its McPherson site to the hospital's second floor. A decade later it closed, but a new clinic opened in 1947 as part of the Washington University Clinics. In a major financial commitment, the Children's Research Foundation

At Christmastime, the Children's Hospital staff worked particularly hard to create a festive atmosphere. As the December 1953 issue of *Small Talk* described it, "...there is a huge Christmas tree on every floor, decorated by the children well enough to be up. These trees are as thickly hung with bright ornaments...as the Christmas tree might be in the child's own home. When the children are 'tucked all snug in their beds,' on Christmas Eve, you can see each night nurse tiptoeing from one little white bed to another — carefully hanging up a Christmas stocking for every patient. In each are included the usual simple candies, fruits, and gifts."

A highlight of the season was the annual children's party on the afternoon of Christmas Eve when Santa Claus made his appearance. For more than 25 years pediatrician Max Deutch played this role, and he was succeeded by Kenneth Koerner, a 1941 School of Medicine graduate and member of the clinical staff since 1947.

Donning a wig and beard, and stuffing his red outfit with a pillow, Koerner went from child to child, handing out toys that the Auxiliary had provided. "It was great to see those little smiling faces," he recalled. "The kids might have been hurting, but they were always glad to see Santa."

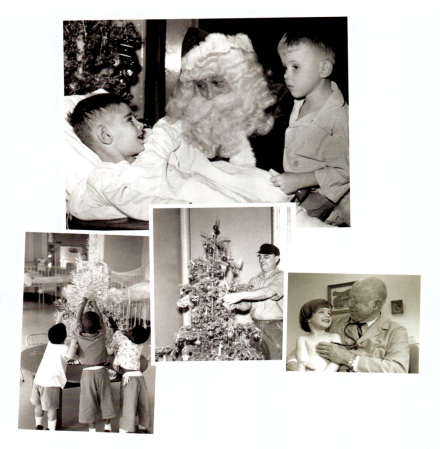

CLOCKWISE FROM TOP **Max Deutch** as Santa; **Kenneth Koerner,** who succeeded Max Deutch as Santa; **Les Plueck,** head of maintenance, helped decorate the trees as Santa's helper; the wonder of Christmas on the ward. Becker Medical Library

HOPE AND HEALING

1944

One hundred infants receive care through the hospital's participation in the Emergency Maternal and Child Care Program (EMIC), a service for the families of soldiers.

1945

The pediatric outpatient department increases its hours to seven days a week with the help of funds from the Children's Research Foundation.

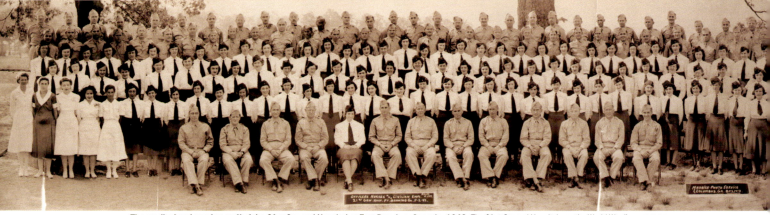

The medical and nursing staff of the 21st General Hospital at Fort Benning, Georgia, 1942. The 21st General Hospital was the World War II successor to Base Hospital No. 21, drawing all personnel from the medical school and its associated hospitals, which remained short-staffed during World War II. The 21st served in North Africa, Italy, and France and treated more than 65,000 patients. Despite battle conditions, the standard of care was so high that the unit received awards from both the French and American governments. Becker Medical Library

> **ST. LOUIS POST-DISPATCH**
> ## New Drug Used to Treat Meningitis Cases Here
> Children's Hospital Reports It Effected Its First Cure of Two Types of Disease by Administering Sulfanilamide.

donated $100,000 over a five-year period to create a training program in mental health issues for University pediatricians and others.

Overall, the hospital census for these years was static — ranging between 3,000 and 3,400 from 1937 through 1939 — though the patient mix was changing. The number of free patients to occupy the 135 beds was diminishing, while the ranks of paying patients swelled from 531 in 1937 to 679 two years later. Although deaths were going down, from 155 in 1937 to 121 in 1939, there were some intractable problem areas. In 1936, surgeon-in-chief Evarts Graham reported sadly a "disappointing mortality" from appendicitis, saying that "because of ignorance on the part of the parents many children are not seen by a physician until after the appendix has perforated. The situation then becomes very much more dangerous to life."

ANTIBIOTIC "MAGIC"

Suddenly, some of these intractable cases became treatable in 1937 when Children's Hospital — indeed, the whole practice of medicine — underwent a momentous clinical shift with the introduction of a new class of drugs. Sulfa drugs, which included sulfanilamide, sulfapyridine and later sulfamethylthiazole and sulfathiazole, had an astonishing impact on children with bacterial infections. The Children's staff joined in testing these promising new drugs as part of a landmark 11-institution study published in *The Journal of Pediatrics*, and the work at Children's "hastened the general acceptance of the drug by the medical profession in the allied group of hospitals and in the city in general," wrote Hartmann in his annual report.

The clinical results of this study became headline news in the *St. Louis Post-Dispatch*, which proclaimed, excitedly: "New Drug Used to Treat Meningitis Cases Here." In this article, the writer reported that 97 patients had received the drug since December 1936 and among them, "the first patient treated with sulfanilamide" — a 21-month-old boy — "was also the first case of streptococcic meningitis in the hospital to make a complete recovery." In April 1937, a nine-year-old girl with pneumococcal meningitis was also the first with that disease to recuperate.

The sulfa drugs and penicillin "were magic drugs as far as infections were concerned. You could see almost instantaneous improvement," said John Herweg, a 1945 medical school graduate, and then later a resident and chief resident at Children's. "Meningitis was very common, both meningococcal and hemophilus influenzae [and]

ABOVE **Headline from the *St. Louis Post-Dispatch*, 1937.** Sulfa drugs, tested at the hospital in 1937 as part of a landmark study, were a boon in the treatment of bacterial infections. Becker Medical Library

1945
20-year president of the Board of Managers, Mary McKittrick Markham, resigns and Alice M. Langenberg takes her place as fifth president of the hospital.

1946
Ridge Farm opens again briefly but, due to a lack of patients and staff, is closed permanently in October and sold to a Catholic order.

memories *Neal Middelkamp*

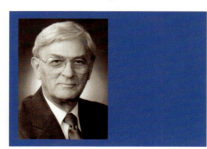

J. Neal Middelkamp, a 1948 Washington University School of Medicine graduate, interned for a year in Washington, D.C., started his residency at Children's Hospital, and then served in the U.S. Navy during the Korean War (1950-52). Back at Children's Hospital, he completed his residency, followed by a co-chief residency with Alexis Hartmann, Jr., M.D.'51. He joined the faculty in 1953; through the 1950s, he headed the Junior Clerkship program and worked with John Herweg, M.D.'45, to establish the hospital's infectious disease division.

"Before desegregation occurred in the 1950s, there were predominantly two medical schools that trained African-American physicians: Meharry in Nashville and Howard in Washington, D.C. Few African-Americans went into pediatrics, however. In 1953, Alexis Hartmann, Sr. received a grant from the U.S. Children's Bureau to establish an expanded pediatric residency at Homer G. Phillips Hospital. Drs. Park White, Helen Nash, and I set it up, and it was further staffed by School of Medicine pediatric faculty. Park White's sister-in-law, Dr. Katherine Bain, was at the Children's Bureau then in the Program Development office, so I think that helped in obtaining the grant.

"For six years, we provided lectures for the residents, interns, and nurses there. At first there was no premature nursery, so we had to send our residents for a month or two to train in the care of premature infants at the University of Colorado or Columbia University in New York. Then, in the mid-1950s, we got funding to build a modern 'preemie' unit in a wing of Homer G. Phillips. Dr. Helen Nash had a special interest in this area, because African-Americans tended to have more premature births than Caucasians.

"During the life of the program, we trained many excellent, board-certified pediatricians: Drs. Homer Nash; C. Ronald Higgins, Jr.; Albert Crocker; Gloria Texauer, George Lowe, John Young, John Hall, and Lincoln Calvin, for example. We really were able to attract fine physicians, who then moved on to programs or practices around the United States."

pneumoccocal meningitis. Children would get an ear infection...then they would get mastoiditis, followed by meningitis, and they would die in the matter of a few days to a week. The sulfanomides were really the first anti-microbial agents that were at least reasonably effective — and if you got the patient early on in the course of the disease, they were very effective."

WORLD WAR II

In the early 1940s, another class of antibiotic — penicillin — became widely available, and Children's adopted its use in 1943 for a case of influenza meningitis. Yet this new wave of change would not take place until another kind of upheaval had occurred: the advent of World War II. In 1942, Hartmann proudly reported that the hospital had had "much less difficulty than most hospitals in appointing and maintaining an adequate house staff for the care of an ever-increased number of patients." To cover the anticipated depletion of men, they appointed three women physicians and had senior medical students double as interns during their elective quarters.

Gradually, though, the privations of war began to take a toll. "It has been extremely difficult to provide the hospital with sufficient, trained, technical assistants for laboratory positions," wrote Hartmann. "Such people are in great demand in the Army and Navy hospitals." Hospital and research equipment were also scarce. Still, Jean V. Cooke managed to study immunization to tetanus, while Russell Blattner and Florence Heys worked to isolate the virus that causes encephalitis, finally succeeding in 1946. In the wake of the war, Gilbert Forbes and instructor Anne M. Perley did innovative work with radioactive tracers as an aid to diagnosing illness, such as thyroid disease.

By 1944, Hartmann was reporting that every department was handicapped because of reductions in personnel and, as it had in World War I, Ridge Farm also closed for lack of staff. Among those joining the armed forces from Children's were: assistant physicians Henry L. Barnett, Max Deutch, Stanley Harrison, Sol Londe, and Bernard Schwartzman; instructors John H. Doval, and David Goldring; chief resident John Ray Powers; and house staff Walter J. Kennedy, Torrence A. Makley, C. Read Boles, Jack

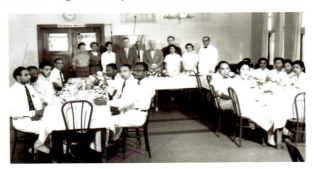

Medical staff, Homer G. Phillips Hospital, 1957. Helen Nash, (standing, far left), Park White (standing, fifth from right) and Neal Middelkamp (standing, fourth from right).
Courtesy of J. Neal Middelkamp

1946

Russell Blattner and Florence Heys isolate the virus that causes encephalitis.

1946

St. Louis experiences a devastating polio epidemic with a huge increase in patients; for the first time, black children are integrated throughout the wards of the hospital.

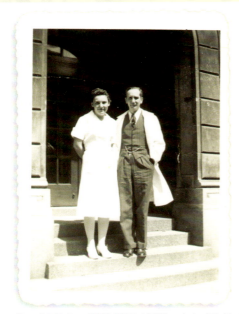

Russell J. Blattner (1908-2002). A 1929 graduate of Washington University and of its medical school in 1933, who served as house officer from 1933-37, Blattner became a faculty member in 1937 and was promoted to associate professor in 1945. A specialist in virus research and infectious diseases, Blattner (pictured here in 1944 with head nurse Irene Schmidt) was appointed head of pediatrics at Baylor College in 1947. Becker Medical Library

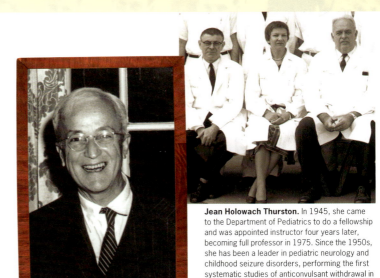

Daniel C. Darrow (1895-1965). A Johns Hopkins graduate who had worked in Boston City Hospital, Darrow was appointed assistant physician at Children's in 1925, specializing in blood-related diseases in children. In 1940 he was president of the Society for Pediatric Research, in 1957 he became president of the American Pediatric Society, and in 1959 he won the John Howland medal. It was often said of him that "All Darrow needed to produce superlative research was a shoestring and a Bunsen burner." The Alan Mason Chesney Medical Archives of The Johns Hopkins Medical Institutions

Jean Holowach Thurston. In 1945, she came to the Department of Pediatrics to do a fellowship and was appointed instructor four years later, becoming full professor in 1975. Since the 1950s, she has been a leader in pediatric neurology and childhood seizure disorders, performing the first systematic studies of anticonvulsant withdrawal in infants and children. In 2004, she received the first life-time achievement award from the Child Neurology Society. Becker Medical Library

Thornton, Leo J. Geppert, George Salmon, and Frank F. Martin. Among the surgeons were James Barrett Brown, Robert Bartlett, Henry G. Schwartz, Brian Blades, Leonard Furlow, C. Barber Mueller, Oscar Hampton, Frederick Jostes, Maurice Roche, and Franklin Walton. Nurses signed up, too, some joining the medical school's General Hospital 21, an Army unit that would staff military hospitals overseas. A few did not return; in 1942, Lt. Rose Rieper, an Army nurse formerly on the Ridge Farm staff, was reported missing in action in the Philippines.

The hospital also participated in a new program, sponsored by the U.S. Children's Bureau under the direction of Martha Eliot. Called the Emergency Maternal and Child Care Program (EMIC), it was aimed at the families of soldiers, offering them medical care at government expense. While not all hospitals took part, Children's signed up immediately, reported Hartmann in the 1944 annual report, "and exactly 100 infants received hospital care in 1944 as a result."

As the war went on, Hartmann re-structured pediatric internships to cope with changing needs. Three of the seven interns did rotating, nine-month internships, spending three months each on the medical service at Barnes, the obstetrical service at the Maternity Hospital, and the pediatric service at Children's. Not only would this attract more recruits, but this broad-based training was also "highly desirable," wrote Hartmann, "since some 95 percent of pediatrics in the United States is practiced by the general practitioner, who for the most part has no opportunity to get pediatric training in a children's hospital beyond what he gets as an undergraduate medical student."

Still, the war placed a heavy burden on the overworked staff. "There were usually three of us first-year people on every other night to take care of about 125-150 patients, many of whom were desperately ill, and often we would have one or more deaths during our evening on....We were all over-worked and most of us had chronic upper respiratory infections," added Herweg. "And the availability of equipment — I don't know whether that was due to the war or the tightness of Miss [Estelle] Claiborne's budget, but when penicillin became available, we had

1946

Hartmann urges the managers to consider the need for "an entirely new hospital" with more room and modern equipment.

1947

The campaign for a new building receives the approval of a sponsoring agency, the St. Louis Community Chest Fund.

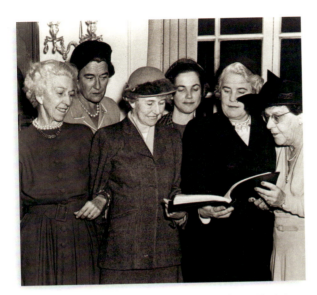

Julia Rumsey Holland. A volunteer with the Martha Parsons Hospital, she served as a board member and vice president of the Children's Hospital Board of Managers. Julia Holland (far right) was a strong proponent of medical social service efforts and integration under President **Alice M. Langenberg** (far left). Becker Medical Library

only two glass syringes in the whole hospital. So they had to be cleaned and autoclaved almost continuously, while the nurses on the infant ward had to take count of all the safety pins....In 1945 and 1946, we began to have returning military physicians and surgeons who came back for a refresher course in pediatrics....They would be on call with a house officer until 11 or so in the evening — so they would learn by doing and we would also get some help."

POST-WAR DESEGREGATION

Along with new faces, the end of World War II brought other changes to the hospital. Ridge Farm — long a haven for children convalescing from rheumatic fever, bone diseases, asthma, and other chronic diseases — re-opened briefly. In January 1946, Hugh McCulloch appeared before the Board of Managers to argue in favor of opening it to "colored patients"; he had already asked the teacher at Ridge Farm, who had said she would be willing to instruct them. On February 15, the first three black children were admitted, but this victory was short-lived. The census at Ridge Farm was dropping, and it was difficult to find personnel willing to travel to Valley Park. Soon the managers began talking about closing the facility — and it did shut its doors on October 15, 1946. "In ink of the reddest hue...was the unfortunate closure of Ridge Farm," said Hartmann, ruefully. The facility was sold to a Catholic order for around $70,000.

At Children's Hospital, the Butler Ward still admitted black children, and all of them "got exactly the same treatment as any other patients on any other wards. That I can assure you," recalled David Goldring once. But many on the medical staff were eager for integration. Park J. White, who also directed the pediatric division at Homer G. Phillips Hospital, was a passionate advocate for change; so was Hartmann himself who "had a strong belief in the rights of people," recalled Lawrence Kahn later. "....Pediatricians tend to be accepting people; as a group they are more tolerant of change than most others. It is integral to their working with children. Children...are a universal society of their own without distinctions or prejudice. Perhaps pediatricians in their association with children reflect some of their candor and straightforward, unadorned look at the world."

The move toward integration had actually begun in the early 1940s, when Goldring was a resident, working in the Children's emergency room one evening. A black infant was brought in, but the Butler Ward had no incubators available, so Goldring sent the child to the white ward instead. At this violation of the rules, the supervisor was furious, and she called Hartmann to back her up — but he supported Goldring instead. In 1946, another impetus to change was a devastating polio epidemic that flooded the hospital with patients. Hartmann used this crisis as an occasion to take over the Butler Ward for polio patients and transfer the black children to wards throughout the hospital. On the Board of Managers, Julia Rumsey Holland championed this change.

"The epidemic of poliomyelitis last summer proved a blessing in disguise," said Hartmann in his 1947 report. "From the standpoint of poliomyelitis, approximately twice the usual number of beds were immediately made available. From the viewpoint of the Negro patient, several very important objectives which I have long sought were met: (1) Negro children were in a position

1947 — Meyer and Regina Waldman establish the Fern Waldman Fund for pediatric cancer research.

1947 — Children's Hospital affiliates with the medical school's Department of Occupational Therapy.

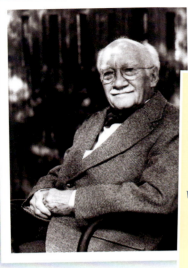

Park J. White (1891-1987).
Becker Medical Library

He Isn't Goin'ta Hurtcha!

"Now, he isn't goin'ta hurtcha!
What an error in child nurtcha —
What lack of parental virtcha
Do those silly words reveal!
I have yet to see a child
Whom they've not made still more wild,
Utterly unreconciled
To the chap who tries to heal.

— by Park J. White
First published in *Hygeia*

Park J. White — or P.J., as he was called — had two lifelong passions: He was a much-loved pediatric practitioner and a lifelong crusader for civil rights and social justice. The two interests often coincided. A *Post-Dispatch* article from 1985 called him "a kind of medical missionary to the urban poor."

A graduate of Harvard, where he joined the Socialist Club, then of Columbia University's medical school, he came to Children's in 1920 as an assistant pediatrician and served on the faculty until 1963. In 1925, he attracted national attention when he published a study comparing black and white infant death rates in St. Louis — pointing out that the death rate for black infants was double that for white babies. At the medical school, he began teaching a course in ethics, which he would offer for 16 years.

From 1945 to 1966, he directed pediatrics at Homer G. Phillips Hospital, training young black physicians who went on to become board-certified pediatricians. His own pediatric practice, which opened in 1924, welcomed white and black children. He took on social causes, such as urging birth control or battling to reduce the impact of lead-paint on inner-city children. In his free time, he was a poet and essayist, whose work appeared in medical journals.

The Park J. White Professorship in Pediatrics, held by F. Sessions Cole, is named for him today.

to get *any* type of service available to white children *without duplication of effort anywhere*; (2) admissions of Negro children became highly elastic, so that no ceiling as to total number had to be considered — the only considerations being desirability of admission and the overall available bed situation; (3) complete abolition of race discrimination was accomplished."

In 1949, the medical staff was integrated, too. With the encouragement of Park White, Helen Nash — who had been a resident and chief resident at Homer G. Phillips — applied to become an attending physician at Children's and was accepted, becoming the first black physician at the hospital. She would serve for more than 40 years on the clinical faculty and attending staff before she was named professor emerita in 1993.

MORE POST-WAR CHANGES

Progress was occurring on several fronts. In 1947, new funding for research into the roots of acute leukemia came available when Meyer and Regina Waldman established the Fern Waldman Fund in memory of their daughter, who had died of leukemia at age 11. A group of volunteer women, some of whom had also lost children to cancer, staged annual benefits to support the fund, which raised more than $18,000 in six years. New therapeutic drugs for children with leukemia were just beginning to emerge, such as aminopterin, administered by Jean V. Cooke, head of the hematology division, and pediatrician William G. Klingberg. Also in 1947, Children's Hospital — which had had an occupational therapist on staff for nearly three decades — affiliated with the medical school's Department of Occupational Therapy. During the early 1950s, Children's acquired its own pharmacy, Mallinckrodt Institute hired its first pediatric roentgenologist, and the hospital's private corridor finally got a small room where doctors could speak confidentially to patients.

The Board of Managers was also in transition. In 1945, 20-year president Mary McKittrick Markham resigned, and Alice M. Langenberg took her place as the fifth president of the hospital, saying that under Markham's leadership "the Hospital has grown in service, responsibility and reputation, and that it will be our obligation to carry on the same high ideals, standards and

1948

The Board of Managers admits men to its ranks for the first time, disbanding the all-male advisory committee.

1949

A 10-bed unit opens for premature infants.

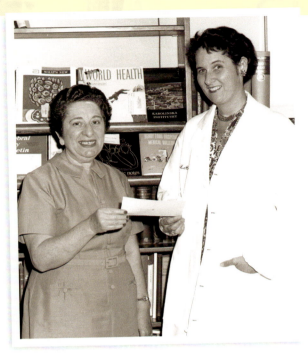

Fern Waldman Fund for research. Established in 1947 by Meyer and Regina Waldman in memory of their daughter, a leukemia victim, this fund was used to support pediatric cancer research. Mrs. Waldman is pictured with Dr. Vietti during the 1960s. Becker Medical Library

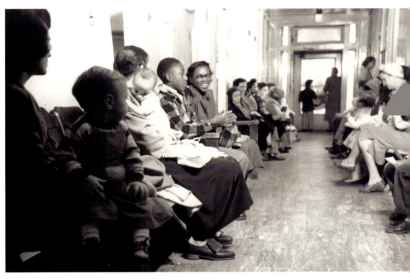

Outpatient department, 1949. Hartmann urged the Board of Managers to begin a campaign for a new building, stating "the O.P.D. is so crowded that often it resembles Union Station during the War." Becker Medical Library

traditions in the same fine spirit." But the historic role of the board — even its composition — was soon to undergo a fundamental shift.

Meanwhile, some talented young physicians continued on staff, such as John Martz as chief resident in 1947 and a house staff that included Kenneth Koerner and Janet Scoville, but other gifted people were leaving. Katherine Bain left to join the U.S. Children's Bureau and, in 1948, Russell Blattner accepted a position as head of the pediatrics department at Baylor University's medical school, taking along his collaborator, instructor Florence Heys, who held the Catlin Fellowship. To replace staff members, Hartmann tended to look within the University's own ranks; little cross-pollination occurred from other schools or departments.

A MUCH-NEEDED NEW BUILDING

Even before Ridge Farm closed — and still more earnestly afterwards — Hartmann began cajoling, pleading, badgering the Board of Managers to undertake a campaign for a new building. More space was sorely needed for inpatient care; "too often children deserving of admission could not be accepted," he lamented in 1948. Frequently, the hospital had to call upon other institutions to help. "The friendly and cooperative, if unofficial, relationships which have been maintained between the St. Louis Children's Hospital and the St. Louis City Hospital, the St. Louis County Hospital, Homer Phillips Hospital and the Jewish Hospital have enabled such children to receive hospital treatment without serious loss of contact with our staff," he added. Further, the still-new Outpatient Department was already bursting at the seams. In 1947, Hartmann reported that admissions had doubled in a year; "the O.P.D. is so crowded that often it resembles Union Station during the War," he wrote, adding: *"Speed is essential."*

In fact, he wanted more than additional room: He also wanted a modern hospital. As early as 1946, he urged the managers to embrace the idea of "an entirely new hospital with adequate provisions for the complete care of the child." That would include such facilities as a division for adolescent children, a larger child guidance clinic, a complete dental outpatient department, and onsite convalescent care.

1949

Helen Nash, former chief resident at Homer G. Phillips, joins the medical staff as the first black physician at Children's Hospital.

1949

The 70th anniversary of the hospital is celebrated at the Chase Hotel, and the board unveils plans for an expanded facility.

memories *Helen E. Nash*

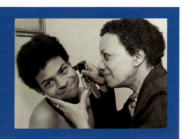

Helen Nash, a 1945 Meharry Medical College graduate, did an internship and then a pediatric residency at Homer G. Phillips Hospital; there she met the supervisor of pediatric training, Park J. White, who became her mentor. With his support, she became the first African-American physician appointed to the attending staff at St. Louis Children's Hospital. Today, the Helen E. Nash Academic Achievement Award is given to a medical student each year. Following is an excerpt from a conversation she had with writer Marion Hunt in 1999:

"Dr. White said if I stayed here, he'd push for me to get me a staff appointment so that I could admit patients at Children's Hospital. Whenever he said he'd do something like that, he always followed through with his promise. I'm sure he kept the pressure on Dean Moore at the medical school. In 1949, I got a notice to come to a meeting in the Dean's office. When I arrived, there were three other black physicians present, all men. The Dean told us we were all being given appointments to the faculty as attending physicians.

"Dr. Hartmann, the head of pediatrics, interviewed me before I took the position….He told me he wanted the Board of Managers at Children's Hospital to see me. That was anger-provoking. What did they think a black woman doctor would look like? But I agreed and went with him to their monthly meeting. Dr. Hartmann introduced me. The gist of what he said was that I was all right and I wouldn't bite. Though the women managers were polite, the whole experience made me feel like an exotic animal. And I guess for women who had never seen an educated black person, I was."

With some trepidation, the managers began to plan, asking a sponsoring agency, the St. Louis Community Chest, to give its approval for a campaign. In March 1947, an aged Grace Richards Jones appeared before the board to give them much-needed moral support and "to assure members of the Board," said the minutes, "that the seeming mountain of expense for enlarged buildings can be moved by faith. Her experience has shown this." Or as she said herself, "People who have money gladly want to give it for something that appeals to them. You have to have faith to move mountains, but the mountains have to be worth moving."

At first, the board set a goal of $1.85 million for a major addition to the hospital that would consist of all the things that Hartmann had asked for, as well as others: laboratories, lecture halls, office space, waiting rooms, a library, larger record rooms, storage, more rooms for house staff. "The list goes on and on," wrote Langenberg. "Our whole problem can be expressed in three words — NOT ENOUGH SPACE." At first, they hoped to gather money quietly by contacting friends of the hospital, in the board's time-honored fashion. As the months slipped by, however, too little accumulated, and behind the scenes they took new measures to calculate the amount they might raise, hiring a New York firm to survey potential donors.

MOVING TOWARD THE GOAL

Just a month later, in December 1948, an epochal change occurred on the board itself: The lady managers decided to admit men to their ranks, thus disbanding the all-male advisory committee. A month after that, the board hired a public relations firm, Fleishman, Hillard and Associates, to lay the emotional groundwork for a more public building campaign. Throughout 1949, heart-warming stories appeared in the press about Children's patients; illustrated brochures came out, vividly describing the need and highlighting children turned away for lack of space. In 1948, they said, the hospital had some 3,351 admissions and served 33,365 outpatients — children with burns, polio, nephritis, or surgical needs, from all parts of the world. "There has been no enlargement of the hospital in the past 27 years," one brochure pleaded.

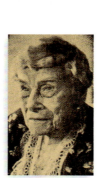

Rose Harsh Fraley (1848-1949). The last surviving member of the original Board of Managers, Mrs. Fraley celebrated her 101st birthday a few weeks before the 70th Anniversary Dinner. Becker Medical Library

1950

A 21-member Board of Trustees is formed, and the Board of Managers becomes the all-women Auxiliary Board, devoted to volunteer activities and fund-raising rather than hospital management.

1950

Roy Kercheval is elected president of the Board of Trustees.

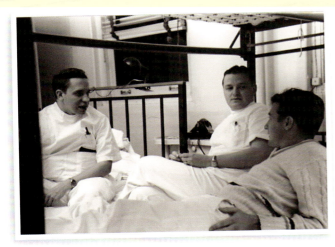

Residents, 1949. More room was desperately needed all over the hospital as the campaign for an expanded facility began in 1949. Even the residents were crowded together in their sleeping quarters. *Becker Medical Library*

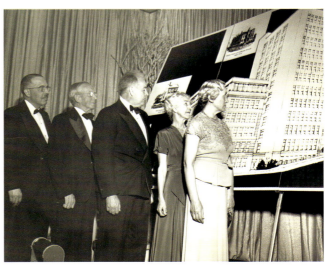

70th Anniversary Dinner. At the dinner, held on May 26, 1949, attendees saw an architect's rendering of the proposed addition to the hospital. From left: Robert Moore, medical school dean; Harry Wallace, board president of Washington University; Alexis Hartmann; Alice Langenberg, president of the Board of Managers; and Estelle Claiborne, hospital administrator. *Becker Medical Library*

> **"A nation is not richer than its children and its future is no richer than its children's health."**

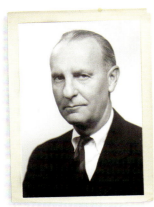

At the hospital's 70th anniversary celebration, held at the Chase Hotel in May 1949, the board unveiled plans for the expanded facility — a new six-story addition to the north and a 10-story tower between the present two buildings — and said the price tag was now $2 million. Soon pledges came in from businesses: $25,000 from Mallinckrodt Chemical, $12,500 from Famous-Barr. Warren T. Chandler, vice president of Mercantile — Commerce and Trust Company, agreed to head the drive, and Jimmy Conzelman, popular former coach of the Washington University football team, volunteered to head a special gifts division.

Amid this giant project, the board underwent an even more tradition-shattering change. In February 1950, a 21-member board of trustees — composed of seven men and 14 women — split off from the 201-member Board of Managers, and the remaining managers now reconstituted themselves as an all-women Auxiliary Board, devoted to volunteer activities and fund-raising rather than hospital management. "Creation of this small body...became necessary because of the continuing rapid growth of the Hospital and widening scope of its services," said a press release. Alice Langenberg remained president of the trustees for several months and then resigned; Royal D. Kercheval was elected in her place, the first man in 71 years to serve as board president.

Just as the fund drive officially began in April 1950, a new factor complicated the picture: a competing fund drive, announced that same April, to construct the six-story, $5 million Cardinal Glennon Memorial Hospital for Children near St. Louis University School of Medicine. This drive, said a newspaper account, "is the largest campaign for capital funds ever undertaken in the history of St. Louis." The article also went on to explain the reason for building this new hospital. "A survey by a New York firm of hospital consultants...showed that there had been no increase in hospital facilities for children in the metropolitan area here since 1930, despite a record-breaking increase in the number of births."

ABOVE **Royal D. Kercheval (1890-1966).** Succeeding Alice Langenberg as president of the new board of trustees was Kercheval, vice president and trust officer of Boatman's National Bank. He also served as treasurer of the building campaign. *Becker Medical Library*

1950
The fund drive for the new hospital officially begins.

1952
Only $350,000 short of the $2.96 million goal, the new building's ground-breaking ceremony takes place on October 22.

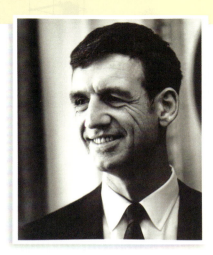

William H. Danforth. A graduate of Harvard Medical School, Danforth did a year's residency training at Children's Hospital before shifting to internal medicine, followed by a cardiology fellowship. From 1965 to 1971, he served as the School of Medicine's second vice chancellor for medical affairs; in 1971, he was named chancellor of Washington University, serving until 1995. Becker Medical Library

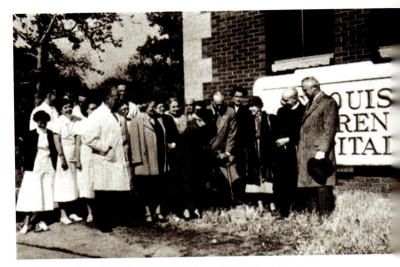

Ground-breaking, 1952. Mary McKittrick Markham and Roy Kercheval wielded the shovel during the 1952 ground-breaking ceremony. Onlookers included Alexis Hartmann and Estelle Claiborne, hospital administrator (front row, left) and Alice Langenberg, president of the Board of Managers; the Rev. Dr. James W. Clarke, pastor of Second Presbyterian Church; and Warren S. Chandler, head of the fund-raising committee (front row, right). Becker Medical Library

So the Children's Hospital campaign labored on. Early on, at least one aspect proved a quick success: attracting $100,000 to endow the "Grace Jones Floor" in the new hospital, as "a living tribute to a great lady and a great benefactress of children," said Chandler. Despite radio pleas from star Eddie Cantor, who quipped "give until it feels good," donations came in slowly as the price tag for construction kept rising; in 1951, newspapers announced that the building campaign had "fallen short," raising only $1.65 million of the total needed, while the cost had risen to $2.78 million. While the Auxiliary held fundraisers, such as fashion shows with gossip columnist Hedda Hopper, Kercheval and the board managed to secure $763,400 in federal funds for the project. As far away as Memphis, one newspaper was touting the project, calling Children's "one of the world's best hospitals dedicated to the treatment and care of children."

By 1952, the board was only $350,000 short of its goal — now up to $2.96 million — but the ambitious project had been scaled back, too. Now they planned to build a six-story wing that would increase the bed capacity to 200, plus renovate the existing hospital. Counting on future donations, the board also borrowed money from the endowment to make up the difference. At last, 100 trustees and staff members came together on October 22 for ground-breaking ceremonies, with Kercheval and Mary McKittrick Markham turning over the first shovels of dirt. Rev. James W. Clarke, pastor of Second Presbyterian Church, spoke, saying: "A nation is not richer than its children and its future is no richer than its children's health."

As the building went up, the board began a second campaign in 1954 to make up the difference, and soon only $240,000 separated them from success. At this point, announced the board minutes, "a kind friend" of the hospital stepped forward — William H. Danforth and the Danforth Foundation — with an anonymous donation of $141,825, stipulating that the remaining $98,175 come from other sources before December 31. With this extraordinary incentive, the board set to work and not only reached the deadline in time, but also raised an extra $67,000.

Even without the new hospital building, the number of patients rose to 42,962 in 1954. The medical staff was not large: 10 full-time members, 40 part-time, six to eight interns, eight to 12 first-year residents. And it was stretched thin, also caring for patients at the St. Louis Maternity Hospital, St. Louis County Hospital, and Burge Hospital in Springfield, Missouri, as well as

1954
The hospital treats 42,962 patients this year.

1954
Jonas Salk's vaccine for polio becomes available.

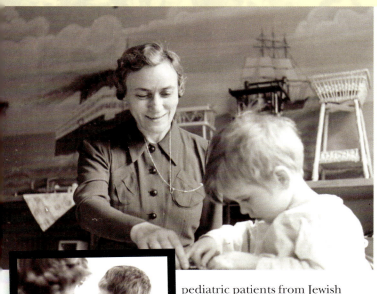

Occupational Therapy, ca. 1950s. Both for healing and for diversion, occupational therapy continued to be an essential part of treatment. Becker Medical Library

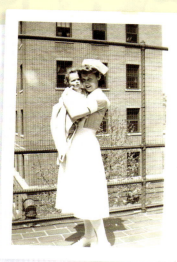

LEFT **Estelle D. Claiborne (1889-1986).** A 1915 graduate of the Washington University School of Nursing, Claiborne served with Base Hospital No. 21 from 1917 to 1919 during WWI. She served as executive assistant at Barnes Hospital from 1921 to 1923 and as administrator of Shriner's Hospital for Crippled Children before her appointment as superintendent of St. Louis Children's Hospital in 1925. Claiborne retired in December 1954. Becker Medical Library

ABOVE **Nursing student with baby, 1944.** Students nurses rotated through each department when they began training, giving them a chance to work with every type of patient at Children's Hospital. After the initial training period, each nurse was permanently placed in the department of her choice. Courtesy of Elizabeth O'Connell

pediatric patients from Jewish Hospital; in addition, the staff participated in the state's Rheumatic Fever Program, Premature Program and the St. Louis Society for Crippled Children. Now changes to the residency program occurred, as more international staff were admitted and the number of chief residents was increased to two in 1953: Alexis Hartmann, Jr., and J. Neal Middelkamp. Estelle Claiborne — hospital administrator for nearly three decades — retired, and in 1955 assistant administrator Lilly Hoekstra took her place.

As it always had, the strong nursing staff formed the backbone of the hospital, working a 44-hour week until a 40-hour schedule was introduced in 1957 — down from 48 hours in 1949. White-capped nurses staffed the various divisions, such as the new toddlers' division, the metabolism ward, or the infants' ward, developing special areas of expertise. In 1955, Children's affiliated with the new Barnes School of Nursing, while continuing to train nurses from the Washington University School of Nursing, in which Children's had played a part for 45 years.

As for the training of student nurses, wrote nursing superintendent Elizabeth O'Connell, the hospital held them to high standards. "During the first two weeks...she will be rotated through all divisions, thus giving her an opportunity to care for every type of patient hospitalized here....She is then assigned permanently to the division of her choice....During the first months, the general duty nurse learns that here the standards of nursing are actually those which comprise good child care. Her performance must always be an example of this care."

In March 1955, the hospital could finally report in its two-year-old newsletter, *Small Talk*, that "with the exception of a few details, our new wing is really complete. Everyone is so proud of the shiny, handsome new quarters, it is really very difficult to take in the enormity of the change." Renovation of the old building would continue, and Hoekstra reported in a 1956 newsletter, a little wearily, that the "architects and contractors... again assure us that the entire building program will be complete by January 1, 1957." When it was actually finished in March 1958, the new building included partial air-conditioning, thanks to a grant from the Ford Foundation.

PROBLEMS GROW DURING THE HARTMANN ERA

From the 1950s onward, the field of pediatrics was undergoing rapid — even breathtaking — change, with the help of the National Institutes

1955	1956	1956
The new wing of the hospital is completed.	More than 500 teenage and adults work as volunteers at the hospital, supervised and trained by a volunteer director hired in 1955.	With an endowment from the Ittleson Foundation, the first chair of child psychiatry in the U.S. is established at the School of Medicine.

memories *John C. Martz*

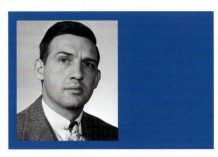

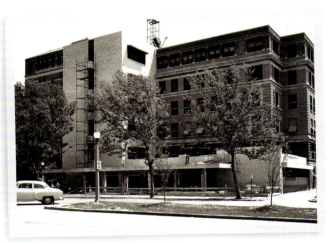

New Wing nearly finished (*Small Talk*, July 1954). Becker Medical Library

John C. Martz graduated from the School of Medicine in 1942, left for military service during World War II, and then returned to Children's Hospital to do his residency from 1945 to 1947. Afterwards, he started his own private practice in St. Louis and became associate professor of clinical pediatrics at Washington University, retiring in 1985.

"On several occasions, when I was a student, I saw McKim Marriott, a man with glasses and a high-pitched voice, but I began my residency under Alexis Hartmann, whom we called "the Chief." Things have changed markedly since then. Incubators — "Hess beds," invented by a pediatrician named Hess — were two layers of metal with hot water in between. They were really just places to keep the kids warm. A 2-pound preemie had very little chance of survival.

After a while, we had sulfa drugs and then penicillin. That made a big different in bacterial meningitis, which was not uncommon in children and was 100 percent fatal. The same was true with pneumonia. At that time, the bacteria were very sensitive to it; we would give 5,000 units of penicillin, and it was really a wonder drug.

After the war, we had lots of older fellows as residents, many of them married; some had been in service for four years as paratroopers and things like that. As soon as my residency ended, I went immediately into private practice, but getting patients was not easy at first. I did much better taking calls on weekends for other physicians, who wanted to have the weekend off.

> **"Everyone is so proud of the shiny, handsome new quarters, it is really very difficult to take in the enormity of the change."**
> — *Small Talk*, March 1955

of Health (NIH) and its generous grant funding for scientific research. At other institutions, NIH-funded researchers were expanding the uses of penicillin and streptomycin into therapies for diphtheria or bacterial meningitis. Chromosomal and metabolic studies were burgeoning; so was scientific interest in hormonal and steroid therapies. Intensive polio research culminated in exciting advances that included Jonas Salk's vaccine, made from killed polio virus, which was launched widely in 1954; Albert Sabin followed with an oral version, created from a weakened form of the live virus. In fact, viral research generally — and scientific understanding of the variety and complexity of viruses — grew as a field. On the psychiatric front, researchers increasingly focused on the psychotherapeutic aspects of pediatric practice, along with the importance of public health and preventive medicine.

While St. Louis Children's Hospital adopted clinical advances, such as the polio vaccine, its staff was not at the forefront of these research discoveries, though some former house officers and faculty members were. At Yale, one-time faculty member Daniel C. Darrow did studies proving the importance of potassium in the treatment of dehydration; Russell Blattner, now of Houston, isolated and identified viruses associated with encephalitis. One-time house officer candidate Edith Lincoln, a researcher in New York City, announced significant findings in the treatment of tuberculosis, while Philip C. Jeans, another former faculty member, now of Iowa City, described the critical nature of folic acid in nutrition. Hugh McCulloch, who had moved to Chicago, continued his work on rheumatic fever.

Still, some progress did occur at Children's Hospital during these years. In 1956, the Ittleson

1957
A 40-hour weekly schedule is introduced for the nursing staff, down from 48 hours in 1949.

1958
Washington University graduate Jessie Ternberg is appointed the first woman chief resident in surgery.

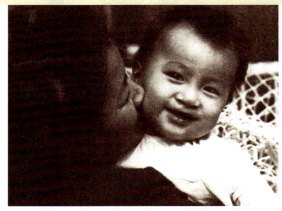

Birth defects center. This child from Hawaii, treated for a cleft lip, was among the hundreds who travelled to Children's Hospital after it opened a birth defects center in 1963. Becker Medical Library

Foundation endowed the first chair of child psychiatry in the United States at the School of Medicine; this chair also inaugurated the Division of Child Psychiatry, which encompassed the Child Guidance Clinic, an affiliated St. Louis County clinic, and a Pediatric Psychiatric Unit at Children's. The Danforth Chapel was constructed in 1955, another gift of William H. Danforth, and two years later, James W. Singer, Jr., was named president of the trustees, followed by Hugh Lewis and then Edwin M. Johnston in 1962. In 1963, a regional birth defects center was established at the hospital.

Volunteers continued to play an important — and growing — role at Children's Hospital. In 1955, a volunteer director was appointed to supervise their training, and by the next year, the roster included 138 teenagers from 19 St. Louis-area schools and nearly 400 adults working as transportation aides, gift and coffee shop assistants, receptionists, seamstresses, doll-makers, and so on. Other visitors made pilgrimages to the hospital: Clarabell, star of the "Howdy Doody" show; Popeye, who talked with the children about spinach; cowboy heroes Red Ryder and the Lone Ranger; skater Donna Atwood. Bob Hope began visiting when his daughter, a Saint Louis University student, worked as a volunteer, and beginning in 1958, he staged benefit exhibition golf tournaments. In 1961, a gala celebration inaugurated the new Bob Hope Foundation, named by the trustees in his honor, which would collect funds to finance research, teaching and building projects.

Some talented people remained on staff, such as a husband-and-wife team: Don Thurston,

memories *Jessie L. Ternberg*

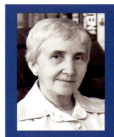

Jessie L. Ternberg, a 1953 School of Medicine graduate, returned to St. Louis as the first woman surgical resident in 1954 after an internship at Boston City Hospital. This achievement initiated a series of "firsts" for Ternberg, a pioneer in pediatric surgery who performed up to 500 operations a year on Children's Hospital patients: first woman chief resident, first woman on the surgical faculty, first woman head of the medical school's faculty council. After helping to establish the Division of Pediatric Surgery, she became its chief in 1972 and stayed on until 1996, when she was named professor emerita.

"In the late 1950s, women residents were housed in what we called the 'convent,' created from the old surgical amphitheatre at Barnes. It was one floor, no windows, and the air-conditioning was so cold that you couldn't sit without some kind of covering on. It was miserable. We were isolated over there — it was like we were behind a concrete barrier.

"On the night of February 10, 1959, I had been working late in the surgery lab, then came back and had just nicely gone to sleep when the phone rang. I was not on call, but here was someone was telling me that a tornado had hit part of Children's Hospital, and that one of the male pediatric residents was badly hurt. I was skeptical, but she was so insistent. Finally, I said, 'If this is a fake, I am going to demolish you when I get there,' and I went over. It was true: In the male residents' quarters, a plate-glass window had fallen in and [later pediatric cardiologist] Tony Hernandez had broken ribs and severe cuts on his chest. We had to deal with him, get the chest wound covered, and try to protect the children as well. We tried to call in [chest surgeon-on-call] Tom Ferguson, but his driveway was blocked by a fallen tree and he couldn't get out; instead, we called the surgery head, Tom Burford, and he came in right away.

"Finally, I could go back to bed, but five to ten minutes later the phone rang again. This time, they were calling from the operating room, where they needed me to assist. Tony was just covered with cuts; I sewed up one of them and it looked a little like a 'J.' I told him, 'Tony, I left my initial on you.' It was a long night."

Jessie Ternberg. Ternberg told students that "surgeons must have the eye of an eagle, the heart of a lion, and the hand of a lady." Becker Medical Library

1958
Bob Hope, already a celebrity visitor for several years, stages the first of several exhibition golf tournaments to benefit the hospital.

MARCH 1958
The new building is completed.

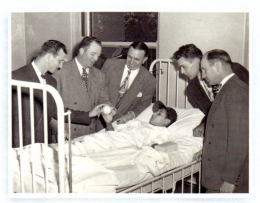

Children with congenital heart disease came to the hospital from around the world for life-saving surgery and treatment. Pediatrician Merl J. Carson, in collaboration with Wendell Scott of Mallinckrodt Institute of Radiology and Thomas Burford of the Department of Surgery, developed a means of determining which of these children could be helped by surgery. Called the "rapidograph," it was an X-ray technique that could visualize the blood vessels within the heart.

One of these "blue babies' was 13-year-old Rudolfo Gutierrez, a baseball fan, who came to Children's Hospital from Colombia in 1949. While awaiting surgery, he enjoyed a visit from St. Louis Cardinals team members, then engaged in a National League Pennant race with the Brooklyn Dodgers.

Rudolfo Gutierrez was visited by five members of the St. Louis Cardinals baseball team: Stan Musial, Manager Eddie Dyer, Coach Terry Moore, Nippy Jones, and Enos Slaughter. Becker Medical Library

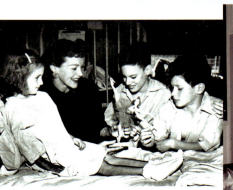

Donna Atwood and patients. Donna Atwood, the skating star, visited children at the hospital before a benefit matinee of the Ice Capades. Becker Medical Library

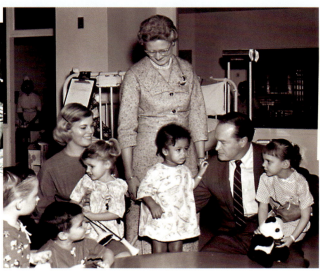

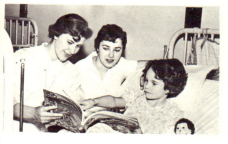

ABOVE **Volunteers, 1956.** High school students were among the many invaluable volunteers at the hospital. Becker Medical Library

LEFT **Bob Hope and his daughter, Linda, visiting hospital patients, 1961**. Comedian Bob Hope was a long-time supporter of the hospital and sponsor of numerous benefits. The Hope Foundation of St. Louis Children's Hospital, established in 1961, was named in his honor. Becker Medical Library

working in the field of allergy, and Jean Holowach Thurston, a pediatric neurologist who founded the Pediatric Convulsion Clinic in 1950. Jessie Ternberg, who had received her medical degree from Washington University in 1953, returned after her internship at Boston City Hospital to become the first woman surgical resident and then, in 1958, the first woman chief resident in surgery. But others, like McCulloch, were resigning to go elsewhere: Merl Carson, who had collaborated with radiologist Wendell Scott and surgeon Thomas Burford to develop the "rapidograph," an X-ray technique that helped determine which "blue babies" could be helped by surgery; Gilbert Forbes and Anne Perley, who left for posts in Dallas. Jean V. Cooke, whose work had focused on infectious diseases, died in 1956. Meanwhile, the house staff was increasingly dominated by international students, some with a limited command of English.

Once again building needs were on the horizon: In 1962, the third floor of the hospital was renovated to accommodate a clinical research center for children with hard-to-treat problems, such as metabolic disorders. The following year saw the start of yet another period of expansion, as Washington University gave Children's a 99-year lease on the land between the hospital and the Barnes Nurses' Home. On this site, Children's hoped to build a five-story addition for research, diagnostic and teaching space, plus renovate two existing floors and enlarge outpa-

1961
The Bob Hope Foundation is established for research, teaching, and building projects.

1963
A regional birth defects center is established at Children's Hospital.

1963
A campaign for a five-story addition to the hospital begins with a dinner honoring Bob Hope.

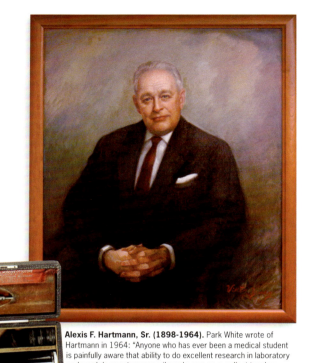

Alexis F. Hartmann, Sr. (1898-1964). Park White wrote of Hartmann in 1964: "Anyone who has ever been a medical student is painfully aware that ability to do excellent research in laboratory and ward does not necessarily make one an excellent teacher. I cannot recall more than six or seven men endowed with the gift of presenting their subjects to the less-informed clearly, progressively, and without notes. At the top of this small list have been Holt, Sr., Marriott, and Hartmann." Viktor De Jeney, Portrait of Alexis F. Hartmann, Sr., 1964. Oil on canvas, 46" x 39". St. Louis Children's Hospital.

Otoscope and Ophthalmoscope used by Alexis F. Hartmann, Sr.
Courtesy of Alexis F. Hartmann, Jr.

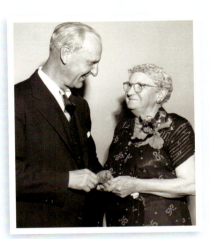

Becker Medical Library

Children's Hospital depended on its faculty and nursing staff, but it also required the devoted efforts of other staff who worked quietly behind the scenes in many capacities such as laundry, maintenance and food service. In 1953, Children's honored 50-year-employee Bertha Ginther (pictured here with Roy Kercheval), who had started in the laundry room of the second hospital building at Jefferson and Adams. Through the years, she became housekeeping director, then semi-retired to take charge of the linen room. From the first, her "cheery smile and quiet efficiency endeared her to the personnel," said the hospital newsletter.

tient facilities. As always, the problem was money. While federal funds would supply $595,000 and $1 million would come from the building fund, the board still had to raise $2 million — and they kicked off this new campaign at a dinner on May 13, 1963, honoring Bob Hope. In 1964, they broke ground for the project.

AN UNCERTAIN FUTURE

The hospital sorely needed strong leadership to rebuild its faculty, establish a stronger focus on research, and guide it through this new construction phase. But Alexis Hartmann, the head of pediatrics for 28 years, was seriously ill, retired early in the year, and then died only months later in September 1964 at age 66. In the latter years of his chairmanship, he had come in for some criticism. Some pointed to his reluctance to apply for those federal grants that were generously supporting researchers at other institutions. As Dean Edward Dempsey wrote testily in 1964 about a grant application they had planned to submit for funds to expand the residency and junior staff, "After all this [preparation], Dr. Hartmann got cold feet and refused to allow the application to be sent in." Still another opinion, voiced by psychiatrist Samuel Guze, was that "the hospital was an extension and expression of his personality; he was just that dominating." Further, he added, "it was primarily a department of pediatrics hospital, not a general children's hospital," and Hartmann couldn't ever make the necessary transition.

Still, Hartmann was a "distinguished physician, a brilliant teacher and an outstanding investigator," recalled David Goldring at Hartmann's 1964 memorial service. Now the pediatrics department — no longer as strong as it once had been — would enter a difficult interim period, led by Goldring, until they could find a new head, who would make the necessary changes to move the hospital forward.

1957

Dr. David Goldring and the Gibbon-Mayo Heart-Lung Pump

In July 1956, 18-month-old Debbie Ballew, a patient of well-known pediatric cardiologist David Goldring, was waiting for a miracle. Born with a hole in her heart, she weighed about the same as her eight-week-old sister; she could not walk, and the least exercise turned her skin a frightening gray. More than 300 other children in the St. Louis area had similar heart defects.

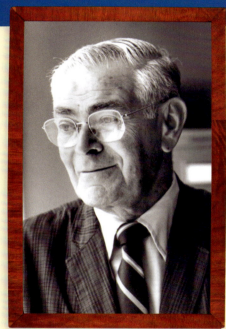

David Goldring (1914-1992).
A 1936 graduate of Washington University and 1940 graduate of the School of Medicine, Goldring spent most of his career at Children's Hospital, where he became "the undisputed paragon of pediatrics," said Lawrence Kahn in a 1992 eulogy, "and a radiant example to everyone who knew him." A pioneer in the field of pediatric cardiology, he founded and then headed the Division of Pediatric Cardiology for more than 30 years, training many fellows, including Alexis Hartmann, Jr., M.R. Behrer, Antonio Hernandez, and Arnold W. Strauss.
Becker Medical Library

For several years, St. Louis Children's Hospital had been searching for a machine that would take over the pumping action of the heart and lungs during delicate cardiac repairs. Carl Moyer, chairman of the Department of Surgery, tried building one of his own, but it broke down during a procedure. Then cardiac surgeon Thomas Burford heard of a new pump, developed by John H. Gibbon, Jr., of Jefferson Medical College and modified at the Mayo Clinic. Teams of physicians from Washington University, including Goldring, visited Mayo to see the machine — and came away impressed.

The problem was the price tag to build one: $65,000. A member of the Children's board was also on the board of the *St. Louis Globe-Democrat*, which decided to take up this cause and launch a city-wide fund drive. The front-page editorial asked: "How much are the lives of 300 children worth to you?" and kicked off the campaign with a $1,000 donation.

"A GLORIOUS DAY"

Money poured in as adults sent donations, children opened lemonade stands, civic clubs and labor groups contributed, even celebrity Eddie Cantor in Hollywood, a heart patient, sent a $100 check. In 12 days, the fund had reached its goal — and still the contributions kept coming. In the end, the campaign netted $102,832.14, and the excess was used to fund the machine's continuing operation. The *Globe-Democrat* jubilantly declared "A Glorious Day for St. Louis," adding that this was "the most spontaneous outpouring of a community's devotion ever recorded in this nation."

The next problem was building the machine, and engineers of the Custom Engineering and Development Company of St. Louis, headed by President Norbert W. Burlis, took up the challenge. Both Jefferson Medical College and Mayo gave their patents on the device to the Research Corporation, a not-for-profit foundation in New York City, which made Burlis' company its sole licensee to do the detailed construction work. Even with its intricate pumps, lines, controls, and vaporizers, the resulting machine was only the size of an office desk.

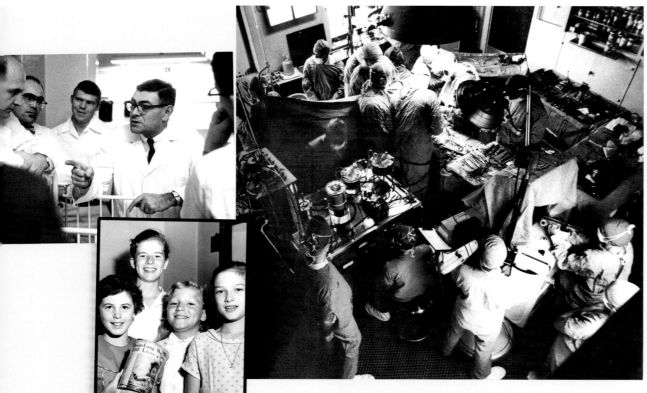

In 1957, at a dedication ceremony, Burlis formally presented the completed pump to Charles E. Pierson, executive editor of the *Globe-Democrat*, who in turn gave it to James W. Singer, Jr., president of the Children's board. "This is truly a heart pump," said Singer. "It came from the heart of the St. Louis community and its neighbors."

At first, surgeons Thomas Ferguson and Charles Roper used the machine to perform open-heart procedures on dogs — and every one died after surgery. "We were not aware," wrote Goldring later, "that the dogs had to be dewormed before the operation, and they died from heart worms which obstructed the pulmonary artery. In desperation Dr. Burford called Dr. [John] Kirklin and learned that they had the same experience at the Mayo Clinic."

THE PUMP SAVES LIVES

Just as Kirklin had, Burford decided to proceed on children with congenital intracardiac defects anyway, and he went on to have "surprisingly good results for those early days of open-heart surgery." The Gibbon Heart–Lung Pump was used from 1958 to 1970 by surgical and medical teams at Children's, assisted by staff radiologists such as Harvey Humphrey, Fernando Gutierrez, and Robert McKnight, as well as anesthesiologist John Shields.

But the *Globe-Democrat* editorial had added, as a caveat, that having this "machine does not, of course, insure that all operations will be successful." Sadly, this proved to be the case for little Debbie Ballew. During cardiac catheterization, wrote Goldring, she "was found to have an absent pulmonary valve and a large ventricular septal defect and died shortly after the campaign."

Still, the fund drive she had triggered did help many others, including Diane Edwards, age 12, of Belleville. Because of the hole in her heart, she could not run or play hard; when she was an infant, her parents were told they would probably find her dead in her crib one morning. Her 1958 surgery, using the new heart–lung pump, saved her life and restored her to normal function. Later articles showed that she grew up to become a nurse anesthetist at Barnes–Jewish Hospital.

ABOVE LEFT **David Goldring, ward rounds, 1949.** "For all of his academic successes," said Arnold Strauss in a 1992 eulogy, "Dr. Goldring never lost sight of the fact that he was a physician, responsible for the care of kids with heart disease. For him, the welfare and wellbeing of the patient *always* came first." Becker Medical Library

ABOVE **Heart-lung machine, Barnes Hospital operating room, 1961.** The Gibbon Heart-Lung Pump, shown here during surgery performed by Thomas Burford and his surgical team, was used from 1958 to 1970 at the medical center. Becker Medical Library

LEFT **Unexpected generosity.** More than enough money was collected by groups across the state to purchase the heart-lung machine, which cost $65,000. These members of the 4-H Club of Murphy, Missouri, proudly donated $82. Becker Medical Library

"For him, the welfare and wellbeing of the patient *always* came first."

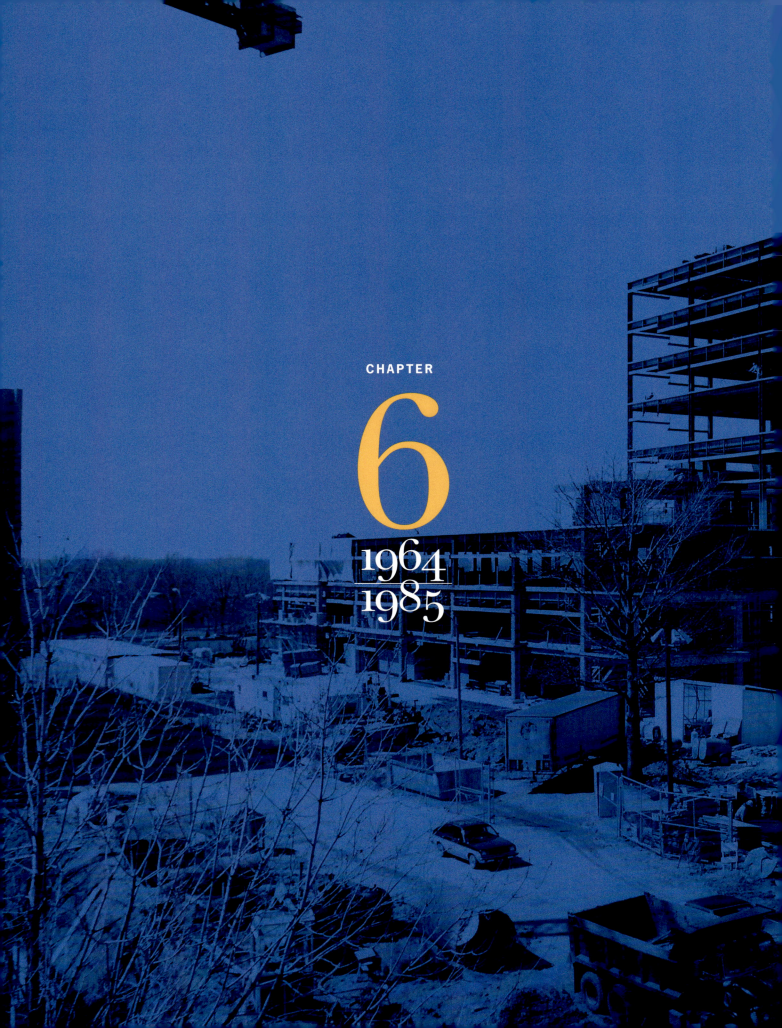

CHAPTER

6

1964
1985

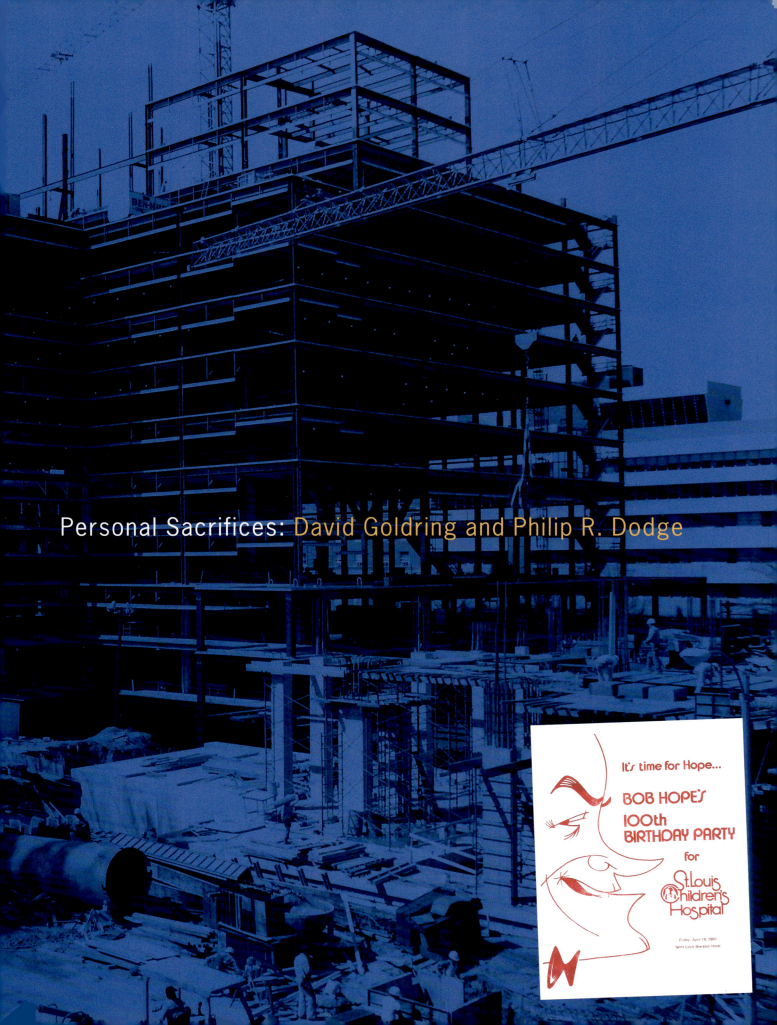

Personal Sacrifices: David Goldring and Philip R. Dodge

CHAPTER SIX PERSONAL SACRIFICES: DAVID GOLDRING AND PHILIP R. DODGE

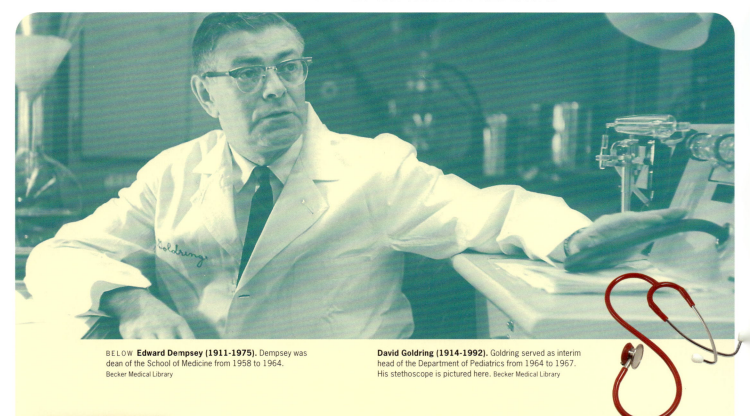

BELOW **Edward Dempsey (1911-1975).** Dempsey was dean of the School of Medicine from 1958 to 1964. Becker Medical Library

David Goldring (1914-1992). Goldring served as interim head of the Department of Pediatrics from 1964 to 1967. His stethoscope is pictured here. Becker Medical Library

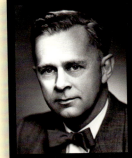

In May 1964, Edward W. Dempsey, dean of the Washington University School of Medicine,

wrote a heartfelt letter of thanks to busy pediatric cardiologist David Goldring for an important "personal sacrifice" he had agreed to make: becoming the acting head of the Department of Pediatrics until a permanent head could be appointed. "I cannot tell you how much I appreciate your taking on this additional work," wrote Dempsey. "…Only one who is going through this difficult time in the Medical School's history can appreciate the loyalty of people like you."

PREVIOUS PAGE **The new hospital building under construction.** Becker Medical Library
INSET **Invitation for "Bob Hope's 100th Birthday Party" for the hospital.**
Becker Medical Library

FEBRUARY 1964
Alexis Hartmann requests an indefinite leave of absence from his position as head of pediatrics.

MAY 1964
David Goldring becomes acting head of the Department of Pediatrics.

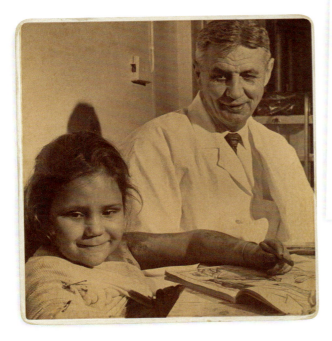

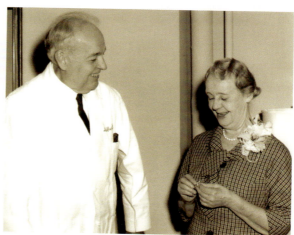

ABOVE **Alexis Hartmann and Margaret Smith.** In May 1964, despite his failing health, Hartmann made a special effort to be present at the retirement party for Margaret Smith, a long-time friend and colleague. He died in September of that year. Courtesy of J. Neal Middlekamp

LEFT **Carl Moyer (1908–1970).** Moyer, head of surgery from 1951 to 1965, discovered that using a weak solution of silver nitrate reduced mortality in pediatric burn victims from 80 percent to around 40 percent, and reduced skin grafts by two-thirds. Becker Medical Library

At this point, Dempsey — who would hurriedly resign later that year to take a job with the Department of Health, Education, and Welfare — must have felt like a man under siege. On the one hand, he was embroiled in a bitter dispute with Edgar M. Queeny, formidable board chairman of Barnes Hospital, who wanted the medical school to provide Barnes with additional income, in part by trimming its house staff and closing clinics that treated the poor. In the new Queeny Tower, which he had funded, he offered space to part-time faculty, a move resented by the full-time faculty, especially the surgeons, who were fighting to maintain their own clinical practices. The Executive Faculty got involved, and one member — Carl Moyer, head of surgery — even resigned in protest.

Amid this growing turmoil, Dempsey had received a letter in February 1964 from Alexis F. Hartmann, Sr., head of pediatrics and a faculty member for 47 years, requesting an indefinite leave of absence without salary beginning on July 1 of that year. His poor health was one reason, wrote Hartmann. "Because of the many hospital problems, particularly centering around a short and poor house staff, I did not feel it possible for me to take adequate vacations for the last three summers." But he also admitted to feeling "farther and farther out of step with the present policies of the Medical School and the attitude of the Board and Administration of the St. Louis Children's Hospital."

In more peaceful times, Dempsey might have welcomed Hartmann's move toward retirement, since the two had already clashed on the issue of government funding for research. Dempsey was an avid proponent, who wanted to garner some of the largesse then pouring from the National Institutes of Health (NIH), while Hartmann was a "state's righter," as one faculty member put it, who did not believe the government should be in the business of subsidizing research.

At this moment, however, Hartmann's move must have been a mixed blessing for Dempsey, who had no time or energy to mount a search. Indeed, as he well knew, such a search was likely to be protracted and difficult for the very reason that Hartmann had noted. The small house staff was now largely made up of international students, many of whom were not fluent in English;

MAY 1964 — Ground is broken for a new laboratory and research building.

SEPTEMBER 1964 — Alexis Hartmann, Sr., dies.

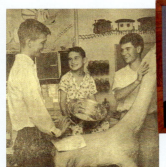 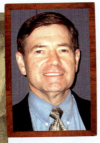

Charles Dougherty as a "candystriper" in 1964, and today. Becker Medical Library

In 1964, five teen-aged boys spent the summer as volunteers at St. Louis Children's Hospital — the first males to hold that position, traditionally the province of female "candy-stripers" and Red Cross volunteers. One of them was Charles H. Dougherty, a senior at St. Louis University High School, who convinced a classmate, Guy Schmitz, to come along. In a newspaper article about these "masculine candystripers," Dougherty said: "I love the work. I guess the biggest thing is the thrill the kids get out of doing things…. There was one little boy — his name was Danny. Guy and I both came in to read to him. He was really sick, although we didn't know what was wrong with him.

"Anyway, I came in after a weekend and Danny was gone; another child was in his room. I asked the nurse what had happened to Danny, and she said he had died. It was a real blow. Nothing like that had ever happened to me before. But against that, there are a hundred things that make you happy — taking the children outside, watching them slide down the slide, watching them playing in the sandbox."

After medical school at the University of Rochester, Dougherty became resident and chief resident at Children's Hospital, then went into private practice in south St. Louis County. He was elected president of the Children's Hospital Medical Staff in 2005.

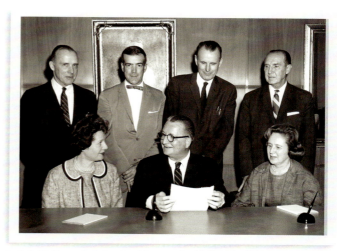

Orrin S. Wightman, Jr. An investment firm executive, Wightman (center) became board president of Children's Hospital in April 1964, after serving as a member since 1957. He was generous, writing a personal check for $15,000 when Dodge needed seed money to improve the pediatrics department. Becker Medical Library

little research was going on, and it was poorly funded. While the hospital continued to attract a growing number of patients — more than 6,000 in 1964, with $400,000 worth of free care — the lean faculty and nursing staff were seriously overworked.

So David Goldring's self-sacrificing acceptance of the department's interim leadership was a godsend to Dempsey, since it bought him additional time. Actually, his own departure would leave the thorny job of finding a head to his successor, former associate dean M. Kenton King. In years to come, King would work closely with the Executive Faculty and with the two men who successively took on the newly created job of vice chancellor for medical affairs, charged with making peace in the medical school's disputes: first Carl V. Moore, head of internal medicine, and then a young associate professor, William H. Danforth.

THE GOLDRING INTERREGNUM

The boundaries of an interim head are narrow and strictly defined. This leader cannot begin recruiting, since the next permanent head may disapprove of the choices or terms of employment. For the same reason, this temporary head cannot try to set a new tone for the department or shake up the staff. Fundamentally, the interim's job is to hold the department together — and that was exactly what the steady, diligent, well-respected Goldring did, with the help of loyal colleagues such as Neal Middelkamp, John Herweg, Donald and Jean Thurston, Antonio Hernandez, and Teresa J. Vietti.

One item that could not be delayed was the ongoing construction of the five-story laboratory and research building. Under the leadership of W. Ashley Gray, Jr., and honorary chairman James S. McDonnell, Jr., as well as enthusiastic new board president Orrin S. Wightman, Jr., the $2 million campaign progressed. Then a stand taken by Goldring changed the scope of the fund-raising effort. "The original plans called for a five-story building," wrote Philip R. Dodge later, "but Dr. Goldring faced the Board of

1964
More than 6,000 patients are treated at the hospital during this year.

1965
The first kidney transplant is successfully completed at the hospital.

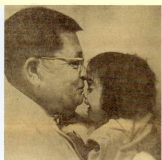

The St. Louis Children's Hospital Birth Defects Center was founded in 1963 by pediatrician and allergy specialist Donald L. Thurston, a 1937 School of Medicine graduate who had joined the Children's Hospital staff in 1947; funding came from the National Foundation–March of Dimes. Its goal was to make children with central nervous system defects "physically independent, mentally competent and socially acceptable," said Thurston in 1966. At first, its emphasis was on children with spina bifida, hydrocephalus, and ecephalocele.

Not only did the Center provide medical assistance to these patients, but it also had social workers on staff to help families and hold group discussions for parents. "This is probably the only instance of group social work in a hospital setting," said social worker Richard Swaine in 1966. "But at the Center we're concerned with the whole child and what he's going home to. No one can really understand what these parents face and what their fears are except other parents with the same problem."

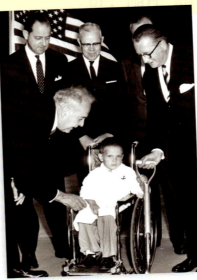

Ground-breaking, 1964. Alexis Hartmann helped patient Billy Turnbaugh break ground for the new wing as W. Ashley Gray, Jr., Chaplain George W. Bowles, Edwin M. Johnston, and Orrin S. Wightman, Jr. looked on. Becker Medical Library

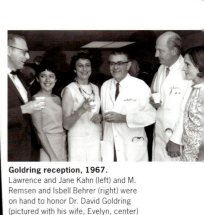

Goldring reception, 1967. Lawrence and Jane Kahn (left) and M. Remsen and Isbell Behrer (right) were on hand to honor Dr. David Goldring (pictured with his wife, Evelyn, center) for his service to the hospital. Becker Medical Library

Trustees and insisted that if they wanted St. Louis Children's Hospital to be once again in the forefront of pediatric medicine, more space was needed. Their faith in Dr. Goldring was such that, with his persuasion, the Tower was extended upward for an additional five floors. His wisdom in pressing for this expansion soon became evident."

In 1965, newspaper articles triumphantly announced that funds for the new 10-story Tower Building and a partial remodeling of the old building were in place, though the cost had risen to $4 million, up from the original $3.5 million estimate. Finally, some $2 million came from the community, $595,000 from the NIH, and $1.4 million from the hospital's own capital fund. By 1967, the building was complete, but its four top floors were left unfinished, awaiting future expansion — and more money. Its dedication, held on November 10, 1968, took place on the empty seventh floor of the building, with much public fanfare, while the remodeling of the old building continued, including the rebuilding of two floors into research facilities.

THE APPOINTMENT OF PHILIP R. DODGE

The year before this happy ceremony, the hospital's new head of pediatrics, Philip Rogers Dodge, had finally arrived. As expected, the search to find him had been arduous and fraught with disappointment, with several strong candidates — among them Lewis Wannamaker, a pediatric professor at the University of Minnesota — turning down the job. Kenton King, who headed the search, tried to recruit an internal medicine professor at Johns Hopkins, the brilliant geneticist Victor A. McKusick, but the pediatric faculty, determined to be led by a pediatrician, dispatched Goldring to the next Executive Faculty meeting to read their resolution opposing McKusick. Seeing failure after failure — Richard Smith and Park Gerald, among others — the Children's Hospital board became fed up; at one meeting, members even asked, in exasperation, whether they couldn't hunt for a head themselves.

Then King hit upon a clever expedient: He realized that the department was inviting a series of pediatric specialists as part of its visiting professor program in 1965. Among them was pediatric neurologist Philip R. Dodge, who had graduated in 1948 from medical school at the University of Rochester; he had also been a resident under Derek Denny-Brown and Raymond

1965 — William Danforth is elected president of Washington University Medical School and Associated Hospitals (WUMSAH), and Vice Chancellor of Medical Affairs.

1965 — Central Institute for the Deaf becomes a member of WUMSAH.

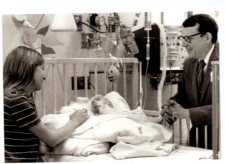
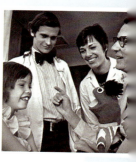

> **"Philip Dodge is one of the heroes of St. Louis Children's Hospital. He worked day and night, taking stints in the emergency room."**

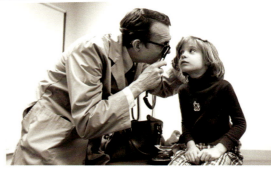

Philip R. Dodge, ca. 1970s. Becker Medical Library

D. Adams at the Harvard Neurological Unit of Boston City Hospital, where he became increasingly committed to neurology and the special needs of children. After Army service and a year-long pathology and neuropathology fellowship, he had joined Adams at Massachusetts General Hospital as chief of the newly established Division of Pediatric Neurology.

By 1965, Dodge was an international leader in his field, with clinical research interests in such areas as bacterial meningitis, neurological complications of fluid and electrolyte abnormalities, and pediatric cerebrovascular disease. As Alan Schwartz would later observe, "Philip Dodge trained nearly all the leaders in the field of clinical neurology — at Johns Hopkins, Boston Children's Hospital, etc. — for the next 25 years. In fact, he is the founder of the field of pediatric clinical neurology."

Further, Dodge was already acquainted with St. Louis Children's Hospital, having met neurosurgeon Henry G. Schwartz and neurologist William Landau at national meetings. During his weeklong visiting appointment, he had also gotten to know the pediatric and neurology faculty. "I had a grand time," he said later. "I liked the people; I liked the environment." When King offered him the job in 1966, he was intrigued, despite the problems that lay ahead. "I was excited; it was a challenge. I wanted to develop an academically oriented department," he said. In November 1966, he accepted the offer to become professor and head of the

Philip R. Dodge was known for his clinical skill, which he used subtly to diagnose neurological disease in children.

"Have you ever seen Dr. Dodge examining a two-year-old in front of an audience?" asked M. Kenton King, then medical school dean. "He had a large basket of toys, a teddy bear, and so on. He would sit on a small stool, and sometimes the mother was present; maybe she even had the child on her lap. Dr. Dodge would do a complete neurological examination of the two-year-old simply by using these toys."

"He was almost magical with patients," added St. Louis pediatrician Charles Dougherty, then a resident at Children's Hospital. "When he walked into a room and did a neurological exam with a patient, you knew you were watching a master.

"He had keen powers of observation. He would reach for things, put them in different fields of vision. The children wouldn't know that he was examining them, but I'm guessing that he knew the answer intuitively to difficult diagnostic puzzles within minutes."

At the October 2005 Second Century Award banquet, neurologist W. Edwin Dodson said this in introducing Dodge, his mentor, who had won an award:

"Phil is a man of great wisdom with many gifts and talents. In my opinion, his unrivaled genius resides in his ability to listen, to observe, and to evaluate. He could perceive causes, relationships, and remedies that others could not discern. And whether the child was sleepy, hungry, reticent, wary, wily, frightened, unruly, or downright hostile mattered little, because Phil would eventually get the information. And he expected us to do so too, though it was largely unspoken. Leading by example, Phil made the difficult and the complex look easy."

NOVEMBER 1966	1967	NOVEMBER 10 1968
Philip R. Dodge accepts the offer to become head of pediatrics.	Alan Robson is named the first head of pediatric nephrology.	Dedication ceremonies for the new laboratory and research building are held.

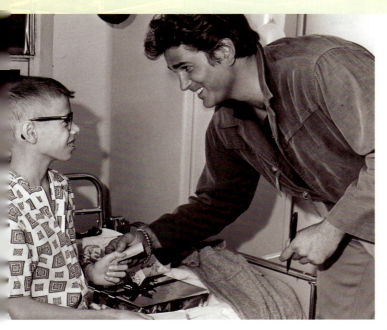

"Little Joe" visits hospital patients. Michael Landon, star of the television show "Bonanza", delighted patients and their parents on his visit to the hospital in 1967. As well as greeting his admirers and signing autographs, he also delivered gifts to several children who celebrated birthdays that day. Becker Medical Library

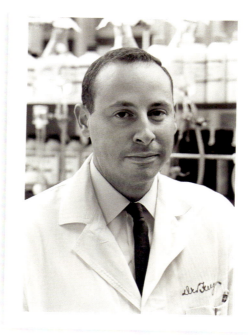

Ralph D. Feigin. During his 1964-65 residency and 1967-68 chief residency of the Children's Service at Massachusetts General Hospital, he met Philip Dodge, who recruited him to come to St. Louis in 1968. He rose to full professor by 1974 and served as director of the Division of Infectious Diseases in the pediatrics department from 1973-77. He left for Baylor College of Medicine in 1977. Becker Medical Library

Department of Pediatrics as well as pediatrician-in-chief (later medical director) at Children's Hospital — only the third in the hospital's history.

THE BEGINNING OF THE DODGE ERA

During the first seven years of his tenure, "Philip Dodge single-handedly brought the department and the hospital into modern medicine," said Kenton King. He threw himself into the task of rebuilding, with little time for himself. Added William Danforth: "Philip Dodge is one of the heroes of St. Louis Children's Hospital. He worked day and night, taking stints in the emergency room. He rebuilt morale and sense of direction. He established good working relationships with the hospital, saving the department and the hospital when it was in need."

Early on, he emphasized the recruitment of new faculty, since the department's roster had shrunk to around a dozen stalwart members, with only eight residents. Clearly, they needed a chief resident who could focus on house staff — and Dodge succeeded in recruiting James P. Keating, who stayed to establish and head one of the top residency training programs in the United States. Although Dodge failed to land Lee Rosenberg from Yale, he did persuade Ralph Feigin to come from Massachusetts General Hospital as an instructor, and David Goldring helped attract nephrology fellow Alan Robson to Children's, where he became the first director of pediatric nephrology in 1967. Perry Schoenecker completed his residency in 1975 and joined the faculty, becoming a leader in pediatric orthopaedic surgery. In 1976, nutrition researcher Dennis Bier also arrived, rising to become professor of pediatrics and medicine, co-director of the pediatric endocrinology and metabolism division, and director of the Pediatric Clinical Research Center.

Not surprisingly, Dodge took a particular interest in developing the pediatric neurology program. Arthur L. Prensky came with him in 1967 as an instructor in pediatrics and neurology and went on to study the neurochemistry of the developing brain. In 1975, Prensky received the

1968
Virginia Weldon, a Johns Hopkins-trained specialist, is appointed in pediatric endocrinology and metabolism.

1970
The structure of care at the hospital undergoes a major realignment, from age-related wards to specialty-related units.

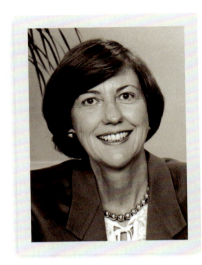

Virginia B. Weldon. Weldon joined the Washington University faculty in 1968, becoming professor of pediatrics, deputy vice chancellor for medical affairs, and vice president of the Washington University Medical Center. In 1989, she left the University for Monsanto, where she was senior vice president for public policy. Becker Medical Library

first chair in child neurology in the United States at Children's Hospital: the Allen P. and Josephine B. Green Professorship of Pediatric Neurology. Within a few years, Dodge had brought in three other stellar recruits: Marvin A. Fishman, Joseph J. Volpe, and Darryl C. DeVivo. Later, they were joined by former Children's Hospital neurology resident and fellow, W. Edwin Dodson.

In 1968, Children's Hospital welcomed a valuable appointment in pediatric endocrinology and metabolism: Virginia Weldon, a Johns Hopkins-trained specialist, who was soon appointed to co-direct that division with Anthony Pagliara, a 1971 recruit. Over time, Dodge asked her to keep track of federal laws that would impact the department; eventually, she expanded this role as assistant and then deputy vice chancellor for medical affairs under vice chancellor Samuel Guze.

"One thing that was obvious from the beginning was that we were primarily a medical, as opposed to a medical and surgical hospital," said Dodge. "We still had no operating rooms of our own, and no on-site X-ray facilities. Really, we only had one person committed to pediatric surgery and then only half-time, and that was Jessie Ternberg." Walter F. Ballinger II, head of surgery, understood the dire need and in 1972 appointed Ternberg as pediatric surgeon-in-chief and director of the division of pediatric surgery. For years, she routinely performed more than 500 operations a year; one specialty was correcting congenital gastrointestinal problems in children.

To add other expertise, Dodge went to each surgical division chief asking him to assign a pediatric specialist within that area. He had mixed results, though a few were instantly cooperative. Bernard Becker in ophthalmology assigned James Miller, who had two grants doing research into strabismus in children; urology head Justin Cordonnier picked Charles Manley, who headed pediatric urology starting in 1975.

Paul Weeks, head of plastic surgery, recruited Jeffrey Marsh, who eventually founded the Cleft Palate and Craniofacial Deformities Institute and developed ground-breaking ways, using three-dimensional computer modeling, of planning and performing corrective surgery.

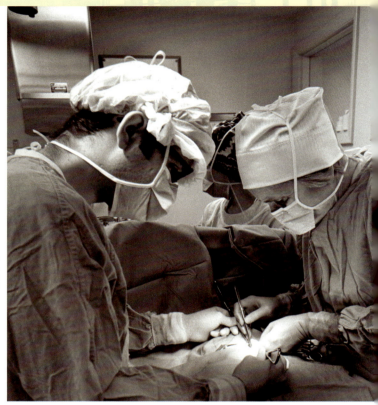

Jessie Ternberg. In 1972 Ternberg (on right) became first pediatric surgeon-in-chief and director of the division on pediatric surgery, performing more than 500 operations year for many years. Becker Medical Library

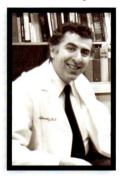

Arthur L. Prensky. Prensky, a pediatric neurologist, joined the Washington University faculty in 1967. In 1975, he received the first endowed professorship in child neurology in the United States, when he became the Allen P. and Josephine B. Green Professor of Pediatric Neurology. His research interests focus on the chemistry of myelin and pediatric headache. Becker Medical Library

FEBRUARY 1970
C. Alvin Tolin is hired by the board to be the first full-time, professional president of the hospital.

JULY 1970
Hospital administrator Lilly Hoekstra retires after 16 years of service.

memories *Larry Shapiro*

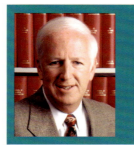

Larry Shapiro, a graduate of Washington University and its School of Medicine, completed his residency at Children's Hospital in 1973, winning the George F. Gill Prize in Pediatrics from the medical school. After serving as research associate at the National Institute of Arthritis, Metabolism and Digestive Diseases, he joined the faculty of the University of California–Los Angeles in 1975, where he was also a Howard Hughes Medical Institute Investigator. In 1991, he moved to the University of California, San Francisco School of Medicine, and became W.H. and Marie Wattis Distinguished Professor and chair of the Department of Pediatrics, before returning to Washington University in 2003 as the Spencer T. and Ann W. Olin Distinguished Professor, executive vice chancellor for medical affairs, and dean of the medical school.

"Today's residents at Children's Hospital probably cannot imagine that much of the technology they use every day did not always exist. In addition to CT scans, PET, and MRI, the residents of the early 1970s did not have e-mail, PDAs, cell phones, or pagers. So the way we were usually summoned was to be audibly paged on the loudspeaker system. Hospital operators, who worked in a windowless basement room of the old hospital, were the intermediaries in this process, and during one's residency, their voices became well known to us and, in some cases, dreaded. If we had time to sleep briefly on nights when we were on call, we told the operator which room we would be napping in.

"For nearly two years, I had the same on-call schedule as one operator, who had a lovely voice and was remarkably kind and protective. More than once, while I was dozing, the telephone would ring, and she would begin by apologizing for waking me, knowing how tired I was. Then she would ask if I was taking care of myself and getting enough to eat. Finally, she would advise me that a) another resident needed to speak with me, b) a patient's parent wanted to ask something, c) a nurse had a question about a medication order I had written, or d) there was a cardiac arrest somewhere in the hospital.

"After two years, we had developed a working relationship and friendship — yet we had never met. On my very last night on call at Children's Hospital, I made a point of finding out where the operators were stationed and arranged to bring her a small gift of thanks.

"Despite the advances in our technologic capabilities during the ensuing 30+ years, the same personal commitment, collegiality, and genuine friendliness of all Children's Hospital staff still persist today."

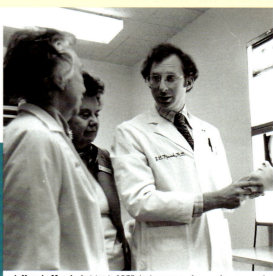

Jeffrey L. Marsh. Arriving in 1978, he became professor of surgery and pediatric surgery in 1986; in 1994, he also became professor of radiology. An international expert on craniofacial reconstruction, he was medical director of the Cleft Palate and Craniofacial Deformities Institute. In 1998, he was named the first Apolline Blair St. Louis Children's Hospital Professor of Surgery. He left for St. John's Mercy Medical Center in 2003. *Becker Medical Library*

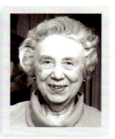

Meanwhile, with the support of pediatrician Dorothy J. Jones, who had given up her own practice to become full-time medical director of the Outpatient Department and head the Junior Clerkship program from 1964 to 1974, Dodge doubled the number of slots available through the residency matching program — and filled every one. In 1967, the total number of house staff, including fellows, rose to 23 from the previous 16. Within several years, top medical students — several of them members of the Alpha Omega Alpha honorary society — began applying to pediatrics.

Among these talented new residents were trainees who went on to prominent positions in academic medicine: Arnold Strauss, who joined Washington University in 1977 as an assistant professor of pediatrics and biological chemistry, was named director of the cardiology division in 1981 and later became pediatric chairman at Vanderbilt; Larry Pickering, editor of the American Academy of Pediatrics, *Red Book*®; Wallace A. ("Skip") Gleason, who became director of the division of gastroenterology, hepatology and nutrition at the University of Texas–Houston

INSET **Dorothy Jeannette Jones (1908-1993).** A graduate of the School of Medicine, she joined the staff of Children's Hospital in 1934 as assistant in clinical pediatrics. In 1963, she was appointed chief of Outpatient Care, a position she held until 1974. From 1979-86, she taught in the Pediatric Nurse Practitioner's Program. *Becker Medical Library*

OCTOBER 1970

Children's Hospital selects Linn B. Perkins to be the first executive director.

1971

The annual report for this year states that more than $1 million out of a yearly budget of $7 million was used for free care for patients whose families were unable to pay.

memories *Susan K. Goddard*

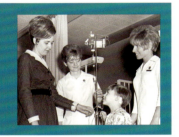

Success stories. Seven-year-old Bruce is pictured here with (from left to right) Doris England, director of patient care; Sue Goddard, nursing supervisor; and Paula Bielefeldt, head nurse. Becker Medical Library

Susan K. Goddard, a Barnes Nursing School graduate, was on the staff of St. Louis Children's Hospital from 1963 to 2000, serving in various roles: as staff nurse, assistant head nurse, nursing supervisor, clinical adviser, manager of the infectious disease unit and of hematology/oncology, and Director of General Pediatric Services.

"In the mid-to-late 1960s, I saw my first child abuse victim; I'm sure we had had abused children before that, but this was the first for me. One morning, I came in — I was on the toddler unit then — and the nurse who was holding him and rocking him had tears streaming down her face. This child was so beaten, with cigarette burns and skull fractures, and he was only about 18 months old. That was a growing up moment. We kept him in the hospital for months because of his head injuries, then he went to foster care.

"Another time a little boy named Bruce from rural southeast Missouri came in as an infant with an abdominal malformation, and Dr. Ternberg took care of him until he was a teenager. He had multiple surgeries, and spent a lot of time at Children's, so we got to know him well. Years later, in the 1990s, I came in to work one day and heard that a father wanted to see me: It was Bruce, all grown up, with his own child. That is the benefit of working in the hospital over a long period of time. You see your success stories."

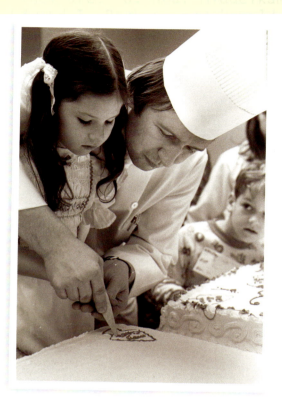

Medical School; Richard L. Schreiner, who would head pediatrics at the University of Indiana; and Larry Shapiro, who had a successful career in pediatric research and administration at UCLA and UC-SF, and then much later became executive vice chancellor for medical affairs and dean at Washington University School of Medicine.

Existing programs were also growing stronger, with a renewed emphasis on clinical research. For example, pediatric oncologist Teresa Vietti, formerly a resident and then chief resident at Children's, was named chief of the division of pediatric hematology/oncology in 1970 and did important clinical research in sarcoma and acute lymphoblastic leukemia. A decade later, Vietti — who became known as the "Mother of Pediatric Cancer Therapy" — would help to found and serve as first chair of the Pediatric Oncology Group, a national collaborative study group that did exciting, innovative work in childhood cancer.

By 1971, four years after he had arrived, Dodge could point to his accomplishments in recruitment and call the department "rich in talent." As he said, most "major specialties are represented within the staff.... During the next phase of our development we hope to strengthen all programs and specialty areas."

THE HOSPITAL IN 1970

For years, the hospital had been organized along age-related lines with an infants' ward, toddlers' ward, and so on; only a few, such as infectious disease and metabolic disorders, did not fit this pattern. But nationally, pediatric clinical care was changing as new sub-specialty boards formed, beginning with cardiology in 1961. Now, under Dodge and nursing head Doris

ABOVE **Dietary Services.** In 1970, the Dietary Department served 107,019 meals and worked with Recreational Therapy in planning parties for children. "Taste and nutrition are important," said the 1970 annual report, "but particular attention is given to how the food looks. Does it have eye appeal to the children?" Children could also choose their own food at a small "Chuck Wagon" cafeteria, decorated in a western theme. Becker Medical Library

1971

A new public relations department is opened, headed by William Keenan.

> "There was little problem finding patients: the inpatient census remained strong and outpatient visits increased in 1969 from 33,000 to 48,000."

England, the structure at Children's Hospital underwent a major realignment to specialty-related units — with a powerful impact on the nursing staff. "On the toddler unit, I had taken care of children with every diagnosis: cardiology, neurology, and orthopaedic conditions. When we went to diagnosis-related units, we had to develop our expertise in the specialty areas we chose," said nurse Sue Goddard, assigned to infectious disease. "Many of us did not care for it initially, but as we learned our specialties and worked with children of various ages, which was a joy, I think we all grew to like it and took pride in knowing our specialties well."

In 1970, these units were scattered among the hospital's six floors. On the first floor was the lobby, along with ambulatory services, the emergency room, and the Auxiliary's coffee shop, known as the "Gingerbread House." The second floor housed the 10-bed Intensive Care Unit, the 25-bed Cardiology Division, and Recreational Therapy, staffed by the "Play Lady" and numerous volunteers. On the third was the 12–isolette Neonatal Unit, as well as the Metabolism Division, Clinical Research Unit, and 23-bed Infectious Disease area. The fourth held the general Pediatric and Surgical Unit, plus Neurology-Neurosurgery, while the fifth and sixth floors housed research. These latter two, said the annual report, were places "where medical history is being made."

A NEW FINANCIAL STRUCTURE

Another structural overhaul was also coming. When hospital administrator Lilly Hoekstra, who had served since 1954, announced she would retire in July 1970, the board convened a committee, consisting of Donald Danforth, Jr., Benjamin F. Jackson, and Charles M. Ruprecht, to plot the future. A prime responsibility of the board, said Neal Wood, who had succeeded

C. Alvin Tolin. Retired corporate vice president for financial services of Ralston Purina Co., became the first salaried president of Children's Hospital in February 1970. Becker Medical Library

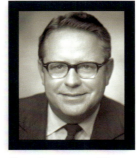

Rolla Streett as president, was to develop cooperative programs with the medical school, but in order to do that the hospital needed "a clear understanding of the means...for financing, directing, controlling and operating them." Within a month, this committee was to produce recommendations for a new organizational framework that could be put into effect at once.

The committee reported back quickly with four sweeping proposals. First, they recommended that the board president become chairman of the board and that Wood should take this job. Second, they argued that the hospital needed a full-time, professional president, who would establish its long-range goals and organization, oversee its finances, and head up public relations efforts. Next, the president and board together would look for ways to strengthen the board's role. Finally, the president would examine how other hospitals were structured, and how best to coordinate planning between the hospital and the medical school.

No sooner had the need for a president been identified than a candidate appeared: C. Alvin Tolin, a former corporate vice-president for financial services at Ralston Purina, who had taken early retirement. He came highly recommended, since Donald Danforth, Jr., executive vice president at Ralston Purina, knew him well. "Al Tolin was the most enthusiastic guy you could imagine," said Dodge. "We spent a whole day talking, and the next morning he told me, 'I accept.'" The board unanimously hired him to begin a month before Hoekstra was due to leave. Over time, he worked closely with the pediatric department's financial manager, hired by Dodge in consultation with the dean of the University's

ABOVE **Linn B. Perkins.** Perkins, who arrived in 1970, became executive director after Alvin Tolin stepped down. His goal for Children's Hospital was: "Healthy children in healthy families." Becker Medical Library

1972
Congress enacts the National Supplemental Feeding Program for Women and Children (WIC).

1972
The medical center, formerly the Washington University Medical School and Associated Hospitals (WUMSAH), becomes known as Washington University Medical Center (WUMC).

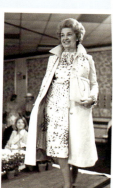
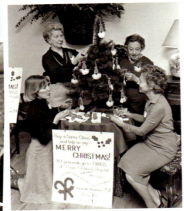
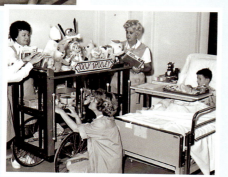

Membership in the Children's Hospital Auxiliary, established in 1954 under the leadership of Cora Lee King Rose, grew steadily, from a starting total of 250 to around 1,000 in 1978. Two offshoots or "Twigs" also formed in the early 1950s: The Women's Association of Ladue Chapel and the Friends of the St. Louis Children's Hospital.

One effort of the Friends was the hospital's gift shop, set up in 1955 and then relocated to the Spoehrer Tower lobby as the "Small World Gift Shop" in 1971. It moved to the new hospital building in 1985.

In 1952, the Ladue Chapel Twig bought a coffee cart and staffed it daily with two volunteers who served juice, doughnuts, and coffee to parents and employees. In 1956, a full-scale coffee shop replaced it, which five years later was serving 800 people a day with the strong support of Twig volunteers. While Miss Hullings, Inc. ran the shop from 1975-78, the Auxiliary returned to manage it in 1979. It closed in 1985 upon the construction of the new hospital.

Lucille Osterkamp, a 1974 *St. Louis Globe-Democrat* "Woman of Achievement," was a long-time Children's Hospital volunteer, who began by staffing the coffee cart and then shifted to the coffee shop. She and volunteer Wanda Shaw re-organized the shop, which began earning nearly $40,000 per year. When Shaw died, Osterkamp and volunteer Margaret Jackes spearheaded a highly successful Children's Hospital cookbook in her memory: *The Confessions of 211 St. Louis Housewives and Bob Hope...or, What's Going on in their Kitchens!*"

Meanwhile, the Auxiliary was instrumental in sponsoring other important fund-raising activities, among them holiday cards, begun in 1954; an annual holiday event in December, the "Children's Love Light Festival," begun in 1985, the "Earn-a-Bed" program, started in 1961. It held "Disney on Parade" benefits in 1970 and 1971 and an annual art and antique auction started in 1972. A trip to Asia in 1966 was followed by a world tour and then a trip to Eastern Europe and Scandinavia, both organized by Laura Gray Jones, who became a *Globe-Democrat* "Woman of Achievement" in 1971.

Auxiliary events. Members of the Auxiliary participated in events such as staffing the "Jolly Trolley," which provided books and toys to patients, walking the catwalk during fashion show benefits, and creating and selling Christmas ornaments for fund-raising. Becker Medical Library

business school: Chester Martin, who was "honest, dedicated, supportive," said Dodge. By October 1970, the hospital also had an executive director: Linn B. Perkins, former assistant director of Christ Hospital in Cincinnati.

HOSPITAL PROBLEMS
The appointment of Tolin had been necessary, said Neal Wood in a February 1970 newspaper article, because of "the growing complexities of hospital management and in particular the mounting financial problems that hospitals face today." That was especially true of Children's Hospital, where the early years of Dodge's leadership were marked by a struggle against deficits and a search for more money. There was little problem finding patients: the inpatient census remained strong and outpatient visits increased in 1969 from 33,000 to 48,000. Despite some reliable funders — such as the Green Foundation, which gave generous, ongoing support to the neurology division — expenditures were high and funding sources generally unpredictable. Even the previously reliable United Way announced it was trimming, and later eliminating, its support for hospitals. In 1970, the board had to use $15,000 in endowment funds to balance the budget, and it projected a loss of $100,000 in 1971.

Worse still, the National Institutes of Health — which in 1968 supplied up to half the research budgets of many American medical

1972

Jessie Ternberg is appointed the first pediatric surgeon-in-chief and director of the division of pediatric surgery.

JUNE 1973

The Tower Building is re-christened the Hermann F. Spoehrer Children's Research Tower.

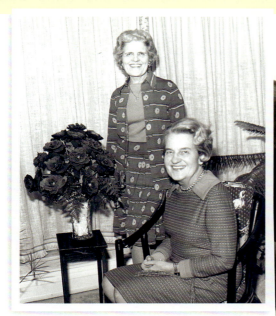

Harriet Baur Spoehrer. A 1928 Washington University graduate and widow of Hermann F. Spoehrer, she gave major gifts to the hospital that made possible the completion of the 10-story tower renamed in 1973 the "Hermann F. Spoehrer Children's Research Tower." Her sister, **Jane Baur Spoehrer** (seated) was President of the Women's Auxiliary for three years, and was named an honorary life member for giving more than 1,000 hours of volunteer service. She also served as a member of the Children's Hospital board. In 1973, both women were named *St. Louis Globe-Democrat* "Women of Achievement." Becker Medical Library

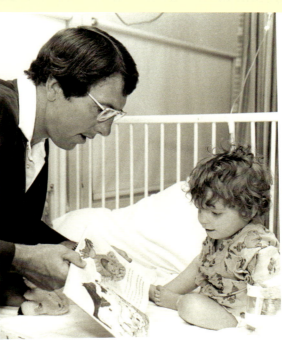

Hale Irwin. In 1976, the first Hale Irwin/St. Louis Children's Hospital Golf Benefit raised more than $74,000, and the number continued to rise over the years: to $100,000 in 1980 and $200,000 in 1985. When in St. Louis, Irwin visited hospital patients in addition to his participation in the benefits. Becker Medical Library

schools through grant support — was also cutting back its funding, largely because of spending on the Vietnam war. In a February 1968 *Globe-Democrat* article, Dean M. Kenton King warned that a dramatic decrease in NIH support would have serious consequences for the University. Further, this reduction came at a particularly bad time, he said, when "a great national effort is being made to produce more physicians."

With the new faculty and staff members, those last four unfinished floors of the new building were badly needed, so the board hired an architectural firm, Hoffmann and Sauer, to draw up plans for them, as well as a long-range study of the hospital's facilities. But how to pay for the changes? One $15,000 grant came from an unlikely source: Ethel Schneider Queeny, the widow of Edgar Queeny, who wished to help fund a new dialysis unit, the first pediatric unit in the Midwest. The ever-helpful Auxiliary, now headed by Jane Baur Spoehrer, made a five-year, $280,000 pledge to finish the seventh floor as clinical and metabolic research space, while the Beaumont Foundation gave $100,000 toward completion of the others, with eight as a metabolic and nutrition research facility and ten as administrative space.

By now, another potential funding source had entered the picture: the Ranken-Jordan Home for Convalescent Crippled Children, established in 1941 to help children disabled by bone tuberculosis, osteomyelitis, or polio. With the advent of antibiotics, this mission had become dated, so Ranken-Jordan administrators discussed funding the development of one or more floors in the Tower Building for genetics research. However, they first had to file suit against Mercantile Trust Co. acting on behalf of Drury College, another potential recipient of the Ranken-Jordan funds, to gain the release of the money. For more than three years, this litigation dragged on, delaying construction of the genetics facility, but in 1968 the Missouri Supreme Court upheld a lower court's ruling in the hospital's favor. In the end, some $500,000 in Ranken-Jordan funds renovated the ninth floor, with a pledge of $50,000 a year for ten years to defray operating expenses. Dodge persuaded genetics researchers William S. Sly and David Rimoin to shift from internal medicine to head a successful new genetics program.

1974

Children's Hospital opens the first pediatric dialysis unit in the Midwest, funded in part by Ethel Schneider Queeny.

JANUARY 1974

The hospital dedicates a new, 30-bed neonatal intensive care unit, and the staff for the unit is expanded to 50.

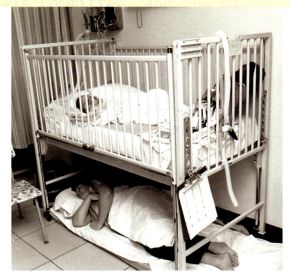

Crowded conditions in the old building. One parent said: "Never have there been adequate facilities for my wife or me to stay overnight or a completely private place where we could talk with doctors, cry, talk with relatives, or discuss our worries without being interrupted or imposing upon some other parents' needs." Becker Medical Library

The generosity of another donor led to a name change for the building. On June 1, 1973, friends of Children's Hospital gathered at the entrance to the Tower Building for a dedication ceremony in which the structure was re-christened the Hermann F. Spoehrer Children's Research Tower in memory of the late businessman, 1924 University graduate, and community volunteer, who had died in 1968. His widow, Harriet — herself an active Children's Hospital volunteer and later a trustee — had made the completion of the building possible with her gifts of more than $600,000.

Energetic new fund-raising efforts were also in the offing. The Auxiliary and its Twig offshoots worked tirelessly to improve the life of patients, making 25,000 puppets in a decade to entertain the children and also sponsoring benefits, such as fashion shows, hat sales, and disco lessons. While the hospital held golf tournaments, including the 1971 Great St. Louis Golf Classic won by Lee Trevino, a new Development Board, led by Harry Hamm and staffed by young executives, undertook St. Louis Blues hockey benefits in 1974 and 1975 as well as the annual Hale Irwin golf benefit, which raised more than $74,000 in 1976 alone. Hospital trustee and St. Louis

memories *Walter Benoist*

Walter Benoist is a 1972 graduate of the School of Medicine; he also was resident at Children's Hospital from 1972 to 1975, and co-chief resident in 1975. Since then, he has been in private practice in St. Louis.

"In 1972-73, the house staff at Children's Hospital covered the well-baby nursery at the St. Louis Maternity Hospital, located off Euclid Ave. If there was a problem, we had to jog through Barnes and up five flights to get to the nursery; if there was a 'Stat' [emergency] we had to run. In fact, you could spend the better part of your day running back and forth through Barnes.

"Relief came in an odd way: a minor fire broke out in the Maternity nursery one evening — lots of smoke but no flames. We had to evacuate the nursery right away and move the babies to a makeshift room at Children's. It was a bit chaotic, but every baby was safe and well.

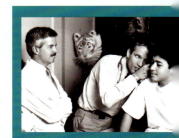

Walter Benoist (left), ca. 1975. Becker Medical Library

"The positive part for us 'worker-bees' was that the nursery was now in our territory, and we didn't have to 'Stat' race through Barnes whenever they needed us. The house staff, of course, tried to talk the administration into maintaining the nursery at Children's — not understanding that Maternity Hospital had an interest in returning the nursery and the babies back to their mothers! So it was a 'no-go.' But we loved the short-lived arrangement while it lasted."

Cardinal football safety Larry Wilson, whose child had been a patient at Children's Hospital, donated $30,000 from a "Salute to Larry Wilson" night at Powell Hall for a new psychology laboratory. To help publicize these efforts and the ongoing work of the hospital, a new public relations department was established early in 1971 and headed by William Keenan.

While Children's Hospital was working to gain wider recognition for its work, so was the medical center, known by the cumbersome title of Washington University Medical School and Associated Hospitals ("WUMSAH"). In 1972, Samuel Guze decided that a new name would explain themselves better to the public, so with the approval of all the constituent institutions,

1974

The Ambulatory Care Department opens.

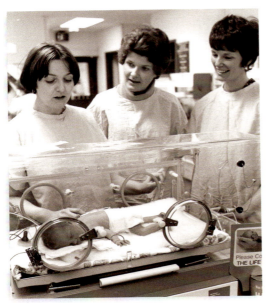

The Life Seekers. This group raised money for a spacious new neonatal intensive care unit (NICU) with room for 30 infants. Becker Medical Library

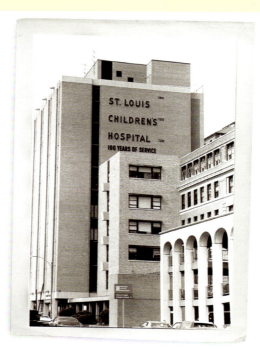

"100 Years of Service" 1979. Becker Medical Library

including Children's Hospital, WUMSAH became simply Washington University Medical Center ("WUMC").

FINANCIAL RECONSTRUCTION

All the while, Tolin, Perkins and a new recruit in 1971 — Ted Frey, fiscal affairs director and the first staff member to come from a strong financial background — were trying to assess the hospital's fiscal condition. "It was in very bad financial shape," said Frey later, "but we couldn't tell you exactly what our position was. Al Tolin told the story that when he went down to talk to the chief accountant, an indication of how good or bad things were was how many unpaid bills were in his drawer....There were a couple of occasions when we had to borrow money to make payroll — and if we didn't have the money, we just didn't pay the bills, especially from Barnes Hospital. We bought a lot of services from them, such as radiology services, and it was easier not to pay Barnes than it would be some outside vendor."

On the revenue side, one major problem was a huge backlog in the billing department, which was not sending out invoices efficiently to insurance companies or self-pay families. Another was the lack of staff to prepare the detailed cost reports required by the states of Missouri and Illinois before they would allocate Medicaid payments that accurately reflected the hospital's costs. In the absence of such reports, said Frey, "they paid us the minimum for our services" — only 63 percent for some indigent Missouri patients in 1972.

Still broader challenges lay ahead, however. Lacking their own pediatrician, too many families used the hospital for basic health services, which caused the number of emergency room visits to skyrocket. Further, unreimbursed care continued to represent a major — and fast-growing — financial burden for the hospital, costing $1.3 million in 1972 and $1.9 million in 1973.

Quickly, the new administrators hired a financial team — in patient accounting, payroll, Medicaid reimbursement — that started to institute sweeping change. During frequent trips to Springfield and Jefferson City, they began an ongoing battle to convince state officials that

1974
The number of positions available through the residency matching program doubles from 1964.

1975
Arthur Prensky receives the first chair in pediatric neurology in the United States: the Allen P. and Josephine B. Green Professorship of Pediatric Neurology.

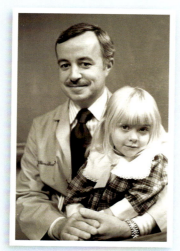

William T. Shearer. Becker Medical Library

In August 1975, Children's Hospital staff physician **William T. Shearer**, director of the division of immunology, performed a thymus transplant on an infant, Krista Sansoucie from Blackwell, Missouri, born with a rare immune system deficiency that left her desperately susceptible to viral, fungal, or bacterial infections. An article at the time said that "fewer than 10 cases of her disorder have been recorded in medical history."

Shearer performed the thymus gland transplant, the first in Missouri, in hopes of conquering the disorder and allowing her to fight routine infections by herself. He was assisted by a medical team that included physicians Donald Strominger, James Wedner, and Ralph Feigin.

After the surgery, Krista had to fight off a series of infections while the new thymus took hold. "She almost died several times but for the heroic efforts of the nursing staff and doctors attending her," said Shearer at the time. But she finally went home and, at 19 months old, was healthy and growing.

they should increase the reimbursement rates. By 1972, Tolin could note hopefully that "we continued to report a loss on operations, but we were closer to the approved budget," with their cost of services not covered by income dropping from $152,000 in 1972 to $65,000 in 1973.

RESEARCH ADVANCES

Through the 1970s, many Children's Hospital physicians and affiliated pediatric surgeons focused on innovative research. Several physicians in different specialties — James Keating in gastroenterology, Morey Haymond in endocrinology and metabolism, Darryl DeVivo in neurology,

"...we have the most wonderful s

and Ralph Feigin in infectious disease — studied the puzzling roots of Reye's Syndrome. Along with pioneers William Daughaday, Mary Parker, and later David Kipnis, other physicians — Virginia Weldon, Sandra Blethen, and Julio Santiago — treated dwarfism in children using human growth hormone, while James Keating and Anthony Pagliara studied children with ketotic hypoglycemia, winning a national award. Joseph Volpe continued to study blood flow in the brains of premature infants, and in 1983 received the department's second chair, the A. Ernest and Jane G. Stein Professorship in Developmental Neurology, facilitated by William Landau's professional association with the Stein family.

Cardiology was an exciting area in these years, led first by David Goldring and later by Arnold Strauss. As Alan Schwartz recalled much later: "David Goldring was an expert in hypertension, and this was the time when Children's Hospital developed its first cardiac catheterization laboratories, sophisticated techniques for diagnosing congenital heart disease, and paired up with the cardiac surgeons at Barnes Hospital for surgery on children with congenital heart disease."

Nursing continued to be the backbone of patient care. As C. Alvin Tolin wrote in 1979, we "have the most wonderful spirit of caring found anywhere. Evidence of this can be seen at nursing stations where the children they brought through a critical illness leave our hospital well, but the nurses have a photograph of the child

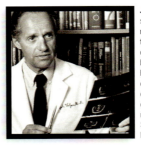

Joseph Volpe. Director of the division of neurology research, then of neurology, he studied blood flow in the brains of premature infants, and discovered that this flow was affected by the mechanical ventilation used to help these babies breathe. With this data, Volpe changed the management of the lung problem so that brain hemorrhages did not occur. He was named to the A. Ernest and Jane G. Stein Professorship in Developmental Neurology. Becker Medical Library

1976
A new building proposed for the hospital is met with criticism; Mayor James F. Conway orders city agencies to stop issuing construction permits on the project.

1977
The auxiliary, with a membership of 1,000, pledges $1 million for one floor of the new building.

aring found anywhere."

on a bulletin board as a constant reminder of those they have helped and cared for." Other staff members were also integral to health care: respiratory care specialists, X-ray technicians from Mallinckrodt Institute of Radiology, pharmacists, social workers, recreational therapists, chaplains, and occupational and physical therapists of the Irene Walter Johnson Institute.

In January 1974, the hospital dedicated a new, 30-bed neonatal intensive care unit (NICU) that nearly tripled the old unit's capacity. This project, which cost $600,000, also provided sleeping areas for three doctors, a nurses' room and a parents' lounge. Much of the sophisticated equipment came from a major donation by Life Seekers, a St. Louis group dedicated to the health of newborns, with other help from the March of Dimes. The staff also grew, as the *Globe-Democrat* reported: "The neonatal unit's nursing staff will be expanded to 50, who will care for the 30 babies in three shifts around the clock. For the most acutely ill babies, there will be one nurse for each infant."

Another 1974 addition was the Ambulatory Care department, designed to handle 5,000 outpatient visits each year, with an emergency room,

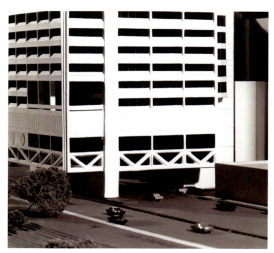

Expansion controversy. This 1976 model shows the proposed 16-story addition to the hospital over Kingshighway. Becker Medical Library

memories *James P. Keating*

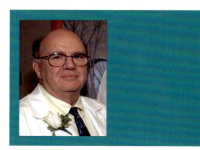

James P. Keating was recruited to Washington University by Philip Dodge in 1968. A founder of the field of pediatric gastroenterology, he also won national acclaim for transforming the Children's Hospital residency program, directing it from 1969-2002. He directed the PICU from 1980-92, and later established the Division of Diagnostic Medicine, which he still heads. In 1998, he was named the W. McKim Marriott Professor of Pediatrics. He was awarded the Distinguished Service Award from the Medical Staff in 2004; the Keating Outstanding Resident Award was established at Children's Hospital in his honor.

"When Phil Dodge came to St. Louis in 1967, he had already grown into a gentle giant of pediatric neurology during his years in Boston, and there was warm acceptance of his humane, inspiring leadership. All the internship slots filled through the match in 1968 and, by the fourth year of his chairmanship, the trainee cohort included more than two dozen who became professors, department chairs, or deans [see list below].

A new hospital building was needed to house the new and expanded programs. Our old buildings had been the scene of many major advances in the care of children from 1910 to 1960. But by the 1980s, the absence of operating rooms, a radiology suite in another building, and a rudimentary emergency department were serious obstacles to growth. The need was recognized by Phil Dodge and, on the hospital side, by Alvin Tolin, president, and Linn Perkins, executive director. Together, they garnered the commitment from the community and created the current building, a block from the old site.

The advent of the new building in 1984 released energy that allowed Children's Hospital to become a true regional center for pediatric health care, as well as a place where knowledge originates. The outstanding leadership provided by Dodge, Harvey Colten, Alan Schwartz, and hospital leaders Tolin, Perkins, Alan Brass, and Ted Frey permitted the blossoming of both the medical school and hospital."

Professors
Donald C. Anderson (Baylor University)
Charles R. Bauer (University of Miami)
Marshall Bloom (Rocky Mountain Laboratories, N.I.H.)
Jane E. Brazy (University of Wisconsin)
Eileen D. Brewer (Baylor University)
Elias G. Chalhub (University, South Alabama)
William L. Clarke (University of Virginia)
Thomas G. Cleary (University of Texas)
Barbara R. Cole (Washington University)
Marilyn B. Escobedo (University of Texas, University of Oklahoma)
Robert S. Greenwood (University of North Carolina)
Laura A. Hillman (University of Missouri)
Georgeanna J. Klingensmith (University of Colorado)
Larry K. Pickering (University of Eastern Virginia)
William T. Shearer (Baylor University)
Michael B. Sheehan (University of Missouri)
Penelope G. Shackelford (Washington University)
Susan K. Ratzan (University of Connecticut)
Kathleen B. Schwarz (Johns Hopkins University)
Dan K. Seilheimer (Baylor University)
Ann R. Stark (Harvard University)
Barbara W. Stechenberg (Tufts University)
Eileen E. Tyrala (Temple University)
David E. Van Reken (University of Indiana)
W. Edwin Dodson (Washington University)
Wallace A. Gleason (University of Texas)

Department Chairs
William M. Crist (Mayo)
Randy A. Kienstra (Southern Illinois University)
Richard L. Schreiner (University of Indiana)
Larry J. Shapiro (University of California-San Francisco)
Arnold Strauss (Vanderbilt)

Deans
William M. Crist (University of Missouri)
Larry J. Shapiro (Washington University)

1977

The World Health Organization (WHO) reports that smallpox has been eliminated from the world.

1978

Jeffrey Marsh establishes the Cleft Palate and Craniofacial Deformities Institute at the hospital.

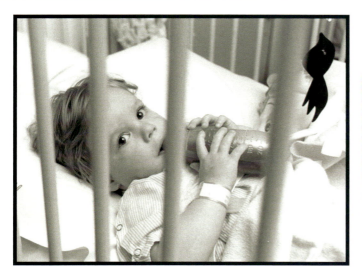

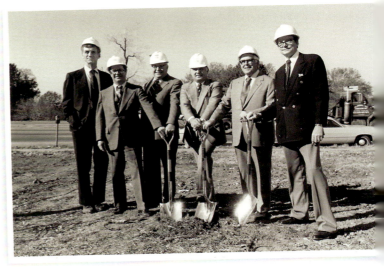

Ground-breaking 1980. (left to right) William H. Danforth, James S. McDonnell III, Linn B. Perkins, James Conway, C. Alvin Tolin, and Philip R. Dodge. Becker Medical Library

acute care clinic, general pediatric clinic, and more than 40 subspecialty clinics such as allergy or birth defects. Later that year, a new division formed: immunology, headed by William Shearer, who received grants from the National Cystic Fibrosis Foundation and the American Cancer Society. Supporting these improvements, and the resulting increase in patient load, was a six-story parking garage that Children's Hospital built in collaboration with Barnes Hospital, then bought from Barnes in 1975 for $1.3 million.

Other ventures were also ahead. In 1979, Children's Hospital voted to participate in the new Washington University Medical Care Group Health Plan with Jewish and Barnes hospitals; Tolin was selected to represent Children's Hospital on that board, and radiologist Ronald Evens was elected to the board's chairmanship. A new Day Care facility, long requested by the nursing staff, was on the drawing board, opening in 1981.

During 1979, the hospital celebrated its 100th anniversary with a special event planned by a Centennial Gala Committee, headed by board chairman William L. Edwards: the Arch Award Fashion Premiere with Henry Mancini and top designers, a benefit for the St. Louis Symphony and the hospital. A sign on the side of the building announced "100 Years of Service," as hospital officials declared their determination to ensure that "Children's Hospital is considered THE outstanding institution of its kind in the nation, not just one of the very best, as at present."

CONTROVERSY OVER THE NEW BUILDING

For years, the idea of building a new hospital had been brewing, since the need for it was increasingly apparent: the five-building campus was aging and overcrowded, the staff had tripled in size over the past seven years, outpatient facilities served some 6,000 patients per month, and inpatient occupancy had exceeded 100 percent on 89 days in 1979 alone. Lacking a modern building, the hospital could not fully realize its potential as a national referral center. In 1978, Children's Hospital was largely a regional center, with fully 75 percent of patients coming from the city and seven surrounding counties in Missouri and Illinois.

Throughout the early 1970s, hospital publications hinted that a new building was coming as a long-range planning committee, established by the board, began meeting with staff to determine future needs. Yet their initial plan was controversial: a 16-story, 215-bed facility with operating rooms and specialty clinics in a most unusual location. As one hospital publication put it: "Five alternative sites were considered and, after great

1979

The hospital reports a 40 percent reduction in childhood cancer since 1970.

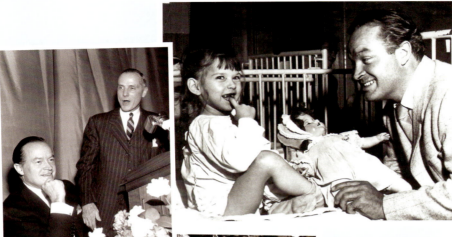

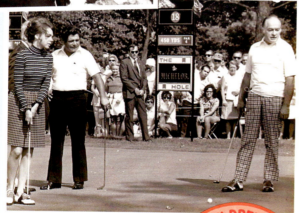

Bob Hope at the hospital, ca. 1960s.
Becker Medical Library

Bob Hope, known as "The King of Comedy," got acquainted with Children's Hospital when his daughter Linda, a Saint Louis University student, was a volunteer. Soon he was actively involved as well, visiting the children, donating his own money, and giving benefit performances. In 1958, he began appearing at exhibition golf tournaments; in 1961, the hospital launched the new Bob Hope Foundation, named in his honor. Two years later, the hospital kicked off its major fund drive at a dinner honoring Hope; and in 1971, Hope performed with Vic Damone, Nancy Ames, and others at a benefit in Powell Symphony Hall that raised nearly $60,000.

When Children's Hospital held a gala benefit on April 18, 1980, both to celebrate its 100th anniversary and to initiate its new fund drive, Hope was again the keynote entertainer. In fact, the dinner was called "Bob Hope's 100th Birthday Party for St. Louis Children's Hospital."

Hope loved making rounds to meet children, and sometimes managed a quip or two along the way. "Once [nurse] Byrd Dell Ohning was taking him around, and they met a child on bed rest," recalled nursing head Elizabeth O'Connell. "When Byrd Dell said, 'This is Bob Hope,' the little girl replied: 'Who is Bob Hope?' And Bob Hope smiled and said: 'I hope Crosby doesn't hear about this.'"

A plaque that once hung in the Children's Hospital lobby read: "Bob Hope has turned the gift of laughter into a promise of health for children." And his slogan appeared on a building campaign report: "If you haven't got charity in your heart, you have the worst kind of heart trouble."

deliberation, we believe the best and most economical solution is a new building west of our Hospital over the north-bound lanes of Kingshighway, cantilevered over part of the south-bound lane to result in 20,000 square feet of space per floor....Such a building could be an architectural beauty with interest almost equal to that shown in the Arch on the Riverfront."

The cost, including equipment, would be around $33 million.

Immediately, this plan ran into criticism. In a March 1976 article, *Post-Dispatch* arts editor E.F. Porter, Jr., called it a "skygrab," while an editorial worried that the "jutting building" would create an urban vista "grotesquely out of harmony." At public hearings, some Central West End residents

1979

The hospital coffee shop, which opened in 1956, comes again under the Auxiliary's management and provides 24-hour service.

1979

Children's Hospital loses the case regarding the new building in the Missouri Supreme Court; a new, more expensive project is proposed.

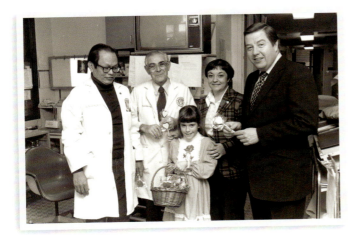

Sorority fund-raising. KSD-TV sports director Jay Randolph (right) was honorary chairman of the 1979 Alpha Phi sorority "Have a Heart" campaign. Antonio Hernandez, assistant professor of pediatric cardiology; David Goldring, cardiology division director; Claire Devoto, president of the St. Louis chapter, Alpha Phi alumnae; and the 1979 Alpha Phi "Heart Child" Elizabeth Fields are pictured with Randolph. Becker Medical Library

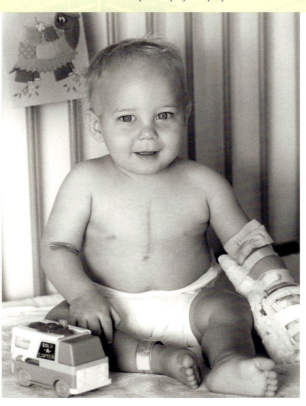

questioned the idea of impinging on Kingshighway, "one of the few nice boulevards we have." Over time, the Victorian Society in America and Mary Stolar, alderwoman for the 28th ward, in which Children's Hospital was located, also challenged the plan, saying they were concerned about the visual impact. Still others worried about traffic snarls or the effect on Forest Park.

Nonetheless, the plan advanced through the Street Department, to the Community Development Commission, to the Board of Public Service, and with support from Mayor John H. Poelker, to the Board of Aldermen, which approved granting the hospital air rights over Kingshighway. Three independent consultants, one of them president of Children's Hospital at Harvard Medical Center, concurred that this expansion plan was the only feasible one, and that two alternatives — acquiring the old Barnes Hospital School of Nursing or the old St. John's Hospital property — were too expensive and would separate Children's from the medical center. The differing opinions of the two St. Louis newspapers mirrored the split in public opinion:

the *Globe-Democrat* called the aldermanic approval a "heart-warming victory," while the *Post-Dispatch* said the measure had "merit[ed] defeat."

Late in 1976, Central West End resident Joseph McKenna filed suit in circuit Court seeking to block the construction, but that suit was dismissed. By then, James F. Conway — an opponent of the hospital's plan — had been elected mayor; he ordered city agencies to stop issuing construction permits on the project. Declaring that delay added $10,000 a day to construction costs, Children's Hospital filed its own suit to overturn Conway's order, while an organization called "the Forest Park Preservation Fund" filed an amicus brief opposing the expansion. In 1978, the hospital won this round with a decision against the city, allowing the hospital to proceed.

But the city appealed and the case went to the Missouri Supreme Court, as did the McKenna petition, which had been revived on appeal. Finally, in June 1979, the long-drawn-out matter came to a halt with the Court's unanimous ruling against Children's Hospital in the city's case. "The practical effect of the Missouri Supreme Court's decision...is quite properly to compel

1979
Children's Hospital celebrates its 100th anniversary with several special events, including a "birthday party" hosted by Bob Hope.

1979
The hospital boasts an 88 percent occupancy rate, "the highest of any children's hospital in this country."

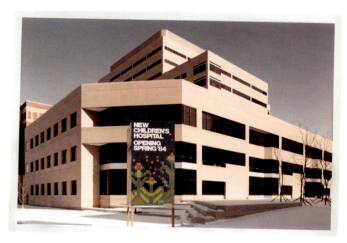

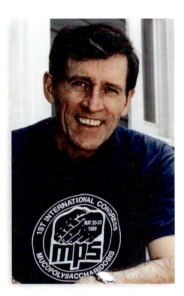

William Sly. Sly, director of medical genetics from 1964 to 1984, was the first to identify an abnormal enzyme in the family of "storage diseases," which includes Tay-Sachs, Gaucher's, and mucopolysaccharide diseases, all associated with skeletal and developmental abnormalities. He was elected to the National Academy of Sciences in 1989. Becker Medical Library

LEFT **Anticipating expansion.** A sign outside the hospital in the winter of 1983 proudly announced the opening of the new facilities in 1984. Becker Medical Library

the hospital to solve its admitted expansion problem by a means other than that of usurping public property," said the *Post-Dispatch*. Said the *Journal* newspaper, ironically, "Children's Hospital Gets 100th Birthday Present from Missouri Supreme Court."

Soon the hospital was talking about a new, vastly more expensive project to be built in a 2.5-acre parking lot at Kingshighway and Audubon, formerly occupied by St. John's Mercy Hospital and now owned by Jewish Hospital and the School of Medicine. This new building would be 12 stories high with 235 beds, while the top three floors would be dedicated to pediatric research. The cost of this facility, designed by the Hoffmann Partnership, Inc., would be at least $80 million: $20 million to come from a public fund drive, $14 million from funds on hand, and $46 million from borrowed money. While Spoehrer Tower would remain for a time as research and support facility space, the other buildings that formed part of the hospital complex would be demolished.

This time, approvals went smoothly, though one *Globe-Democrat* article noted with some concern that "the project is the largest in actual dollars ever considered by a health planning agency in Missouri." On November 10, 1980, came the ground-breaking for the new building, a day that staff called "the beginning of a new era for the healthcare of kids in St. Louis." Dignitaries present included James S. McDonnell III, chairman of the Children's Hospital board; University Chancellor William Danforth; and Mayor James Conway, the man who had worked so hard to block the project over Kingshighway. This new structure, people hoped, would not only give the hospital a state-of-the-art space; it would allow Children's Hospital to remain competitive with Cardinal Glennon and a growing number of county hospitals, including the relocated St. John's Mercy Health Center and DePaul Health Center.

FINANCIAL GAINS AND LOSSES

A gala dinner on April 18, 1980, kicked off the major campaign that would raise the hospital's portion of the funds for the new hospital. As he had often done in the past, Bob Hope provided the entertainment; in fact, the evening — which raised $70,000 — was called "Bob Hope's 100th Birthday Party for St. Louis Children's Hospital." Under the chairmanship of Richard F. Ford, president of First National Bank, and Donald Danforth, president of Danforth Agri-Resources, Inc., the $20 million campaign began. By October, more than $9.4 million had been

NOVEMBER 10
1980

Ground is broken for the new building.

1981

A day care center for the children of hospital staff opens its doors.

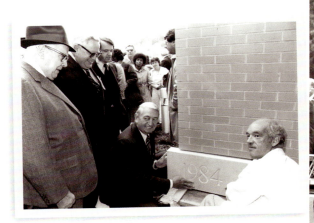

Cornerstone-laying, 1984. Donald Schnuck (kneeling left), chairman of the Board of Trustees, and Alan Robson (kneeling right), director of pediatric nephrology, made final adjustments to the cornerstone as Alvin Tolin and Linn Perkins (standing left) looked on. Becker Medical Library

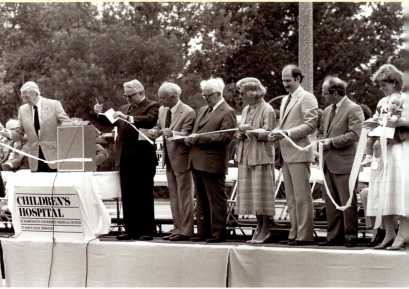

Dedication ceremonies for the new Children's Hospital. Cutting the ribbon that signified the formal opening and dedication of the new hospital were (from left): Donald Schnuck, chairman of the Board of Trustees; Linn Perkins, president and chief executive officer; Alan Robson, president of the Children's Hospital Medical Society; Alvin Tolin, president emeritus; Jo Throdahl, chairman of the pre-opening events committee and secretary of the Board of Trustees; Andrew Newman, first vice chairman of the Board of Trustees; James McDonnell III, past chairman of the Board of Trustees; and Lisa Holly and her daughter, a graduate of the Children's Hospital Neonatal Intensive Care Unit. Becker Medical Library

" Today represents a reminder that our dreams are one step closer to reality."

pledged, including $1.5 million from the Spencer T. and Ann W. Olin Foundation — though the expected price of the hospital had also risen, to $85 million.

To complete the financial package, the hospital hoped to issue $61.8 million in tax-exempt revenue bonds at 10.4 percent interest, payable over 25 years, through the Missouri Health and Education Facilities Authority — but there was a serious problem. Midway through the review process, it became clear that Children's Hospital — in large part because of its continuing burden of unreimbursed care — only had a BBB investment rating, the lowest of four investment grades. On the other hand, Washington University would be a tenant in the new project, leasing the top two floors of the hospital for research laboratories — which would provide 20 percent of the income needed to support the bond issue. Best of all, the University had a AA credit rating, which gave lenders more confidence in the deal.

Somehow, though, the University never discovered the extent of its annual financial commitment in interest and operating expenses to this giant project — $2.5 million in 1984,
$2.65 million in 1985, $2.8 million in 1986, and a continuing lease for 30 years in all — until the bonds were on the verge of release in New York City. An indignant University board found itself reviewing the medical school's rental agreement on the very day of the bond sale, when their negative vote would condemn the whole deal to certain collapse. They did approve their piece of the project, but with considerable resentment. At the November 13 meeting of its executive committee, the board continued to feel unhappy, as the minutes reflected. "It was recalled that the Trustees had not been given adequate time to review and study the contract because those involved were unaware of the hospital's financial expectations of Washington University until the demand for immediate action was upon them."

At the same meeting, they discussed who was at fault and what action to take. First, said the minutes, "The basic question to ask is: Was the lack of advance warning a fluke unlikely to happen again, or was it the result of a basic organizational inadequacy? The Chancellor and his colleagues at the Medical School feel that the latter is the case." Next, they proposed a remedy: a new structure

1983
Joseph Volpe in neurology receives the department's second chair, the A. Ernest and Jane G. Stein Professorship in Developmental Neurology.

1984
The cornerstone is laid for the new building, which contains a half million square feet.

memories *Julie Moschenross*

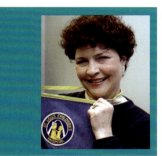

Julie Moschenross came to Children's Hospital in 1970 as a staff nurse on 4C, a new general pediatric unit. Since then, she has held various positions for the hospital and later for Barnes-Jewish Hospital: clinical instructor in nursing education, coordinator and manager of staff development, manager of hospital-wide education and training, and the director of risk management through 2005.

"Over the years, I have held many roles. Altogether, I have worked for two chief operating officers, four chief executive officers, and five presidents; and done this in six office spaces, including a converted bathroom. More importantly, I have taught over 3,500 pediatric nursing students; oriented hundreds of new employees, volunteers, and nurses; trained vice presidents, managers, and supervisors; and planned the first full-blown risk management program.

"One memorable experience was as a young staff nurse on 4C, a brand-new unit that had a low census at first, especially on weekends. One Sunday morning in 1970 or 1971, Dr. Philip Dodge, the chief of the Department of Pediatrics, was making rounds on 4C when he walked into a patient's room; I was sitting on an unoccupied bed watching a moon walk with the patient and family. As Dr. Dodge greeted us, I jumped up from the bed, embarrassed that I wasn't hard at work and expecting to be admonished. To my surprise and relief, Dr. Dodge took one look at the TV and pulled up a chair to join us for this historic moment! To this day, I can still remember the yellow uniform I wore that day and the whole experience — which told me this was a cordial and friendly place to work, without the burden of unnecessary formality."

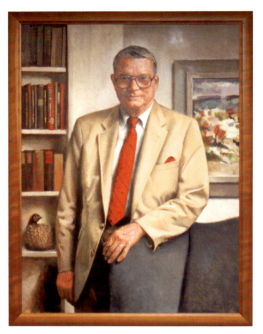

Philip R. Dodge. Dodge, a pioneer in the field of pediatric neurology who received his medical degree from the University of Rochester in 1948, served as head of pediatrics and physician-in-chief at Children's Hospital for 19 years. Among his other commitments, he was chairman of Missouri's Mental Health Commission for four years, and a member for five. Gilbert Gordon Early, Portrait of Philip R. Dodge, 1991. Oil on canvas, 50" x 38-1/4". St. Louis Children's Hospital.

for information-sharing throughout the medical center. Further, "the administration of Children's Hospital now understand that they must negotiate with the Vice Chancellor for Medical Affairs on matters that affect the hospital and the School of Medicine."

DEPARTURES
After years of success, including an anniversary celebration of his leadership in 1977, Dodge's last few years were difficult ones. Several of his stellar recruits had left, among them Ralph Feigin, who in 1977 was named professor and chairman of the Department of Pediatrics at Baylor College of Medicine, physician-in-chief at Texas Children's Hospital, and in 1996 president and chief executive officer of Baylor. Like other past and future faculty members, he was moving to a post that would give him the chance to head a department himself.

Feigin took with him some key people, especially Marvin A. Fishman and William Shearer. Other departing faculty members were Darryl DeVivo, who left in 1979 for Columbia Presbyterian Medical Center, and William Sly, who left in 1984 to become chairman of the Edward A. Doisy Department of Biochemistry and Molecular Biology at Saint Louis University. Hospital administrators Alvin Tolin and Linn Perkins had also faced an increasingly hard time because of the expensive, long-drawn-out failure of the first hospital plan and the precarious funding for this new project.

FEBRUARY 1984

Linn Perkins, executive director since 1970, is appointed president and chief executive officer. Alvin Tolin becomes president emeritus.

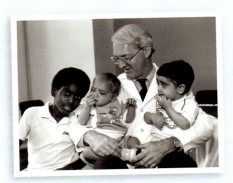

On September 28, 1985, Mustafa Sharafi, only three months old, became one of the youngest patients in the world to undergo a liver transplant. His parents, who had emigrated to Michigan from Jordan, had brought him to Children's Hospital because he suffered from hereditary tyrosinemia, an enzyme disorder that can lead to liver failure. A four-year-old sister had already died of the disease, and Mustafa needed a transplant to survive.

Transplant surgeon M. Wayne Flye performed the successful eight-hour surgery at Barnes Hospital, and afterwards Mustafa was transferred to Children's Hospital for follow-up care. His jubilant parents, who had at first asked to remain anonymous, agreed to share their story. "I had already decided to bury my son in St. Louis," said Rafik Sharafi, Mustafa's father. "What did I have to talk about?"

M. Wayne Flye. As liver transplant surgeon and head of the medical center's transplant program, Flye was always delighted by visits from his previous patients. Here he greeted (from left) Frank Owens, 13, Brandon Riddle, 1, and Mustafa Sharafi, 1. Becker Medical Library

A new concern had also come to the fore: the nation was in the grip of a recession, and this affected the patient load at Children's Hospital, especially the number of children admitted for elective surgery. Suddenly, the hospital — which had in 1979 advertised an 88 percent occupancy rate, "the highest of any children's hospital in this country" — had an explicably low census. By March 1981, patient days were down seven percent from budget and down 15 percent compared to the same two months of the previous year, noted Tolin, adding that they had reduced the staff proportionately. While the Building Fund pledges had exceeded the goal — up to $20,350,000 in January 1982 — unreimbursed care continued to increase as the patient census kept dropping: by March 1984, Children's Hospital "for the first time in many years" had an "occupancy of less than 70% of capacity."

Changes in key personnel followed the move to the new building. Effective February 1, 1984, Alvin Tolin became president emeritus, while Linn Perkins took his place briefly as president and chief executive officer, leaving the following year when the financial crisis persisted. For a time, Dodge had the assistance of a new Children's Advisory Committee headed by Ronald G. Evens, radiologist-in-chief at Children's Hospital and also head of Mallinckrodt Institute of Radiology. Then, after nearly two decades of service, Dodge announced in May 1984 that he would give up his post, after the Executive Faculty requested that he step down.

THE "PREMIER" HOSPITAL

Meanwhile, Children's Hospital held a cornerstone-laying ceremony for a spacious, up-to-date building that its founders could never have imagined. Nephrologist Alan M. Robson, Medical Staff president, spoke with feeling about it: "In recent years...it has become apparent that no matter how much ingenuity we use

APRIL 14 1984	MAY 1984
The new Children's Hospital opens its doors, with NICU patients and their nurses leading the way at 5 a.m.	Dodge resigns from his position as medical director of the hospital.

> "...while we have served thousands and will serve many thousands more when we are needed, it has been a great first 100 years."

— or how much we rebuild — the present hospital can no longer meet the needs of modern medicine. For example, we have insufficient space around each bed to accommodate all the life support equipment that modern medicine demands....Today represents a reminder that our dreams are one step closer to reality."

Another momentous event took place on April 14, 1984, as the new Children's Hospital — one half million square feet in all — opened its doors. The move, which began at 5 a.m. on a Saturday morning with the NICU nurses and their tiny patients leading the way, also included a ribbon-cutting ceremony featuring board chairman Donald O. Schnuck and state officials, along with open houses attended by 12,000 people. The building won high praise for its innovations: a 52-bed NICU; a 16-bed psychiatric unit; a rooftop heliport; a new Adolescent Unit; a state-of-the art pediatric intensive care unit (PICU) with sleep-in features for parents; two oral surgery operating areas. Hospital brochures declared it the "'premier' children's hospital in the nation."

The long rides that patients had once taken through corridors and tunnels to get to essential services were a piece of the hospital's past. At last, Children's had eight surgical suites of its own, supervised by Richard Bower, surgeon-in-charge. In April 1984, 12-year-old Howie Sutton became the first surgery patient at the new hospital, inaugurating the new "Short Stay Surgery" program. Finally, too, Children's had its own radiology facilities, satellite locations of Mallinckrodt Institute of Radiology, as well as anesthesiology and pathology services.

But how to pay for this facility, now that the optimistic projections for its use were proving inaccurate? Surrounding hospitals were also becoming nervous. In November 1983, at a retreat attended by representatives of all the Medical Center institutions, wrote Tolin later, "it became evident that there was an underlying concern about the financial future of Children's Hospital and how its failure to meet its $60 million debt would affect the other Medical Center institutions."

New leadership was ahead and, despite these tough times, a future that would vindicate the decision to construct this costly building. First, on May 16, 1985, a party on the Goldenrod Showboat marked the contributions of Dodge, who was returning to teaching and clinical research. Despite the financial woes, the hospital had a good deal to celebrate. The academic staff had nearly quadrupled in size during Dodge's period of leadership; its research grants had also burgeoned to a peak of nearly $13 million. As Alvin Tolin said once, "while we have served thousands and will serve many thousands more when we are needed, it has been a great first 100 years."

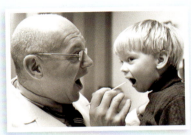

Donald Strominger (1928-1983).
Becker Medical Library

In the 1960s, pediatrician Donald Strominger, a 1953 graduate of the School of Medicine, ran a well-known cystic fibrosis (CF) clinic at Children's Hospital that attracted children from a wide region. A 1969 *St. Louis Globe-Democrat* article described the scene: "If you look into the CF clinic at Children's Hospital on Friday afternoon, it might seem that fate cruelly picked only beautiful children to have the dread disease. They love to tease and cuddle up to 'Dr. Don.' He invites them to his home for swimming parties and hamburgers...and [with] his common-sense approach [he] refuses to allow them to feel sorry for themselves..." His treatment program included new antibiotics and postural treatments. And to the assembled crowd in the clinic, he said: "Just don't forget. If you have enough faith and work hard, you can move mountains."

Today, asthma specialist Robert Strunk is the Donald Strominger Professor of Pediatrics at Washington University School of Medicine.

Children's Hospital Nurses: "Devoted to the Care of Children"

"Do you want to go back to work?" whispered one retired nurse to another. In October 2005, some of Washington University School of Nursing alumnae, on a tour of Children's Hospital, were so taken with the exciting facility and innovative equipment that they were tempted to dig out their white caps and start all over again. Giraffe beds that fold into isolettes. Computers on wheels, known informally as COWS. Blanket warmers, meal carts, up-to-date supply stations.

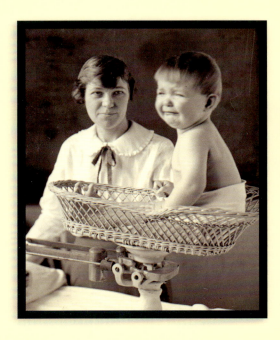

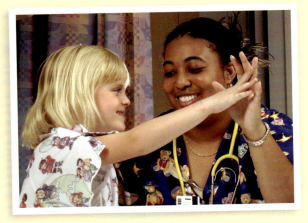

Nursing then and now. Although the nursing profession has changed dramatically since the hospital was founded, the level of compassion and quality of care has remained high. Becker Medical Library

Not that nursing today is easy, despite these advances. "With all the new technology, as well as the many kinds of illnesses and their complexity, our nurses are constantly facing challenges," says Velinda Block, vice president of Patient Care Services. "They are the eyes and ears at the bedside of patients, 24/7, and they need critical thinking skills and the ability to assess subtle changes, rapidly and accurately. Our nursing team also spends a tremendous amount of time as advocates for families. Since we see patients from all over the world, family dynamics and cultural needs are far different than they were years ago."

The field was not always so sophisticated. When the hospital opened in 1879, it had one matron, paid $20 per month, and no nurses at

memories *Janice McKiernan Rumfelt*

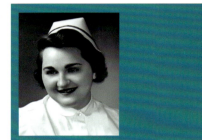

In 1959, Janice McKiernan Rumfelt — a new R.N. — joined the Children's Hospital staff at a salary of $310 per month. Like others, she supplemented her pay with private-duty nursing for critically ill patients: $16 for an eight-hour shift. Over the next 11 years, she held various positions: assistant head nurse, head nurse, staff development coordinator, and instructor in the nursing education department.

"On July 1 every year, interns change and then nurses have a great responsibility to help the new staff along with pediatric dosages and the way things are done. One day, Dr. Vietti came on the unit; we had a child with hemophilia who needed to have his leg wrapped with an ice pack and ace bandage. Dr. Vietti came to me and said 'Miss McKiernan, this child does not have his leg wrapped with ice pack.' I said, 'But Dr. Vietti, the intern didn't write an order.' She replied: 'You know that is what I expect and if he didn't write an order, you should have gotten it from him!' We nurses always joked and groaned when July 1 came.

"When I was at Children's Hospital, the physicians and nurses always worked as a team; we ate lunch together, even had birthday parties. It was a real comradeship that evolved. Today, the nurses still round with the teaching team on the floor and have a lot of input into the child's care."

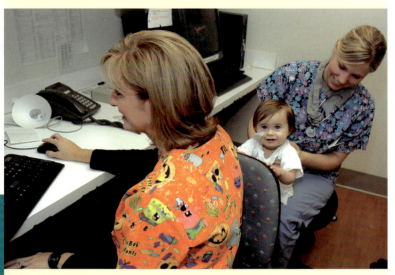

Velinda Block. As vice president of Patient Care Services, Block shadows staff a few times a month. Here she was following nurse Erin Fowlkes, right, on the 12 West neurorehabilitation unit and meeting patient Sarah Coomer, 1. Becker Medical Library

all. Soon nurses came on board, but they were not formally trained and were classed with housekeepers in the hospital hierarchy. Over time, the Board of Managers encountered problems with lightly trained and supervised nurses; in 1884, some of them, on their own authority, put the healthier patients to work. "It was resolved," reported the board minutes sharply, "that the children should not be compelled to work in any way and that all of the nurses should take their orders from the matron and physicians." The next year, the board enforced the rule that nurses wear uniforms — another step toward formalizing their status.

In 1907 the board took a giant leap of faith: They established their own nurses' training school, staffed by members of the homeopathic staff, which would "grant diplomas to graduate Students upon completion of a satisfactory course of study and experience in the Medical and Surgical Nursing of Children." The first superintendent of this school, Anna L. Wood, oversaw six paid nurses and seven trainees in a two-year program, heavy on lectures, long hours, and grueling practical experience. Three of the first 16 enrollees dropped out during the year.

NURSING GAINS PRESTIGE
When conventional physicians took over from the homeopaths in 1910, nursing was one of the first areas tackled by head physician George Tuttle. Each of the five departments in the 110-bed hospital needed two day nurses and one night nurse, he insisted — a jump from the previous eight nurses and one probationer. The contagious ward was especially short-staffed, he said, and baby nurses should have a graduate nurse to supervise them. The board capitulated, leaving decisions about the nursing staff entirely up to the physicians. Also in 1910, the young nursing program was absorbed by the new Washington University nursing school, in which "the requirements for admission are a good common school education, good moral character, and a sound physique."

By now everyone realized the importance of nursing to Children's Hospital — especially, as so often happened, when they were short staffed. In 1912, the board decided to reward graduate nurses with five-dollar gold pieces for

1879	1885	1888	1892	1907
The hospital opens with two patients under the care of a "matron." Gradually, nurses — with uncertain training — join the staff.	The Board of Managers decides to enforce the rule that nurses must wear uniforms.	The minutes first mention the fact that the small nursing staff is overworked, with 34 patients.	The minutes states that the monthly nurses' salaries were raised "to $18, for those who have been working for more than a year."	A school for the training of nurses is founded at Children's Hospital, a superintendent is hired, and students enroll in the program.

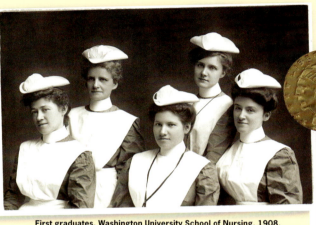

First graduates, Washington University School of Nursing, 1908.
Becker Medical Library

LEFT Christmas bonus. The 1912 graduate nurses were rewarded at Christmas with a five-dollar gold coin from the Board of Managers. Courtesy of Mike Hardbattle

Nursing students in an anatomy class, ca. 1925
Becker Medical Library

Nursing students in laboratory, ca. 1920s. Dean Marriott determined that the nursing program must "assume more thoroughly the responsibility for the scientific teaching of these nurses" if the nursing shortage of the 1920s and 1930s was to be remedied.
Becker Medical Library

Christmas, "this gift being so satisfactory it was decided to establish it as a precedent," said the minutes. By 1913, the board was contacting orphanages around the city, trying to recruit baby nurses 16 and over, who would earn eight dollars per month during the training period.

The following year, the head of the nurses' school — Miss Darling — resigned, so the board combined nurses' training with social service under one head: the remarkable nurse Julia Stimson, who had joined the hospital staff in 1910. Reported the board minutes: "This new arrangement, which is somewhat of an experiment, is undertaken to enable a three-year's training course to include Social Service work, equipping the nurse for public as well as private nursing." Now the trainee had to have at least one year of high school work in order, added the minutes, "to attract a more intelligent class of women to the Profession of Nursing in this city."

The "experiment" lasted until 1916, when Stimson gave up social service to focus on the nursing staff and nursing school. But at the start of World War I in 1917, she left to take charge of a large nursing contingent — including some from Children's Hospital — bound for overseas service with Base Hospital No. 21. Stimson did not return; she was promoted to head of the Army Nurse Corps and dean of the Army School of Nursing. Back at home, the 1918 influenza epidemic presented a new crisis, as the depleted nursing staff bravely managed to care for gravely ill children in the contagious ward.

MORE NURSING SHORTAGES

With the 1920s and 1930s came a continuing scarcity of nurses, and an increase in the head nurses' salaries to a minimum of $70 per month. The nursing shortage, said W. McKim Marriott, head of pediatrics and dean of the school, was caused by several critical needs: "better education, better training, better living conditions…. The future policy of our training school, it seems to me, should be to establish the school on a much firmer basis with a better curriculum, and to assume more thoroughly the responsibility for the scientific teaching of these nurses."

With the start of World War II, nurses again left for overseas assignments, many with Washington University's own 21st General

1910	1910	1914	1917
St. Louis Children's Hospital discontinues its training school and affiliates with the Washington University Hospital Training School for Nurses.	The hospital begins training babies' nurses for service in private families. Students have six months in the hospital and two months training in homes.	Julia Stimson is appointed head of two newly joined departments: nursing and social service.	Julia Stimson leaves for active duty with a cadre of nurses, and Helen L. Bridge is named acting head of nursing.

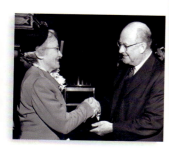

Two graduates of the Washington University School of Nursing served the hospital as its administrators. Estelle Claiborne, once a nurse with Base Hospital No. 21 during World War I, was hired in 1925 by lady manager Mary Markham to succeed Louis Burlingham, and remained in that role until 1954. Upon her retirement, she received a sapphire-and-gold pin from the trustees, and in 1956 won an alumni award from Washington University for outstanding achievement.

LEFT **Estelle Claiborne (1889-1986)**. RIGHT **Lilly Hoekstra (1908-1981)**. Becker Medical Library (both)

Her successor was Lilly D. Hoekstra, who had served as student nurse, general duty nurse, then the hospital's assistant administrator from 1940-43 and again from 1951-54. In between, she spent two years as chief nurse of the 106th General Hospital in England during World War II and also was general administrator of Puerto Rico's government hospitals. She once said that the mission of the hospital was: "the best care of the greatest number of children in a manner satisfying to the children, to their parents, and to all who have a part in their care in the hospital." She retired in 1970.

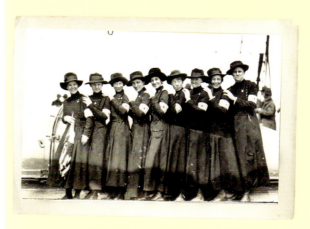

Base Hospital No. 21. A group of nurses from Base Hospital No. 21 on the deck of the S.S. St. Paul in May 1917, while en route to Liverpool, England. Chief nurse Julia C. Stimson is at far right. Becker Medical Library

Hospital group. Physician Harry Agress, MD'32, later recalled the work of nurse Lucille S. Spalding with hungry children at Bou Hanifia, a medical outpost in Algeria, where part of the group was stationed. "The Americans were sending over canned milk for feeding infants, but they didn't know how to use it and Spalding was our head nurse. She had trained with McKim Marriott, who had worked out all this formula business. So off she trotted with a bunch of cans of milk" — knowing exactly what to do.

Back in St. Louis, the hospital was critically short staffed. "Yet (head nurse) Marjorie Moore never flinched when staff nurses came down and said: 'I want to go with unit 21,'" recalled Elizabeth O'Connell, head of nursing from 1946 to 1957. "If you had to single out nursing's finest hour at Children's Hospital, it really was that period. Although our staff was so meager, we continued to provide quality care." Volunteers helped to fill the void: grandmothers from the community, American Red Cross nursing aides, and the Gray Ladies.

Other crises posed challenges to the nursing staff in those years: polio outbreaks that meant use of the iron lung and hot packs during steamy summer months; tetanus patients, with padded beds, the ever-present smell of formaldehyde, and darkened rooms to prevent convulsions; meningitis patients and their daily antibiotic taps. "Since the parents were not permitted into the children's rooms, the nursing staff played a major role as parent substitutes," said nurse Virginia Hagemann. "We became very attached to those children."

By the 1950s, many nursing students and new alumnae were circulating through the hospital's wards. "We assure the young graduate that she will have a very comprehensive orientation during the first two weeks spent in our hospital," said a 1955 *Small Talk* article, "and that she will

Timeline

1919 — Children's Hospital affiliates with the training schools for nurses of the U.S. Army.

1924 — Washington University School of Nursing establishes a five-year course leading to a bachelor's degree in nursing. The three-year diploma course continues.

1925 — Nurse Estelle Claiborne is hired as hospital administrator.

1934 — Marjorie Moore is named superintendent of nurses, serving until 1957.

1946 — The Division of Graduate Nursing Education is founded to meet need, following World War II, for nurses with specialized training.

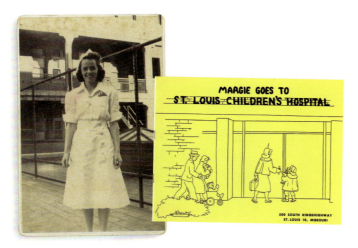

An article in the 1954 *Post-Dispatch* described Elizabeth O'Connell, 1943 graduate of the Washington University School of Nursing and nursing superintendent from 1948 until 1957 at Children's Hospital, and a new coloring book she had developed for prospective patients. Called "Margie Goes to St. Louis Children Hospital," the book used pictures drawn by a student nurse to describe a typical hospital stay, from little Margie's exam in the Admitting Room to her wave good-bye when she is released, well again.

Head nurse Elizabeth O'Connell, 1944.
Courtesy of Elizabeth O'Connell and Betty V. Reinke

This coloring book, continued the article, was one in a series of innovations intended to reduce the strain on patients and their families. Others included longer visiting hours and an improved understanding of children's emotional reactions to hospitalization.

The article said: "Responsible for much of this common sense consideration is a tiny, wiry dynamo named Elizabeth O'Connell…[who] makes up for her size, managing to be everywhere at once, to fill her own job and fill in for others, without losing her concern for every patient and every parent."

memories *Virginia Hagemann*

Virginia Hagemann worked at Children's Hospital from 1948 to 1961, with an educational leave from 1956-57. Her positions included: staff nurse on the surgical ward, assistant head nurse in the isolation unit, head nurse for the preschool unit, and director of nursing education.

"From 1951 to 1956, I was head nurse for the preschool unit, and during this period we had very hot summers in St. Louis. Without air-conditioning, we resorted to placing large blocks of ice around the ward and kept fans blowing over the ice to try to cool the children. Another fond memory was serving meals. The food was delivered to the unit in food carts, and the charge nurse was responsible for portioning out the food for each child. At least once a week dessert was chocolate ice cream. This meant a second bath after lunch because chocolate decorated every child!

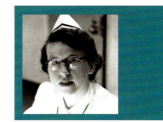

Virginia Hagemann. Courtesy of Elizabeth O'C[onnell]

"Various celebrities would visit the hospital and stop by to see the children. A few I remember were Cardinals team members, James Arness, Margaret O'Brien, Bob Hope, and Red Skelton. We had a little girl with terminal cancer, and Red Skelton was very taken with her. He spoke with her mother and invited both to visit his home in California. They did, and he gave the child what she had dreamed of — her very own organ. Her mother later reported that when they returned, and her daughter knew she was going to die, she wrote a will giving her organ to her church."

be rotated through all divisions, thus giving her an opportunity to care for every type of patient hospitalized here. When she has completed this rotation process, she is then assigned permanently to the division of her choice."

SWEEPING CHANGES

Soon a quiet fashion revolution occurred among the nursing staff. White uniforms and starched caps gave way to colorful, more casual dress, including multi-colored shoelaces. "To the best of my recollection," recalled Susan Goddard, nursing staff member from 1963 to 2000, "we stopped requiring nurses' caps in the late 1960s and began allowing white slacks instead of the traditional skirt uniform. By the mid 1970s, colorful smock tops started appearing with the white pants, and white athletic shoes replaced the white leather 'duty shoes.' By the late 1980s, scrubs were becoming popular and still seem to be the 'uniform' today. Our nursing department was always open to these changes and preferred to stress neat, clean (and modest) rather than dictate style."

Nursing was greatly affected by changes made by new pediatric head Philip Dodge in switching age-based wards to disease specialty units. Even the terminology changed, from "nursing" units to "patient care" units — to indicate that units focused on patients and their treatment. At first

1949	1949	1949	1953
gram in psychiatric nursing ablished with funding from S. Public Health Service.	The 48-hour nursing work week is reduced to 44 hours.	The University approves plans to found a master's program in nursing.	The Washington University School of Nursing affiliates with Jewish Hospital School of Nursing so that students can have four months of pediatric training.

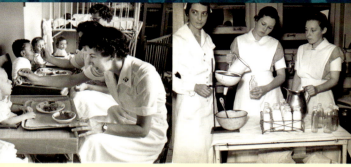

Lunchtime on toddlers' ward. Dorothy Greendonner, head nurse on the Toddler's Ward, feeds a young patient a bit of lunch. Becker Medical Library

Unidentified nurse and two nursing students in the Milk Lab of St. Louis Children's Hospital, 1936. Becker Medical Library

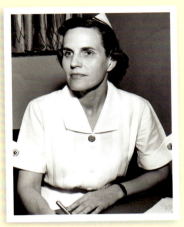

Mary Elizabeth Beckman. She served as director of nursing from 1957 to 1964. Recalled Byrd Dell Ohning: "We had a little girl by the name of Ina Going, who was severely burned. Anybody would do anything for Ina, and if she wanted some food she got it. One day, Mary Liz had brought her some lunch and put it in the nurses' refrigerator; that was fine, except that later she brought her own sandwich and put it there — then couldn't find it. We said, 'oh, oh, Ina had it; Ina got your sandwich.' And that's what I think is so great about the nurses at Children's: We'd do anything for the children." Becker Medical Library

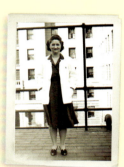

these changes were unpopular, but gradually most nurses came to like them. All the while, remembered pediatric surgeon Jessie Ternberg, Children's Hospital nurses were "all the most fantastic people. I always found them to be superlative caretakers." Added pediatrician Lawrence Kahn: "I think it is the pediatric nurses who fulfill the institution's objective. They often have the acrid odor of babies' burps, look and are tired — but radiate saintliness."

Other changes redefined the nursing staff. Into the 1980s, Children's Hospital employed registered nurses (RNs) only, who performed every task, said Goddard, "changing diapers, carrying food trays, making beds. Everything done to the patients, other than what the physicians did, was done by the nurses. When the nursing shortage began and salaries began to rise, Children's Hospital brought in nurses' aides to help take care of patients, doing non-technical things."

"DEVOTED TO THE CARE OF CHILDREN"

During these decades, said Doris England, head of nursing from 1965 to 1987, the Children's Hospital nursing staff promoted a number of ground-breaking initiatives: open visiting hours for parents, the hiring of master's-level clinical nurse specialists, a clinical nurse program for

INSET **Grace Yesley (1907-1993).** During World War II, she volunteered at Children's Hospital as a Red Cross nurse's aide during the nursing shortage, then worked as ward clerk on the infant ward before becoming secretary of the Nursing Department, a position she held until retirement. "Grace Yesley made a tremendous contribution to Children's Hospital over the years. There was no one I thought of more highly than her, and many others shared my feelings," wrote Elizabeth O'Connell. Courtesy of Elizabeth O'Connell

memories *Cathy Zeuschel*

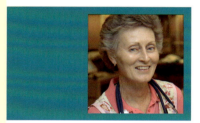

In 1963, "Z" — as she is known on her floor — began as a staff nurse in the old hospital building; five years later, she became head nurse of the neurology unit. In 2005, she celebrated 42 years at Children's Hospital. "My favorite position is being a plain old lowly staff nurse," she says, "because I like working with patients and their families best."

"As a nursing student at Lutheran Hospital, I took a three-month pediatric rotation at Children's Hospital, living in the old nursing dormitory. In those days, student nurses ran the floors at night because of the nursing shortage. When I started work there the day after I graduated, I was one nurse with 28 patients! To this day I don't know how I did it. Each night, the charge nurse had to give a rundown to the nursing supervisor on every child. If you tried to bluff your way through, they would catch you. Florence McQuarter and Jean Starkey were my supervisors, and I learned a lot from them.

"I wore a cap until we moved to the new building in 1984. I was one of the last to quit; I just felt I worked so hard for my cap, I didn't want to give it up! Now I have my own uniform: white pants and an apron that I made from children's-type material. Altogether, I have over 100 of them, with Spider Man, Sponge Bob, dogs, cats. The girls tell me that, when I retire, they each want one.

"Over time, the relationships I have had at Children's Hospital have been a major part of why I love to work there. Patients come back to see me after they have grown up; one man, who had leukemia when he was five, is now a paramedic and stops by every time he brings in a patient. My friendships with other nurses are also so important — they are very important people in my life."

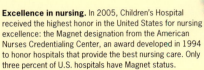

1953 The first African-American student enters the Washington University School of Nursing in the basic nursing program.

1954 For the first time since World War II, the hospital is able to attract a full complement of nurses.

1955 Washington University School of Nursing's diploma course ends. Children's Hospital affiliates with the newly organized Barnes Hospital School of Nursing.

1955 Lilly Hoekstra, an R.N. with a bachelor's degree, becomes administrator of Children's Hospital, replacing Estelle Claiborne. She stays until 1970, replaced briefly by Frieda Enns.

1961 A clinical instruction program for student nurses is initiated with five instructors, to teach students, work with them on divisions, and advise them when needed.

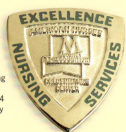

Excellence in nursing. In 2005, Children's Hospital received the highest honor in the United States for nursing excellence: the Magnet designation from the American Nurses Credentialing Center, an award developed in 1994 to honor hospitals that provide the best nursing care. Only three percent of U.S. hospitals have Magnet status.

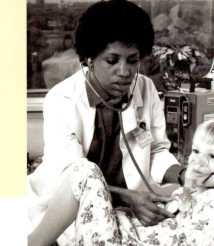

Denise Rodgers, Respiratory Care. Philip Dodge initiated a major change in the hospital when he shifted the unit from age-based wards to diagnostic categories. Becker Medical Library

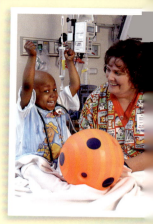

A smile during treatment. Four-year-old cancer patient Alexa King shares a smile with nurse Maureen Seper during her chemotherapy treatment in 2003. Becker Medical Library

memories *Marie Oetting*

Between October 1954 and October 1955, James Oetting, an infant suffering from a life-threatening form of Hirschsprung's disease, was admitted five times to Children's Hospital — spending five months there in all — as a patient on the old Private Corridor. His mother, Marie Oetting, stayed in his room with him. After surgery and extensive treatment, including extraordinary nursing care, he survived; after 20 years with IBM, today he is a computer consultant.

"The Private Corridor was the only place in the hospital where mothers could stay with their children. There were 16 rooms with one toilet and bathtub among them; we had only one public telephone on the floor. Each room had a bed for the child, a cot and rocker without arms for the mother, and a washstand for the staff. That was it; they were all as barren as that.

"Yet I cannot tell you how much I loved that place for the care and concern of the staff. It had a special environment: the way in which nurses took care of patients and the way doctors — your own and others — came back to see every child. Our surgeon was C. Barber Mueller, and he was absolutely incredible. The head nurse was Betty Vallero — or 'Betty V,' as we called her — who was a most remarkable person. Like the others, she was paid a pittance; their hours were hard and they often worked overtime. But their reward was in their lives of service, and they asked nothing for themselves.

"That year, Jimmy had major surgery on December 7, and we got home on the 23rd to a new house with no rugs and white walls. That day a dozen roses arrived from Betty V. for us. Later, Jimmy had another crisis, Barb Mueller did emergency surgery, and Betty V. was there. She finished work but never went home that night, because she knew this time was so critical for Jimmy.

"For five weeks it was touch-and-go, and Betty went to mass every morning before she came to work. Jimmy made it, but when we came home from the hospital we still had to care for him around the clock. We never went out; my parents did all our grocery shopping. One evening, Betty came by with her sister, saying, 'We're going to baby sit; we want you to go out for dinner.'

"I've always felt, ever since then, that I couldn't do enough or live long enough to give back to the world what those people at Children's Hospital did for our family."

> "It was — and still is — a family devoted to the care of children."

nurses in subspecialty areas, a nurse technician program for nurses' aides, and one of the first risk management programs in the country. The hospital's Child Life Program was a pioneering effort; in partnership with the Auxiliary, the program also introduced a children's garden. Patients sometimes returned after their release just to harvest the vegetables they had planted.

Today, Children's Hospital's large nursing contingent is organized within a shared governance model, with five nursing councils — research, education, clinical practice, professional development, advanced practice, plus an executive council — providing guidance on nursing issues. More than 500 students use Children's Hospital as their clinical site, including students from the Barnes-Jewish College of Nursing and Saint Louis University. Altogether, more than 800 nurses on staff care for some 275,000 patients annually.

The quality of the nursing staff has received national recognition. In 2005, Children's Hospital received the highest honor in the

1963	1975	1988	2004	2005
A student nurse affiliation with Missouri Baptist Hospital begins. This program also includes Barnes, Jewish, Lutheran, and St. Luke's Hospitals.	The Children's Hospital board approves the reorganization of the nursing staff for each of the seven nursing units, resulting in 92 more employees.	The Center of Nursing Excellence is established to develop programs that will improve the quality of patient care and assist in the career development of nurses.	Some 850 nurses are on staff at Children's Hospital in a variety of roles, from NICU to the Family Resource Center to Healthy Kids Express.	Children's Hospital receives the highest honor in the U.S. for nursing excellence: the Magnet designation from the American Nurses Credentialing Center.

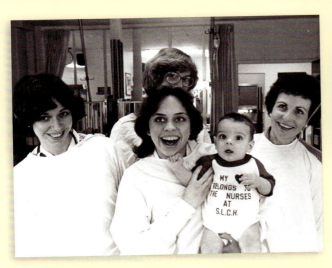

Nurses, 1980s. Elizabeth O'Connell said of the hospital, "It was — and still is — a family of professionals and non-professionals, devoted to the care of children." Becker Medical Library

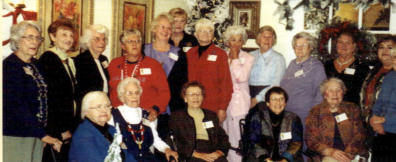

Nursing alumnae. These women were already long-time members of the Children's nursing staff when they began meeting for an annual luncheon in the 1960s, and have continued the traditional gathering every year since. Pictured left to right (seated): Byrd Dell Ohning, Mary Beckman, Dorothy Herweg, Shirley Nienhaus, and Norine Sgarlata; (standing) Roberta Middelkamp, Betty Reinke, Elizabeth O'Connell, Jane Girand, Doris England, Mary Naehr, Sue Goddard, Alice Roam, Virginia Hagemann, Betty Whitener, Carol Luckey, Janice Rumfelt, and Lois Niehoff. Courtesy of Elizabeth O'Connell

essionals and non-professionals,

United States for nursing excellence: the Magnet designation from the American Nurses Credentialing Center, an award developed in 1994 to honor hospitals that provide the best nursing care. Only three percent of hospitals nationally have Magnet status.

Over the years, nursing has changed dramatically, but at least two things have not. "Children's Hospital was like a family, and a family will make sure every child gets the best of care. If the hospital had had a mantra, that would have been it," said Elizabeth O'Connell. "It was — and still is — a family of professionals and non-professionals, devoted to the care of children."

Those children always have come first. In a 1989 *Post-Dispatch* magazine supplement, one mother summed up the personal attention given to her son, Cedric, who had spent nearly three months in the NICU with a dangerous lung disease: "Our nurses gave Cedric the best of care," she said. "They loved him as much as I loved him. They were more than nurses. They were beautiful people."

memories *Doris England*

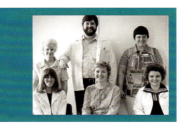

Doris Asselmeier England graduated from the University of Missouri in 1960 with a BSN and earned an MSN from Washington University in 1965. While in graduate school, she worked at Children's Hospital as a staff nurse and clinical instructor. Hospital administrator Lilly Hoekstra offered her the director of nursing position immediately after graduation, when she was only 26. Later, she was named vice president of patient care and worked at the hospital until 1987, when she was recruited to Children's Hospital of Michigan. She retired in 2000.

"In graduate school, because of some compassionate and caring faculty, I became very interested in child/parent relationships among hospitalized children. Not long after my appointment as director of nursing, I began to test the waters to see whether we could institute open visiting hours for parents. At that time, visiting hours were only 2 to 4 p.m. and 6 to 8 p.m. My idea was not that popular with physicians or nurses, and progress on it was slow.

"Then along came Dr. Phil Dodge as chief of pediatrics, and we began talking about expanded visiting hours. He was also interested in reorganizing the patient units from age groupings to major diagnostic categories — another unpopular idea with doctors and nurses. After many discussions, it became clear that we could help each other, so after a few negotiation sessions (always friendly) we accomplished both our goals. As I recall, it took some time for the staff to get used to the open visiting because of the sheer number of people. The nurses and physicians soon realized, however, that having parents — who know their children best — close at hand, far outweighed any inconvenience."

Doris England (center) with members of the Patient Care Team, 1979. Becker Medical Library

CHAPTER

7

1985
1995

"Much Stronger National Force": A New Era of Leadership

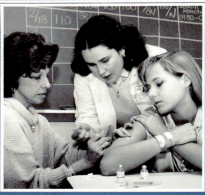

CHAPTER SEVEN "MUCH STRONGER NATIONAL FORCE": A NEW ERA OF LEADERSHIP

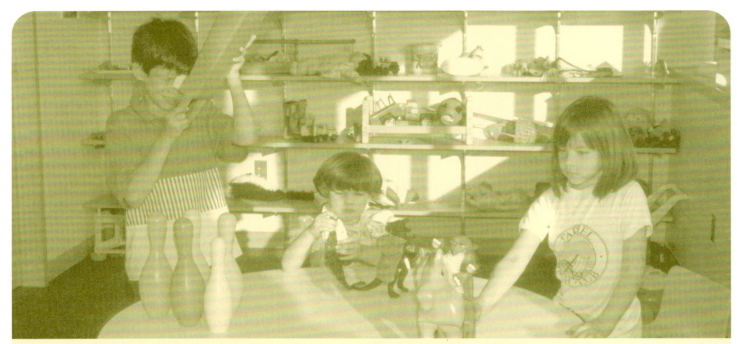

BELOW **Photo of NICU.** By 1993, some 15 neonatologists worked in the division of newborn medicine, and the nurse-to-patient ratio was one to one or one to two. Becker Medical Library

Recreational therapy. A large space for recreational therapy was one of the many advantages of the new hospital facilities. Becker Medical Library

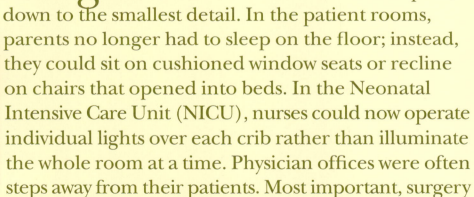

Everyone — the children, their families, and the long-suffering staff — loved the new hospital, down to the smallest detail. In the patient rooms, parents no longer had to sleep on the floor; instead, they could sit on cushioned window seats or recline on chairs that opened into beds. In the Neonatal Intensive Care Unit (NICU), nurses could now operate individual lights over each crib rather than illuminate the whole room at a time. Physician offices were often steps away from their patients. Most important, surgery and X-ray facilities were located in the hospital itself, along with a new adolescent unit, one-day surgery unit, recreational therapy area, psychiatric unit, Center for Communications Disorders, and heliport. The only problem, said patient care manager Charlene Cooney in a 1984 *Post-Dispatch* article, was that the building might be "too beautiful."

PREVIOUS PAGE **The new building after completion in 1984.**
INSET **The first edition of Children's Hospital Magazine, 1986.**
Becker Medical Library

OCTOBER 1984

The hospital's financial concerns, exacerbated by the recession and reduced occupancy, are the subject of an article in the *St. Louis Business Journal*.

1984

Unreimbursed care at the hospital reaches nearly $10 million.

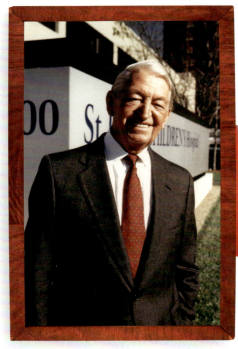

Donald O. Schnuck (1922-1991). Schnuck was a longtime supporter of Children's Hospital, serving as a member of the board from 1976 to 1986 and as chairman from 1982 to 1984. He and his wife, Doris, also served as honorary chairs of CAROUSEL, the gala benefit. Becker Medical Library

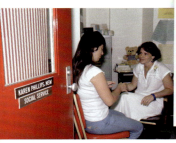

Social Work. In 1985, the Children's Hospital social work department celebrated its 75th anniversary, its role vastly different than it had been in 1910. Then social workers visited homes to teach families good diet and hygiene; by the 1980s, the service had evolved into a highly trained team of professionals, often working with the seriously ill. Becker Medical Library

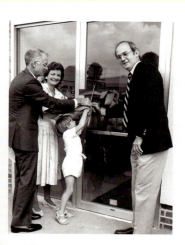

Child Development Center. This day care center, operated by Children's Hospital for the children of Washington University and hospital employees, renovated a building and more than doubled the number of children it could accept in 1987. Ronald Evens (left), Rosalyn Kleinberg, director of the child development center, and Philip Stahl assisted Kathleen Griffin in the ribbon-cutting ceremony. Becker Medical Library

Behind the scenes, however, there was no shortage of serious worry, primarily about money. Not only did the new hospital more than double the available floor space, but it also required a much larger staff — up from 900 nurses, housekeepers, maintenance, and dietary workers to a new total of 1,200. Somehow the projected income to meet these higher expenses had not materialized: In July 1984, the sleek new beds were only 70 percent filled; in October, the hospital was averaging around 60 percent of capacity — well below the 75 to 80 percent they needed. By November 1985, the Executive Faculty minutes reported that "Children's Hospital is losing money associated with reduced occupancy of beds, unreimbursed care, and certain expenses that are out of control. Last year, the loss approximated $7 million. Currently, the loss is projected at $4 million. Thus, Children's Hospital remains in financial trouble and can certainly use help."

Concerned, the University began searching for ways to supply this help. To reduce the hospital's heavy debt service, Lee Fetter, assistant dean for finance, proposed one solution to the University trustees in October 1985: refinancing the hospital's $61.8 million in tax-exempt bonds at lower interest rates, with the University guaranteeing the hospital's credit. The board's executive committee decided not to pursue the proposal, but did say they were "considering every possible avenue to provide non-cash assistance to Children's Hospital in the quest for an improved financial condition."

Rumors began to circulate about major changes at the hospital, even its acquisition. Already in 1983, the Executive Faculty minutes reported an "instance of a question raised by a member of the part-time staff as to whether or not Children's Hospital would any longer actually be intended for children. Obviously, such a perception was associated with the concern that Children's Hospital was being converted into something else." Late in 1984, the hospital quelled another rumor by stating firmly, in a memo: "Children's Hospital is not now, and has never been, involved with Barnes Hospital or any other organization exploring the potential of merger or takeover."

And the hospital's financial problems began to surface in local newspapers. In October 1984,

1985
The Children's Hospital social work department celebrates its 75th anniversary.

1985
Ronald Evens becomes president of Children's Hospital.

memories *Ron Morfeld*

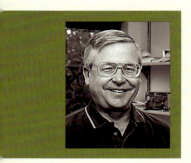

Ron Morfeld — who earned a B.S. from the University of Missouri-St. Louis and an M.B.A from Southern Illinois University-Edwardsville — was hired by Ted Frey in 1974 to help set Children's Hospital on a new fiscal course, especially in the area of reimbursement. Over the past 30 years, he has been accounting manager, director of financial planning, director of managed care, and now director of payer development.

"Not all of it was easy but it was very interesting: When I came, we were converting from a volunteer-dominated and supported organization to a business-like structure. We were also moving from having no systems to developing a strong automated system for the hospital. Except for one doctor, I had the first PC in the hospital! When I started, we only had the old-fashioned 10-key manual calculators.

"In the 1970s and 80s, I remember going to Jefferson City and cajoling, wheedling, begging for increased Medicaid reimbursement. We had some good success over time. When I started here, Medicaid was in its infancy, and we were paid only $28 a day for services up to a maximum of 10 days per patient, even though many children, especially in the neonatal unit, actually stayed 70 or 100 days. Eventually, the length-of-stay limit was eliminated and our payment rate went up to $489 per day! Once we were in the new hospital, they went up still higher to $659 a day, reflecting our increased costs.

"But I always thought of us — Ted Frey, Mike Wuller, who was the controller, and I — as strictly behind-the-scenes people. No patient came to Children's Hospital to see me! Like everyone else at the hospital, everything we did was for the kids. Ted Frey emphasized that for years: Doing what was right for the kids."

the *St. Louis Business Journal* ran a long article titled: "Children's Hospital Finances Ill," with the subtitle, "Annual debt payments of $6.7 million." In it, the writer quoted Ted Frey, then executive vice president, bemoaning the confluence of circumstances — the recession, the new emphasis by insurers on outpatient care — that made the hospital's situation more precarious.

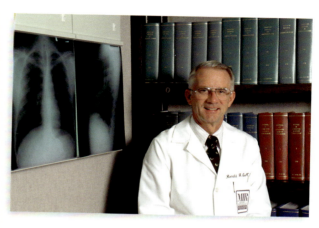

Ronald G. Evens. Evens was Elizabeth Mallinckrodt Professor, head of radiology and director of Mallinckrodt Institute of Radiology from 1971-1999, also serving as president and chief executive officer of Children's Hospital from 1985-88. Vice chancellor for financial affairs from 1988 to 1990, he became president of Barnes-Jewish Hospital in 1999, retiring in 2005. Becker Medical Library

"You couldn't have written the scenario any worse," said Frey in the story.

Yet on the hospital side, some staff members believed that a sense of panic was unwarranted: The financial problems were temporary, they thought, probably the result of a cyclical economic downturn, and were already yielding to various remedies, such as increased advertising. They agreed with Lee Fetter's assessment in his October 1985 proposal: "The Hospital has been able to pay all debt service during the last year throughout its most difficult period of operations. While they still rely heavily on non-operating revenue (gifts and interest income) to accomplish this, the net revenue from operations continues to grow stronger. I think the 3–5 year prognosis for the Hospital is improving and the risk of the University guarantee being exercised is minimal."

RE-STAFFING THE HOSPITAL

Nonetheless, the Children's Hospital board, headed by Andrew Newman, was shocked by the losses. After Linn Perkins' abrupt departure, Newman approached radiology head Ronald G. Evens, known as a strong operations manager and a tough negotiator, about becoming hospital president. Evens was intrigued but wanted to keep his position at Mallinckrodt Institute, so he

1985

An extracorporeal membrane oxygenation (ECMO) unit is added to the hospital.

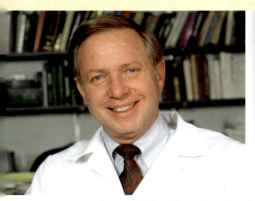

Harvey R. Colten. After receiving his medical degree in 1963 from Western Reserve University, he did his residency at University Hospitals in Cleveland and Children's Hospital in Washington, D.C. Following military service from 1964 to 1968, then five years at the National Institutes of Health, he served on the Harvard faculty from 1970-1986 before becoming head of pediatrics at Children's Hospital. His research interests included surfactant protein B deficiency, genetic control of complement proteins, and genetic deficiencies of proteins important in pulmonary diseases. Becker Medical Library

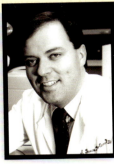

LEFT **S. Bruce Dowton.** From 1986 to 1997, he was director of the Division of Medical Genetics, with appointments in pediatrics and genetics. During his tenure, he also served as associate dean for medical education and associate vice chancellor. He left in 1998 to become dean of the Faculty of Medicine at the University of New South Wales, Australia. Becker Medical Library

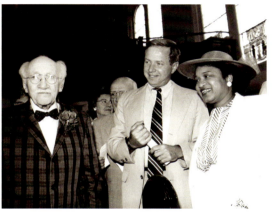

BELOW **Tribute to Park White.** Three weeks before his death on August 6, 1987, at age 96, White was honored as "an original, a pioneer, an intellectual, a master physician, a man of compassion, and a Christian" in a special worship service at Pilgrim Congregational United Church of Christ. Pediatricians Harvey Colten and Mary Anne Tillman were among the professionals who attended the tribute for Park White (left). Becker Medical Library

reluctantly refused. Undeterred, Newman came back again with another offer: What if Evens took the job half-time while retaining his post at Mallinckrodt, as well as his clinical appointments and faculty position? This time, Evens accepted, becoming president in 1985.

At the same time, a search also began for a new head of pediatrics and pediatrician-in-chief, and in 1985 members of a search committee appointed by the Executive Faculty stopped off at Harvard Medical School to pay some calls. Chief among them was a visit to Harvey R. Colten, head of the cell biology and pulmonary divisions at Boston Children's Hospital, whose research had focused on the genetics, biochemistry, and cell biology of such disorders as cystic fibrosis, arthritis, and asthma. Among those supporting his candidacy was Emil Unanue, appointed head of the Department of Pathology in 1985, who had known and admired him at Harvard. Over time, he says today, Colten vindicated his confidence: "He blended the clinical academics with the practitioners, added an academic dimension, and respected and supported the faculty, old and new."

Some two years earlier, Colten had decided that he would be receptive to an offer to head a department, and a number had already approached him. From the start, this opportunity felt unusual. "It was a very flattering thing," he said later. "These were giants in academic medicine — Sam Wells, Joe Davie, and others — who were coming to see me. We talked about the future of academic medicine and pediatrics, about the importance of balancing serious research and clinical expertise, and the value of this in developing future physicians and physician scientists. It was a spectacular visit, just terrific, and I enjoyed it very much."

Several weeks later, while on a medical exchange program in Japan, Colten received a phone call from Dean M. Kenton King inviting him to St. Louis as soon as possible for an on-site visit. When he arrived, he had stimulating conversations with search committee members, such as pharmacology head Philip Needleman. By the time Colten returned to Boston, "it was clear that I was hooked," he said. "Here was a department in distress, but distress surrounded by a tremendous school that would appreciate what I had in mind. I love to build...the thrill is in the development of people and programs, and this was a golden opportunity." He accepted the offer and arrived on staff in July 1986.

ST. JUDE CHILDREN'S RESEARCH HOSPITAL

During the search that ended in the hiring of Colten, the citizens of Missouri and Tennessee were confronted with the possibility of an unexpected, but well-publicized, hospital move.

JULY 1986

Harvey Colten becomes pediatrician-in-chief and the head of pediatrics at the hospital.

1986

Talks begin between St. Jude Children's Research Hospital in Memphis and St. Louis Children's Hospital, about the possibility of St. Jude's moving to St. Louis.

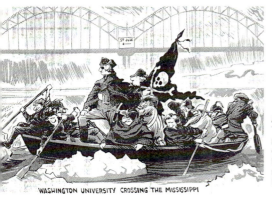

A possible move from Memphis. This cartoon from the Memphis newspaper *Commercial Appeal* demonstrated the negative opinion that some Memphis residents had about the proposed move of St. Jude Children's Research Hospital to St. Louis.

St. Jude Children's Research Hospital in Memphis, founded in 1962 by entertainer Danny Thomas, announced that it was engaged in talks with Children's Hospital about shifting its research operations, including some $80 million in National Institutes of Health (NIH) grants, to St. Louis. The board of St. Jude's was eager to expand its facilities; coincidentally, its former board chairman, who had been instrumental in locating the hospital in Memphis, had just died, thus weakening its ties to that city.

Leaders in both places quickly spoke out about the proposal. In St. Louis, Chancellor William H. Danforth called the discussions the "beginning of what could be a great opportunity....Combined, these institutions would provide the opportunity to mount world-class research programs for the last decades of the 20th century." But in Memphis, a dismayed mayor, business leaders, and state officials met quickly to decide how to keep St. Jude's in town, while the chancellor of the University of Tennessee Health Science Center, St. Jude's institutional research partner, admitted that Washington University researchers "are at the cutting edge of their field — biomedical research."

In the end, after year-long negotiations, Memphis won. While St. Louis was reported to have offered a $125 million incentive package to attract

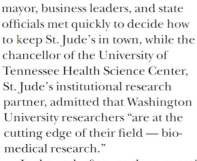

Julio V. Santiago. Co-director of the division of pediatric endocrinology and metabolism from 1985 to 1993, then director from 1993 until his death in 1997, Santiago was its leader when much of its diabetes-related, clinical research base developed. Santiago also held other prominent roles:

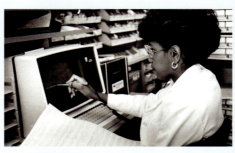

Pharmacy technician Trudy Miller in the Children's Hospital pharmacy. Becker Medical Library

By 1988, the Children's Hospital pharmacy was a very busy place, dispensing some half million doses of medication to patients inside the hospital each year. On staff were 17 pharmacists and 11 technicians, who had the challenging job of providing the dosage sizes needed for children of all ages, from premature infants to burly adolescents. For babies, they might have to convert the medication from capsule to liquid form.

Some of the drugs were invented at Children's Hospital, such as "Thurston's Cocktail," a concoction of antihistamines developed by pediatrician and allergy specialist Donald L. Thurston for children with allergies. Among the 2,000 items that the pharmacy had in stock was at least one surprise: old-fashioned leeches, rediscovered by plastic surgeons for improving circulation after a child's severed limb was reattached. "The only pharmacy prescription ever known to have been nicknamed by a Children's patient was a leech, dubbed 'Larry,'" said a 1988 Children's Hospital magazine story.

St. Jude, there was even stronger pressure on the other side. Danny Thomas weighed in with his support for the hospital's native city, Memphis officials made attractive offers of help, and Tennessee Governor Lamar Alexander proposed spending $25 million to improve research facilities at the University of Tennessee. Perhaps most importantly, Memphis gave St. Jude a large area for expansion, while St. Louis could only offer three smaller sites of largely "vertical space" on the close-packed medical center campus.

MAKING CHANGES

Meanwhile, Evens moved ahead with his own list of changes for the hospital. With the strong support of the Children's Hospital board, he quickly targeted new cutbacks in expenditure, such as layoffs, and renewed marketing efforts, especially to referring physicians in the community. Some of these admitting doctors felt alienated, Evens said later, and had been sending patients to other hospitals. Now Children's Hospital began treating them more courteously than it

director of the Diabetes Research and Training Center at Children's Hospital, editor-in-chief of *Diabetes,* and a principal investigator and national leader for both the Diabetes Control and Complications Trial and the Diabetes Prevention Program. Becker Medical Library

AUGUST 1987

Pediatrician Park White dies at the age of 96.

1987

The hospital's Child Development Center renovates its building and doubles the number of children it can accept.

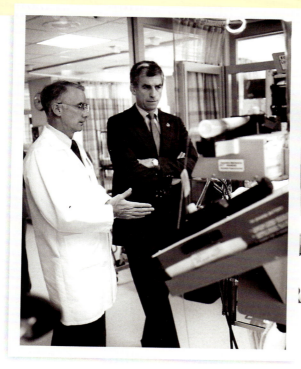

Senator John Danforth at Children's. Among the many guests and visitors to the hospital was Senator Danforth, who was accompanied by Ronald Evens on his tour of the facilities. Becker Medical Library

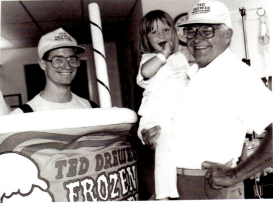

Ted Drewes Day. Ted Drewes visited the hospital in 1991 and distributed 250 mini-concretes to patients. He also donated the frozen treats for sale in the gift shop, which helped raise $700 for the hospital. Becker Medical Library

had; he also made successful overtures to longtime friends of the hospital, such as Harriet Spoehrer, James McDonnell III, and Dana Brown, about considering sizeable donations.

Like his predecessors, he also focused on the area of unreimbursed care, which had reached nearly $10 million in 1984. The *Business-Journal* article on hospital finances had reported that Medicaid patients made up some 30 percent of patients at Children's Hospital. To garner more Medicaid revenue from these patients, especially premature infants in the NICU, Evens stressed the need to work with Missouri's new governor, John Ashcroft; Ted Frey and his staff — now with strategic assistance from board member Norman J. Tice, executive vice president of The Boatmen's National Bank of St. Louis — continued their efforts, which had begun to bear fruit under Missouri's former governor, Christopher Bond, and his director of the Department of Social Services, Barrett Toan. In 1988, Children's Hospital joined in a petition drive to place on the ballot the MedAssist Program, which would give uninsured and underinsured Missouri residents affordable health care.

Various fund-raising initiatives also paid off. In 1983, the Children's Miracle Network Telethon was founded by the Osmond Foundation to benefit pediatric hospitals across the nation. Broadcast locally on KPLR-Channel 11, this annual program garnered $678,000 for St. Louis pediatric hospitals in 1988, a total that was split equally between Children's Hospital and Cardinal Glennon Children's Hospital. The Auxiliary, Twigs, and Development Board continued to be active, sponsoring such benefits as the "April in Paris" fashion show and later the CAROUSEL Auction Gala. The Hale Irwin Golf Tournament, begun in 1975, was still an annual event, realizing some $365,000 in 1988.

"It was relatively soon that these strategies began to work," said Evens later. "Within 18 months, we had good enough numbers that we not only went to the bank and showed them that we were on the road to recovery, but we were also able to re-negotiate the loan, because there were better interest rates." This refinancing, which took place in 1986, was not underwritten by the University; Children's Hospital itself purchased bond insurance from an insurance company —

1988

The hospital's financial position improves dramatically, and it reports an $8 million net gain.

FEBRUARY 1988

Alan Brass replaces Ronald Evens as president and chief executive officer.

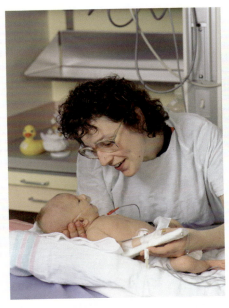

ECMO success. Born in Wyoming, Kyle Hansen (pictured here with physician Joan Rosenbaum) was transferred to Children's Hospital when he was 24 hours old after showing signs of breathing difficulties and a bacterial infection. At Children's he received an advanced new treatment available only at a few medical centers in the country: extracorporeal membrane oxygenation (ECMO) and began the process of full recovery. Becker Medical Library

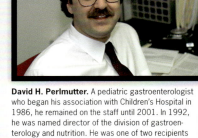

David H. Perlmutter. A pediatric gastroenterologist who began his association with Children's Hospital in 1986, he remained on the staff until 2001. In 1992, he was named director of the division of gastroenterology and nutrition. He was one of two recipients to win the 1994 E. Mead Johnson Award for Pediatric Research from the Society for Pediatric Research; other winners from the Department of Pediatrics had included: Alan L. Schwartz, Harvey R. Colten, and Arnold W. Strauss. Becker Medical Library

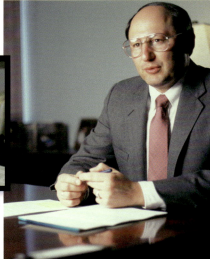

Alan Brass. Brass, who served as president of St. Louis Children's Hospital from 1988 to 1995, had previously worked as director of corporate services at Children's Hospital in Columbus, Ohio. Becker Medical Library

and the lower interest rates more than offset that cost. By 1988, Evens said, the hospital's financial position had dramatically changed: from a $1.5 million net loss to an $8 million gain. "I felt comfortable enough then that things were in shape that I asked them to search for a new president," he said.

During this three-year period, research and clinical work also made progress. Joseph J. Volpe, chief of pediatric neurology and a recruit of Philip R. Dodge, continued his ground-breaking research into the cause and prevention of brain injuries in premature babies, while Jeffrey Marsh did internationally acclaimed work in correcting severe craniofacial deformities. A new pediatric dentistry division began, providing the first dental services in the St. Louis area for children with serious medical problems, and in 1985 the hospital added an extracorporeal membrane oxygenation (ECMO) unit, a device that did the work of the lungs by sending oxygen into the blood artificially.

ALAN BRASS JOINS CHILDREN'S HOSPITAL

The search to replace Ronald Evens ended in the recruitment of Alan Brass — formerly director of corporate services at Children's Hospital in Columbus, Ohio, and executive director of both its foundation and research foundation — who took over as president and chief executive officer in February 1988. "Children's hospitals represent something very special to me," he said then. "Working for children is infectious."

With the help of Neal J. Farrell, chairman of the Children's Hospital board, Brass launched the development of a strategic plan for the hospital's next three to five years. How to cope with changes in reimbursement and new legislation? How to compete with local hospitals moving into the pediatric field? How to deal with the population shift westward, away from the Central West End? To gather information, they spent a year interviewing more than 200 full- and part-time faculty, as well as nursing staff, trustees, community leaders, and legislators.

The result was a strategic plan that called for stronger department chiefs, surgical expansion, more ambulatory care, and community education services. Just as important, it outlined ways

MAY 1989

Children's becomes one of a handful of pediatric hospitals in the U.S. to offer home health care as an extension of their in-patient and out-patient programs.

1989

Major donors to the Golf Tournament raise over $350,000 for the purchase of a pediatric mobile intensive care unit for the hospital, the first in the St. Louis area.

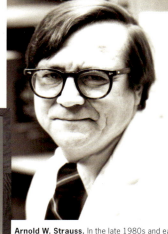

BELOW **Bradley T. Thach.** In the area of newborn medicine, Thach — a 1968 graduate and then resident at the medical school — continued his research into Sudden Infant Death Syndrome. Becker Medical Library

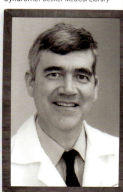

Arnold W. Strauss. In the late 1980s and early 1990s, cardiologist Strauss made a significant contribution to the understanding of Sudden Infant Death Syndrome when he and colleagues identified two gene mutations that cause an enzyme deficiency linked to these deaths. Strauss came to the University in 1977, was named director of the Division of Cardiology in 1981, professor of molecular biology and pharmacology in 1992, and Alumni Professor of Pediatrics in 1998. He received the E. Mead Johnson Award for Excellence in Pediatric Research in 1991. Becker Medical Library

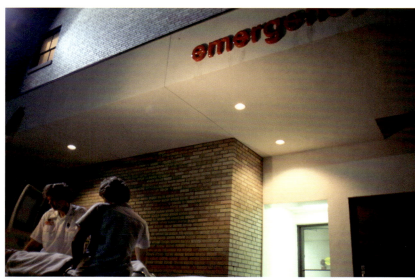

to improve the hospital's finances, such as increased productivity and fund-raising, and a better articulation of financial needs to legislators. It also developed a revised mission statement that reflected an international focus — and a growing recognition that the hospital should not only care for children but also advocate for child-related causes, such as disease prevention and health care reform:

> *"St. Louis Children's Hospital is an internationally recognized center dedicated to excellence in patient care, research, education, and advocacy for children and adolescents."*

Or, as Alan Brass put it later in the 1993 Annual Report, "Our commitment to serve as a standard-bearer for children's well-being is the core of our ongoing efforts. We are dedicated to assuring that their interests and needs are heard in the local and national clamor for health care reform."

COLTEN UNLEASHES "WHIRLWIND"

Even before Brass arrived, Harvey Colten had unleashed a "whirlwind of activity," said one staff member, primarily in the area of faculty recruitment. While some divisions had strong leadership, Colten said later — notably infectious disease under Dan Granoff, cardiology under Arnold Strauss, endocrinology and metabolism under co-directors Dennis Bier and Julio Santiago — others would need fresh recruits. From Harvard, he brought key division directors, all physician-scientists: Alan L. Schwartz in hematology and oncology; S. Bruce Dowton in genetics; David H. Perlmutter, who became head of gastroenterology and nutrition in 1992; and F. Sessions Cole in newborn medicine, charged with revitalizing that program. In 1991, Louis Dehner became pathologist-in-chief, while Jonathan Gitlin was named director of the immunology division. In 1989 alone, Colten added 16 pediatricians for a total of 214 on the full-time staff.

Never before had Children's Hospital had a pulmonary division, but Colten — a specialist in this area, who in 1989 had been named to the prestigious Institute of Medicine of the National Academy of Sciences — established one, and hired Robert C. Strunk, an asthma expert, as its director. Rheumatology also developed from scratch. Recognizing the growing importance of emergency medicine, Colten scouted for a head and in 1991 successfully recruited division director David M. Jaffe, among the first physicians in the United States to have done a fellowship in pediatric emergency medicine. Immediately,

Emergency services. Recognizing the importance of emergency medicine, Harvey Colten recruited division director David M. Jaffe in 1991. Colten also focused on building one of the first multi-specialty pediatric ambulatory departments in the country. Becker Medical Library

1989

The Omnibus Budget Reconciliation Act is passed, requiring increased reimbursement for pediatric services.

1989

William Peck becomes dean of the Washington University School of Medicine.

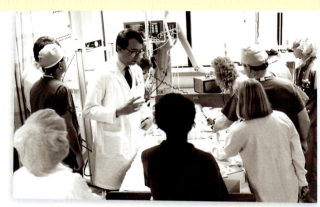

PICU. Doctors, nurses, and respiratory therapists work around the bed of a patient who has arrived in the PICU following heart surgery. Becker Medical Library

BELOW **T.S. Park.** Park was named neurosurgeon-in-chief at Children's Hospital in 1990. Becker Medical Library

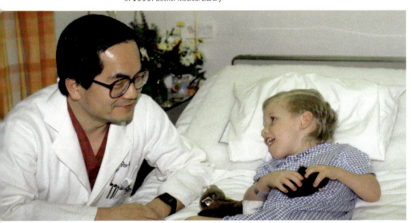

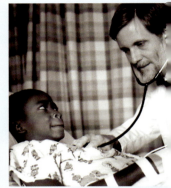

Robert Strunk. Becker Medical Library

An asthma expert, Robert C. Strunk — director of the division of allergy and pulmonary medicine — and pediatrician Elliot Gellman launched the Childhood Asthma Management Program (CAMP) in 1992. This eight-center, NIH-funded trial was aimed at determining the long-term effects of such therapies as anti-inflammatory agents on pulmonary function. Its staff also included physician Gordon Bloomberg.

Among his patients was 15-year-old Lucious Rogers of East St. Louis, who had suffered from bouts of asthma for most of his life, but then passed out during a more serious attack. Physicians at Children's Hospital revived him, and he left the hospital after a week. Meanwhile, the asthma management team worked with Lucious and his family on ways to control the risks of the disease. They educated "the family on how and why things needed to be different and ways we could help them incorporate these differences into their lives," said nurse Sue Green, a team member.

Jaffe began adding staff, improving triage, and developing research. Recruiting John B. Watkins to head ambulatory services, Colten also focused on building one of the first multi-specialty pediatric ambulatory departments in the country. With the addition of Julio Pérez-Fontán, he created the post of director of the division of critical care medicine, with oversight of the PICU and a fellowship program.

Colten received help from other departments in strengthening pediatrics. On the surgery side, neurosurgery head Ralph G. Dacey, Jr., recruited neurosurgeon T.S. Park in 1990 from the University of Virginia to establish a top-notch pediatric neurosurgery program; Bruce Kaufman also joined the pediatric neurosurgery staff, initiating brain tumor research. Also in 1990, Robert P. Foglia came from UCLA to become surgeon-in-chief and director of pediatric general surgery. Lawrence Tychsen, a specialist in the cause of crossed eyes in babies, was appointed head of pediatric ophthalmology in 1989, while in the following year, Richard E. Mattison became psychiatrist-in-chief, greatly expanding the services in this area by focusing on such issues as eating disorders and adolescent suicide.

Attracting more patients to the full-time and visiting staff was crucial, and one way to do that was the new Children's Hospital Answer Line (454-KIDS), which doubled referrals to affiliated physicians during its first few weeks; another was a strong public relations effort under corporate director, Nancy W. Litzinger. Making better guest relations a priority, the hospital initiated new services, such as valet parking. More intensely than ever, Colten focused on community physicians, trying to build strong ties. Certain benefits were now available to them, including a group purchasing program and patient home health care services. In 1990, Children's Hospital began outreach seminars that sent staff members to meet with physicians in rural Missouri and southern Illinois; it began teleconferencing its "Early

1989
Harvey Colten is named to the Institute of Medicine of the National Academy of Sciences.

1990
Children's Hospital offers the Answer Line (454-KIDS) as a free community service to provide answers to parents' questions.

> **"By the end of 1991, Children's Hospital had a roster of 312 full-time physicians and 249 community pediatricians..."**

Bird Rounds." In 1990, a "locum tenens" program, staffed by former chief resident Gregory J. Schears, was added.

By the end of 1991, Children's Hospital had a roster of 312 full-time physicians and 249 community pediatricians — 516 in all. In that same year, the hospital formed an important new committee: the Children's Medical Executive Committee (CMEC), as the chief policy-making and action committee of the Medical Staff. At monthly meetings, CMEC members — elected Medical Staff officers, department chiefs, the hospital president, executive vice presidents, and Medical Staff services manager, and four elected private practice physicians — would regularly oversee functions of the Medical Staff and provide input to the hospital in its effort to meet community needs. Early leaders of the CMEC were elected Medical Staff officers F. Sessions Cole, president; Steven I. Plax, president-elect; and Jeffrey L. Marsh, treasurer; as well as elected private physicians Charles H. Dougherty, Katherine L. Kreusser, Mary A. Tillman, and Patricia B. Wolff.

Appreciation of the community physicians — and the need to improve the residents' training — were both strong motives in the development of a new program: Community Outreach Practice Experience (COPE), in which residents were matched with working pediatricians to serve in their offices one half-day a week for all three years of their residency. In its first session, under the leadership of Teresa Petross, this program attracted 18 physicians; by 1992, some 60 community physicians were participating. Eventually, the program won awards for its innovation, and it was emulated by hospitals around the country. Colten also established the Part-Time Advisory Group (PTAG) of part-time private physicians associated with Children's Hospital.

Facilitating all these changes was the strong working relationship between Colten and Brass.

memories — *F. Sessions Cole*

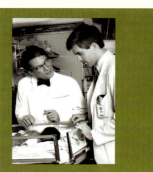

F. Sessions Cole (left). Becker Medical Library

F. Sessions Cole did his residency at The Children's Hospital Medical Center in Boston, followed by a research fellowship in neonatology and cell biology at Brigham and Women's Hospital. In 1986, he came to Children's Hospital, where he is now Park J. White, M.D. Professor of Pediatrics and professor of cell biology and physiology, vice chairman of the Department of Pediatrics, and director of the Division of Newborn Medicine. A primary research interest is surfactant protein B. deficiency (SP-B); in 2001, he received a five-year, $3.6 million grant from the NIH to study genetic variations in the SP-B gene in some 50,000 children worldwide.

"On June 4, 1997, I was at the Saint Louis Club with other members of the department; we were hosting a dinner for pediatricians taking part in the COPE program. It was 7:30 or 8:00 and dinner was about to be served, when we looked out the window toward Children's Hospital and saw smoke rising. Simultaneously, Alan Schwartz's beeper and my beeper went off — with the news that there was a fire at the hospital. Alan stayed to talk to the private pediatricians, and I came back to the hospital to see what was going on.

"When I arrived, I found that an evacuation of the entire hospital was in progress. By then, things were under control. Fortunately, this happened at a time when two shifts of nurses were there, as well as many parents who could help. Unlike an adult, to whom you can say 'please go to the stairway,' you can't tell that to a two-year-old. You need nearly one adult per child to get the children out.

"It was one of those experiences that prompts the development of trust and provides the substrate for improved understanding among all of us."

memories *Michael R. DeBaun*

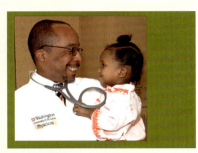

Michael DeBaun.

A St. Louis native, DeBaun graduated from Howard University in 1982 and Stanford University Medical School in 1987, and then became resident, chief resident, and fellow in hematology/oncology at Children's Hospital. After receiving a master's degree in public health from Johns Hopkins and a clinical epidemiology fellowship at the National Cancer Institute, he joined the Washington University pediatric faculty in 1996, focusing his research and clinical work on sickle cell disease. In 2003, he received the largest grant ever awarded to a pediatric faculty member at Washington University, $18.5 million, to lead an international multi-center trial in sickle cell disease funded by the National Institute of Neurologic Disease. With asthma specialist Robert Strunk, he also received a four-year $8 million grant in 2005 from the National Heart, Lung and Blood Institute to investigate asthma and nocturnal hypoxia in sickle cell disease.

"I chose to come back to St. Louis after medical school because of the spirit of intellectual entrepreneurship that Harvey Colten and his recruits brought to the department. Rather than receiving lectures with free lunches daily, the house staff was expected to learn pediatrics at the bedside and was constantly challenged to evaluate their thoughts and patient management strategies. Every other week, Dr. Colten did rounds himself with the house officers, and he peppered us with questions designed to initiate a critical thought process — even in cases where there might not be any clear-cut answer. He wanted to stimulate us to think about questions that could be answered not only for this one patient, but also for the specific group of patients from which this one had come. With us, he was immaculate, punctual — a model of professional integrity — and he expected no less from his division heads and chief residents.

"I will always be grateful that Dr. Colten, and Dr. Schwartz after him, embraced the concept that clinical investigation can be done with the same level of rigor with which they and others had pursued basic science research. That is a tribute to their common vision that science can be initiated both in the basic science laboratory and at the patient's bedside."

"It was a true partnership," said Alan Brass later. "We did not let issues come between us. We had a pact from day one: If there was a problem, we would go into each other's office to figure out a solution, so we could maintain total harmony in the system." They also shared a new vision for the hospital: as more than a regional referral center, but increasingly a center that deserved national — even international — recognition.

CHILDREN'S HOSPITAL REFLECTS NATIONAL TRENDS

Just as they were doing across the country, women physicians were playing a growing role at Children's Hospital, with some — such as Barbara Cole, who became director of the division of nephrology in 1988 — serving as division directors. Others headed programs, including Dianne F. Merritt, director of pediatric gynecology. Key women faculty members joined the staff, among them Susan Mallory in dermatology, Susan Mackinnon in plastic surgery, and Angela Sharkey in cardiology. This trend was also apparent in the composition of the residency staff: In 1991-92, for example, two out of three chief residents, Kimberly S. Quayle and Kimberlee Coleman Recchia, were women; the third was Michael R. DeBaun, who would go on to join the staff and become a leader in sickle cell therapy and research.

Like the country in general, Children's Hospital was also involved in the debate over health care reform, taking an advocacy position for children and for a basic benefit safety net that would emphasize prevention and primary care. To help community physicians, a new program began in 1994: The St. Louis Children's Pediatric Physician Hospital Organization (PPHO), which gave pediatricians a unified voice in addressing concerns generated by health care reform proposals. "The reform debate will be particularly pivotal for institutions

1991

David Goldring becomes the first recipient of the St. Louis Children's Hospital Medical Staff Distinguished Service Award for exemplary service and dedication.

memories *Harold S. Morse*

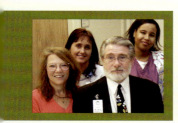

Rev. Hal Morse with the staff of the PICU.

In 1979, the Rev. Harold S. ("Hal") Morse, a United Methodist minister, became the first full-time chaplain employed at Children's Hospital. A graduate of Colgate-Rochester Divinity School, he was previously a parish minister for five years in Michigan and did a two-year residency at the University of Kentucky Medical Center. Today, the chaplaincy staff includes three chaplains of various religious faiths.

"At Christmastime 1984, we had a marvelous, real-life Santa Claus come to help the children and staff celebrate. However, he had never been in Children's Hospital before, and he was not used to seeing sick children. By the time he got to the ninth floor, he could hardly go on — he was so sad. So the person escorting him, Peggy Dolan, called me: Would I come quickly? I had to hurry over and cheer up Santa Claus."

"Over the years, I have seen how much spirituality, not religion, has grown here. Once parents and patients would ask me to pray for them 'later', but today, I have been physically dragged into a room to pray with a family. We have continued to get better at caring for whole patients and families — me included."

"Through the years, I have also noticed that sick kids seem to fall into three categories. First are the ones who are treated and go home all better. Second are those who receive the best treatment but, tragically, die anyway. Third are those who are treated but never get well or die. These are the chronically ill whom we sometimes call 'frequent fliers.' They are the ones we see again and again, and they are the ones people tend to forget when they think about the critical work of a pediatric hospital."

---

such as St. Louis Children's Hospital that provide highly specialized services available at only a handful of medical centers worldwide," said the 1992 annual report. "If we cannot dedicate resources to maintain these programs at a level of excellence, many children will be left with no care alternatives."

Also in line with a national trend, rehabilitation services and facilities were growing, thanks to a more comprehensive program of physical and occupational therapy, along with speech and language pathology. "Rehabilitation is an integral element of patient care in almost every department of the hospital," said Michael J. Noetzel, medical director for therapy services. Neuro-rehabilitation services, involving help from various disciplines, were added to help children with brain injuries or neurological disease.

Another crucial emphasis was the hospital's continuing reaction to the national AIDS epidemic, which had affected children as well as adults. Among the 200,000 AIDS cases diagnosed nationally, said Gregory Storch, medical director of infection control in 1992, some 4,000 pediatric cases had been identified, with still more HIV-positive patients. At Children's Hospital, the staff had seen 49 patients since testing had begun and they were following 30, with seven deaths, said Storch. Later, he was joined in this effort by Kathleen McGann, who would help coordinate the pediatric component of the Washington University Family HIV Clinic.

A RISING TIDE OF CHANGE

The effects of these efforts soon became apparent, when *U.S. News & World Report* named Children's Hospital one of the top pediatric hospitals in the United States. "Prominent physicians, nursing staff quality, technological sophistication, research, clinical trials and support services were cited as the leading factors in determining the excellence of the hospitals surveyed," noted *Doctor's Digest*. Next, a poll

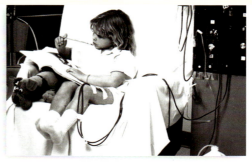

Homework at the hospital. Cassie, a dialysis patient, works on her schoolwork while undergoing treatment at the hospital. Becker Medical Library

1991
The Children's Medical Executive Committee (CMEC) is formed to be the chief policy-making and action committee of the medical staff.

1991
The Community Outreach Practice Experience (COPE) is formed to allow residents to serve with working pediatricians one half-day a week for all three years of residency.

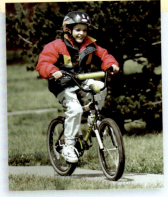

Tyler Robertson. After his diagnosis with leukemia, Tyler became the first patient in Children's new bone marrow transplant unit with a donation from his sister Britany. Becker Medical Library

Starting in the 1980s, Children's Hospital began building its transplantation programs into international prominence, with the addition of resources and new staff, such as Charles Huddleston in 1990, Surenda Shenoy in 1993, and Jeffrey A. Lowell in 1994. In 1993, Blue Cross/Blue Shield designated the hospital as a national pediatric organ transplant center. From 1990 to 1993, the number of organ transplants increased by 156 percent, with 64 children receiving them in 1993 versus 25 in 1990.

- The liver transplant program began in 1985 and celebrated its 20th anniversary in 2005. Through the years, it pioneered various procedures: The first split-liver transplant, which gave a new liver to a five-month-old baby, took place in 1993, while the first living donor transplant occurred in 1994.
- In January 1986, three-year-old Willow Lamoreaux from Montana — born with a rare heart disorder — underwent cardiac transplantation by a team of surgeons headed by Morton R. Bolman III. However, her lungs were badly damaged by her defective heart, and she died of pneumonia a week later. In 1990, a 33-day-old boy became the youngest Missourian to have a successful heart transplant.
- Corneal transplants also took place, such as one successful procedure in 1987, performed by ophthalmologist Lawrence Gans on a six-year-old girl.
- By 1989, the kidney transplant program was well established under the leadership of Douglas Hanto. In 1987, 17 transplants were performed, and the Transplant Clinic was following some 50-60 patients. Thanks to the advent of new immuno-suppressive drugs, the two-year graft survival rate had risen to around 90 percent.
- In 1990, the only pediatric lung transplant program in the United States at an all-pediatric institution began at Children's Hospital, and it eventually became the most active pediatric program in the nation. Later that year, surgeons performed a double-lung transplant on a 12-year-old patient, the youngest to have successfully undergone the procedure.
- Tyler Robertson, an eight-year-old leukemia patient, was the first admitted to the bone marrow unit at Children's Hospital when it opened in 1991.
- In 1995, 10-year old Gabriel Webb of Morrisonville, Illinois, underwent transplant surgery to replace his small intestine. He had been born with gastroschisis, in which the intestines develop outside the abdominal wall. His surgery was performed by Jeffrey Lowell and Todd Howard; his gastroenterologist was Robert Rothbaum.

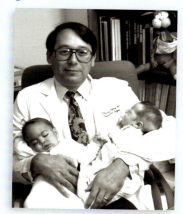

Tiny transplant patients. Thomas Spray, director of cardiothoracic surgery, received a visit from two healthy girls who received heart transplants when they were both less than two weeks old. Becker Medical Library

of pediatric department heads placed the Department of Pediatrics among the top three in the United States, while a 1993 *Child* magazine article named Children's Hospital as one of the 10 best pediatric hospitals in the U.S.

The reimbursement issue had marked an encouraging milestone, with passage of the 1989 Omnibus Budget Reconciliation Act that required increased reimbursement for pediatric services. At the maximum, fees had increased 100 percent for office and outpatient visits of children with complex medical issues, though they had gone up only five percent for the evaluation of healthy children. Still, these new rates, said government relations director Charles Swisher in the hospital newsletter, "improve Medicaid patients' access to care...Medicaid payments to hospitals are as close to maximum as we can reasonably expect to receive in either Missouri or Illinois."

The patient census had also been increasing. In 1991, the number of patients was up to a record 175,000, or 4.9 percent growth over the previous year. Overall, occupancy had risen to 80 percent, up from 73 percent in 1990 — and these increases marked a 2.5 point increase in the hospital's share of the local pediatric market. With this improvement came more money: Children's Hospital realized a $4.6 million operating gain that year against $126.8 million in operating revenues, while investment income and fund-raising efforts exceeded projections.

1992

Alan Brass is elected chairman of the board of the National Association of Children's Hospitals and Related Institutions (NACHRI).

MAY 1992

David Goldring dies at the age of 78.

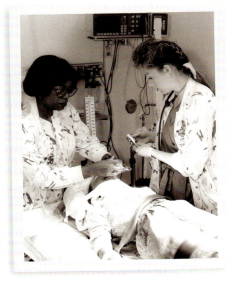

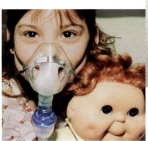

Becker Medical Library

LEFT **Emergency room nurses.** "The nurse is probably the critical individual in the interface between the health care team and the patient," said Harvey Colten in 1990. "The nurse spends the most time with the patient and has the greatest opportunity to support the efforts of the whole team."
Becker Medical Library

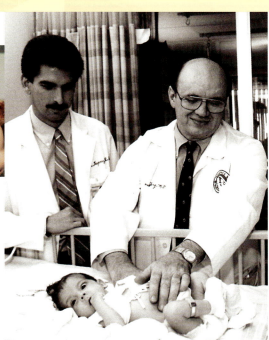

James P. Keating. In 1992, James Keating (right) became director of the division of medical diagnostics, heading up the new Diagnostic Center.
Becker Medical Library

NEW SPACE, NEW RESOURCES

Soon Children's Hospital felt enough financial confidence that it began looking toward expansion, even developing a five-year plan for growth. By 1990, it was involved in modest new construction projects, including a pedestrian bridge across Audubon Avenue and an expanded garage. "Today," said a 1991 newsletter, "there are pleas coming from nearly every corner of the hospital, 'We need more space.'" Spoehrer Children's Tower was renovated for support personnel, and a courtyard enclosure was created for a larger cafeteria; soon two off-site facilities, in the Central West End and in West County, had opened. By 1992, Alan Brass was even speaking of "some instances of overcrowding" at Children's Hospital itself.

To keep abreast of changes in medicine — especially the growing importance of imaging technologies for diagnostic precision — the hospital acquired a Magnetic Resonance Imaging unit, so heavy that several floors of the hospital needed shoring up to accommodate it. At the same time, it became only the second pediatric institution in the nation to install a spiral CT scanner. Within the area of oncology, a small bone marrow transplant unit was added; ophthalmology got specialized equipment for intro-ocular surgery; and cardiology received new cardiac catheterization equipment, which gave the hospital the only pediatric cardiology intervention program in the region. Now there were two Mobile Intensive Care Units (MICU) to transport critically ill patients to the hospital, two additional operating units, a Motion Analysis Laboratory for children with disabilities, and another inpatient unit. In 1992, James P. Keating (a "phenomenal diagnostician," said Alan Brass later) took on a new role: as director for the division of medical diagnostics, heading up the new Diagnostic Center.

With this financial stability, Children's Hospital began developing unique capabilities that would attract patients from around the world. Soon it was enlarging its pediatric transplantation program, begun years earlier with liver and kidney transplants and now adding heart, corneal, and lung. Between 1986 and 1991, 27 heart transplants took place with a survival rate of 88 percent. In its first year of existence, the new lung program — begun in 1990 under Thomas L. Spray, director of cardiothoracic

DECEMBER 1992

In collaboration with the Mallinckrodt Institute of Radiology, the hospital installs its first magnetic resonance imaging (MRI) unit.

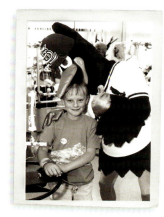

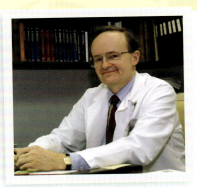

RIGHT **William H. McAlister.** In 1992, long-time staff member McAlister was appointed radiologist-in-chief of Children's Hospital, succeeding Ronald Evens, who had served since 1971. Becker Medical Library

LEFT **A welcome visitor.** Fredbird, the mascot for the St. Louis Cardinals, greets a patient with his signature style. Becker Medical Library

surgery — did 14 transplants, with 64 percent survival. Between 1990 and 1992, pediatric kidney and liver transplant surgeon Samuel S.K. So performed eight transplants among children under two-and-a-half years of age — at a time when only two U.S. centers were working successfully on children under a year old.

In fact, surgery as a whole was expanding, with the number of cases jumping 71 percent from 1986 to 1992 and the number of operating hours up 97 percent. To support this expansion, Gary Hirshberg joined the medical faculty in 1992 as the new anesthesiologist-in-chief and director of the division of pediatric anesthesiology. Surgery head Robert Foglia oversaw a move into new areas, such as fetal research by surgeon Jacob C. Langer, who joined the staff in 1992. In 1998, the first cochlear implant at Children's Hospital — and in the St. Louis area — was performed in 1989 on 17-year-old Sally Waltz of Kirkwood. By 1993, otolaryngologists, among them otolaryngologist-in-chief Rodney Lusk, had done more than 50 such procedures at the hospital.

AFFILIATIONS BEGIN

During these years, the chairmanship of the Children's Hospital board had shifted to William Cornelius, president of Union Electric Co., while the leadership of the medical school had also changed with the retirement of Dean M. Kenton King in 1989 and the accession of William Peck. Then, in 1993, Children's Hospital underwent a restructuring as well. Now there would be a new parent company — Children's Health Services — overseeing three entities: Children's Hospital; the Children's Hospital Foundation, a fund-raising subsidiary; and Children's Health Network, a new organization charged with developing off-site facilities. While Alan Brass remained as head, Vincent J. Cannella now became chairman of the board and of Children's Health Service.

Affiliation agreements were becoming more common nationally, and Children's Hospital and the Department of Pediatrics began taking tentative steps in that direction. In 1989, they made an agreement with St. Luke's Hospital to

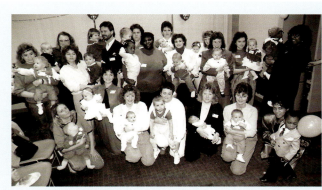

First annual ECMO reunion. Becker Medical Library

On Valentine's Day in 1990, a special party was held at Children's Hospital: a reunion of young patients who had spent some life-saving time on Extracorporeal Membrane Oxygenation (ECMO), a kind of long-term heart-lung bypass used in cases of cardiac or respiratory failure. The reunion was organized by Thomas Spray, the cardiothoracic surgeon in charge of ECMO since the program started in 1985.

One of these patients was a healthy infant, Nathan Anderson, who had been only weeks old when he became the 95th and then the 100th baby on ECMO in fall 1989. His mother, Lori, wrote a note to the hospital staff after he was released: "There hasn't been a day pass since Nathan has been at Children's that I haven't thought of everyone there with a special thanks in my heart. Words just do not express our feelings or how grateful we are."

JUNE 1993
BJC Health System forms.

1993
Child magazine names Children's Hospital as one of the 10 best pediatric hospitals in the U.S.

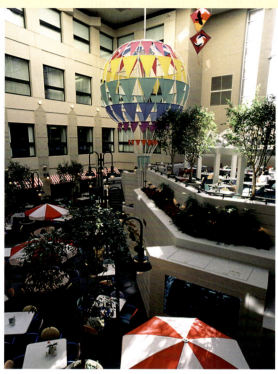

Edison Center Atrium Cafeteria.
In 1992, this new cafeteria provided more space for dining and food preparation.
Becker Medical Library

provide neonatal care for premature babies at St. Luke's. In the next year, they signed an agreement to help support the newborn nursery at Christian Hospital Northwest; two years later, they affiliated with Springfield (Missouri) Hospital. Children's Hospital also partnered with Cardinal Glennon Children's Hospital in a program, Health Care for Kids, aimed at providing access to health care for inner-city children.

In January 1990, the Children's Hospital board looked over a confidential report, "A Case for Centralized Pediatric Care in Metropolitan St. Louis," which urged the board to explore the centralization of services and facilities in light of the critical issues of "ongoing quality of care, increasing costs, and a growing scarcity of highly trained and experienced pediatric health care professionals." As the report outlined, St. Louis was one of only four U.S. metropolitan areas with two comprehensive, free-standing children's hospitals. Together with St. John's Mercy Medical Center, Children's Hospital and Cardinal Glennon Children's Hospital provided some 76 percent of the pediatric care in their market; the remaining 24 percent was divided among 18 other area hospitals, including Shriners Hospital, an orthopaedic facility that relied heavily on Washington University faculty. The report concluded: "because fragmentation is a contributing factor to a less efficient and possibly lower quality health care environment, the mandate exists for the St. Louis community to begin working now toward the consolidation of pediatric beds over the next decade."

These findings, however, did not result in a major consolidation. Twice in the 1990s, the board investigated the possibility of a full-scale merger with the 190-bed Cardinal Glennon, administered by SSM Healthcare Corporation. Despite intense discussions and the approval of community leaders, the merger never took place, derailed mainly by irreconcilable cultural differences. Still, said Lee Fetter much later, such a move would have had some advantages. "There are things we could do together better than separately, such as coordinating our fund-raising or our government relations efforts," he said.

BJC: "A MILESTONE IN OUR HISTORY"

Other, even broader, changes were in the offing — particularly the proposal of a merger with the BJC Health System, which had formed in June 1993 and was one of the largest nonprofit healthcare organizations in the United States. Already it included Barnes Hospital, Jewish Hospital, Christian Health Services, Missouri Baptist Medical Center, and various other health care entities: 15 member hospitals in all, with seven nursing facilities, and one retirement center. BJC also provided medical services throughout a 150-mile radius of St. Louis with 22 hospitals in its Regional Healthcare Network and relationships with 12 hospitals in the VHA Great Rivers Network.

The rationale for this proposed merger was a changing economic picture nationally. Overall, children's hospitals were booming during the late 1980s and early 1990s — on average showing a 22 percent increase in admissions and a parallel increase in revenues. But a declining

1993

Children's Health Services is formed as a parent company to oversee Children's Hospital, the Children's Hospital Foundation, and Children's Health Network.

1994

The St. Louis Children's Pediatric Physician Hospital Organization (PPHO) is established to give pediatricians a unified voice in addressing concerns generated by health care reform proposals.

" ...a common commitment to excellence in all aspects of care..."

census followed, reinforced by pressure from insurers to limit costs. In St. Louis, BJC argued that its network would offer Children's Hospital four major advantages: access to newborns through its obstetrical network, access to a fully integrated health system, greater geographic coverage, and more leverage for managed care contracting.

While some employees supported the idea of joining BJC, others expressed doubt on opinion surveys; they were especially concerned, said one newsletter, that "BJC Health System's top management didn't understand pediatrics" and that there might be "a reduction in pay and benefits as a result of the merger." These divergent opinions were reflected in management as well, with Alan Brass strongly favoring the change, but with executive vice president, Ted Frey, believing that Children's Hospital would do better by remaining independent. Meanwhile, the BJC board of directors, under chairman Charles F. Knight, was applying strong pressure to join.

In August 1994, BJC Health System and Children's Hospital announced the signing of a merger agreement. The hospital would continue to operate under its own name, and five hospital directors would join the BJC board. Fred Brown, BJC president and chief executive officer, called this merger "a milestone in our history, because it expands our ability to deliver leading-edge medical services to every member of the family." Brass agreed, saying: "Integrating Children's pediatric programs with BJC will allow us to create innovative models for women's and children's health services focused on prenatal care, diagnosis, and earlier pediatric intervention." Knight added that "the organizations are natural partners because we share a common commitment to excellence in all aspects of care, as well as a mutual interest in changing the way health care is delivered, making it more affordable and accessible."

memories *Teresa J. Vietti*

Teresa J. Vietti, a 1953 graduate of the Baylor University College of Medicine, was a resident and chief resident at Children's Hospital. After a fellowship and positions elsewhere, she returned to join the pediatric faculty in 1961, becoming full professor in 1972. She served as chief of pediatric hematology/oncology from 1970 to 1986. From 1980 to 1993, she also was the first chair of the Pediatric Oncology Group, a national cooperative study group that she helped to found. She was named professor emeritus in 1998.

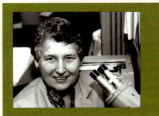

Teresa Vietti. Becker Medical Library

"One thing I have always appreciated so much at Children's Hospital is the extremely friendly attitude here. When I was first on the house staff, making only $10 a month, the nurses were always so nice — they even took me out to some baseball games, which I couldn't afford.

"When I was chief resident, I took half my salary — I made $300 a month — and some of the residents' money to hire a lab technician to work at night. Prior to this, the residents had to spend much time every evening doing the lab work for their patients. Since they worked every other night, this meant that they would sometimes be up all night or only get two or three hours sleep. Dr. Hartmann, 'the Chief,' chewed me out for this, but he kept the technician and paid for a night technician after that.

"I'm not sure how it developed, but I know that the outlook of the staff has always been that the child comes first. This attitude drew all the departments and divisions together; this was our joint goal. I didn't appreciate it until I worked elsewhere — there was just not the same spirit. This attitude is still here. If you want to do something else, forget it if it interferes with the care of the child. The sick child comes first."

DEPARTURES

Coincidentally, Harvey Colten and Alan Brass — who had worked so effectively as a team — both stepped down from their posts in 1995. Colten had declared from the outset that he would not stay more than 10 years, saying "That's about the length of time one could make a substantive contribution and not get stale in the job." He was true to his word; he returned to teaching and research, then two years later left Washington University to become dean at Northwestern University. Brass continued for a time on BJC's senior management council as executive vice president of operations, spearheading health-care delivery initiatives.

AUGUST 1994

BJC Health System and Children's Hospital announce the signing of a merger agreement.

1995

Harvey Colten and Alan Brass both step down from their positions.

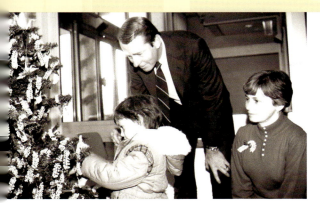

A Christmas tradition. Warren and Marni Hauff, who lost their son Gavin to leukemia in 1986, established a Christmas tradition at the hospital in 1988. Each year a "Canes to Cranes" tree was erected and decorated with candy canes. As the canes were sold they were replaced with a folded paper crane, the Japanese symbol for good health, long life, and peace. The proceeds from the sale of the canes were donated to the Children's United Research Effort (C.U.R.E.). Becker Medical Library

Steven Rothman. A pediatric neurologist and former resident at Children's Hospital, Rothman received the prestigious Javits Neuroscience Investigator Award in 1989 that would provide $1.1 million of NIH funding over seven years. In 1992, he was named neurologist-in-chief. Becker Medical Library

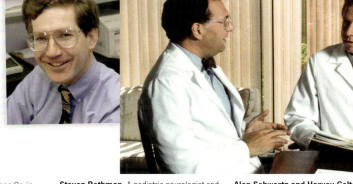

Alan Schwartz and Harvey Colten. Schwartz (left) said that Colten "brought a reinvigoration to the department." Becker Medical Library

Together, Brass and Colten had enlarged the scope of the hospital and defused sensitive problems, particularly the well-publicized case of an anesthesiology fellow, accused by a nurse of hastening by several minutes the death of a child on the verge of dying from muscular dystrophy. They had worked together to replace departing faculty members, such as well-known neurologist Joseph Volpe. Most of all, they had given the hospital a national outlook, while also deciding to forego independence in favor of a network that they saw as securing its future.

Even more new programs were just beginning: a comprehensive eye movement disorder center, a neuro-oncology service, a pain management program, and an expanded epilepsy program under Blaise F.D. Bourgeois. By 1994, the staff included 628 full-time and part-time physicians, with 1,794 employees and 817 volunteers. Operating revenue was up to $155 million, with 11,774 admissions in 1993. Now Children's Hospital had new locations, as well as an after-hours emergent care program. Thanks to Brass, the hospital had a fine cadre of nursing heads and effective line managers.

As for Harvey Colten, said hematologist/ oncologist Alan Schwartz, he "brought a reinvigoration to the department, focused on the pathophysiology of disease." While some key staff members had left, Colten had recruited physician-scientists who brought new energy to research, especially basic research. Arnold Strauss was doing important work in the genetic underpinnings of Sudden Infant Death Syndrome, F. Sessions Cole was investigating the genetics of surfactant protein B. deficiency, and Jonathan Gitlin had just discovered the gene that causes Wilson's Disease. At the same time, Steven Rothman had won major grants for research on excitatory amino acids, Julio Santiago had become nationally known for his work on diabetes, and Robert Strunk was continuing his multi-institutional studies in asthma management. Altogether, NIH support had tripled under Colten's leadership.

Further, the quality of the house staff had improved, thanks to his intense efforts to attract, as he put it later, "the crème de la crème" of medical graduates. The COPE program was also a stunning success, strengthening both the residency program and the relationship of Children's Hospital with its community physicians. Altogether, said William Peck, who had become dean of the medical school in 1989, Harvey Colten "took the department academically and clinically to a new high level; you could call him a quadruple threat. He was an outstanding researcher, clinician, teacher, and administrator. Pediatrics became a much stronger national force while he was head."

With its two top leaders gone, both Children's Hospital and the School of Medicine had to face the difficult task of replacing them, of adjusting to a wholly different administrative hierarchy — and of continuing to build on their success in a future filled with new challenges.

A Roundtable Conversation with Eight Community Physicians
St. Louis Children's Hospital: Building "A Big Something"

In late August 2005, eight community physicians — many of them former Washington University medical students or residents and all currently on the clinical staff of Children's Hospital — sat down to reminisce about changes at the hospital and in medicine.

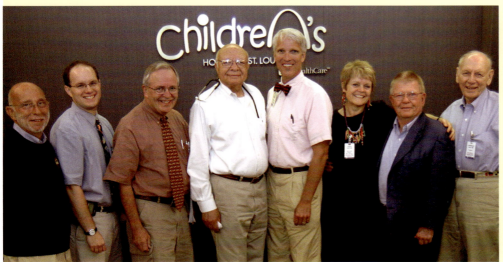

Lawrence Kahn. A 1945 graduate of Louisiana State University School of Medicine, he interned at City Hospital #1 in St. Louis. After Medical Corps service in the U.S. Army, he returned in 1948 for two years as a house officer at Children's Hospital, followed by a one-year research fellowship. In private practice from 1951-1969 he then joined the full-time faculty until his retirement in 1992.

Homer E. Nash, Jr. A 1951 Meharry Medical School graduate, he did an internship at Mt. Sinai Hospital in Chicago. From 1952 to 1955, as a pediatric resident at Homer G. Phillips Hospital, he first came to Children's Hospital for Friday conferences. He was appointed to the Medical Staff in 1955; he and his sister, pediatrician Helen Nash, were the first African-American physicians on staff at Children's Hospital. He has been in private practice in St. Louis since 1955, and won the Distinguished Service Award in 1998.

Paul Simons. A 1967 School of Medicine graduate, he did his residency training, followed by a one-year chief residency, at the Bronx Municipal Hospital Center from 1967 to 1971. After a stint with the Public Health Service in New Orleans, he came back to St. Louis in 1973, practicing at Forest Park Pediatrics.

Asked about their recollections of Children's Hospital:

Dr. Nash: One of my most vivid memories is that cage elevator in the old hospital. You got on it and just hoped it ran. We got stuck once between the second and third floors, and it took a while to get us out.

Dr. Kahn: Notable people used to come, as they still do, to visit children on the floors. One day, Stan Musial, Red Schoendienst, and two or three other star Cardinals came to the hospital, got on that elevator — and the future World Series contenders were stuck.

Dr. Wool: I don't know if any of you younger people know what an iron lung looked like. When I was a resident, we had an Infectious Disease Ward that had six or seven iron lungs with polio victims inside.

Dr. Kahn: The infants ward on the third floor was the nerve center of the hospital. It was the largest ward, and a woman named Dottie Glahn, now Herweg, was the chief nurse on that ward. She was an extraordinary nurse, with three to four nurses under her, and they were all amazing.

Dr. Lonsway: Do you remember the summers at Children's Hospital? Only about four rooms were air-conditioned. In June 1951, when I started, we had by my actual count 15 days in a row over 100 degrees! The cystic fibrosis (CF) patients would come in sweating and dehydrated, so they got the air-conditioned rooms.

Dr. Simons: I came in the middle 1960s, and Spoehrer Tower hadn't even been built yet. We were in the old facility, with really cramped wards, and the space was terrible. Everything was jammed together.

Dr. Wolff: Remember the winters with a whole room full of croup tents — and you couldn't see any of the kids? Were the patients inside alive or dead? There were no monitors, no anything.

Dr. Lonsway: My father [physician Maurice Lonsway, Sr.] told a story from 1917. There was only a 25-watt bulb in the ER and you couldn't even see the patients, much less diagnose what was wrong with them. Well, he lost his head and bought a 100-watt bulb with his own money and put it in. The next day, someone came down with two employees and a ladder, took out the 100-watt bulb, and put back a 25-watt bulb.

Dr. Wolff: I notice that the people around the table, older than I, are all men. Were there any women then?

Dr. Lonsway: Yes, there were lots of them. Hulda Wultmann was a chief resident when I was here in the early 50s.

Dr. Kahn: One intern at Children's Hospital during the 1930s was Helen Aff-Drum, and a chief resident during the 40s was Jane Erganian. I think the hospital was notable for having women.

Dr. Wool: Jessie Ternberg was the first pediatric surgeon. They were all good.

Dr. Putnam: Times have really changed! My class of interns was 75 percent women: five men and 15 women.

How has the role of the clinical faculty changed? And relations between Children's Hospital and its clinical faculty?

Dr. Wolff: In 1979, I had just finished my residency and they asked me to be an attending. It was a huge amount of work. One time my son, who was two, was sick and couldn't go to the babysitter, but I still had to come, make rounds, and give a talk to the house officers. He had a little blanket and was lying on the ground; halfway through, he got up and threw up in the wastebasket, then lay back down. It was what you had to do to survive as a mother and a doctor; kids had to be extremely low maintenance.

Dr. Kieffer: One memory from my training is the esteem that Children's Hospital had for our foremothers and forefathers in medicine, so I had a chance to work with doctors who had been in practice a long time, like Dr. Goldring, Dr. Kahn, Dr. Nash and his sister, Dr. Ternberg, and so forth. When I was a student, these physicians were still teaching; and despite the burgeoning of technology in our era, the 1980s and 90s, we got to listen to heart murmurs with Dr. Goldring and talk about how to make diagnoses the way they did in the old days. That is still a reasonable way to practice medicine, as a community pediatrician, because you don't have every new gadget in your office.

Dr. Putnam: I'm listening to these good stories and, though I'm a doctor too, it's a totally different experience now. Some of the procedures and diseases you guys dealt with I have read about in history books. I think Children's Hospital has become a place where kids that the house staff takes care of are often sicker, with more unusual problems, whereas community pediatricians can handle things that once landed children in the hospital. With new technology, better diagnosis, and better treatment, these kids now get oral antibiotics and stay home. At the same time, I think the hospital is still a welcome place for a person like me. A primary care doctor can come in and rub elbows with people who spend a lot of time in the labs to see where we are going next.

Dr. Simons: It's interesting to see the transition we've gone through, in looking at the different chairmen and their philosophies. Harvey [Colten] was very interested in pulling community physicians in: I remember his once-a-month meetings, having community physicians come and tell him their complaints. He was sensitive to that.

Dr. Lonsway: Let's talk about Philip Dodge. When he came in, it was a joy; I watched him handle the other heads of the departments in the medical school, and he was smooth. The whole atmosphere here changed because of him. He brought in Dick Marshall, and we had a newborn nursery because of him. He brought in Jim Keating.

Dr. Wool: I loved Phil Dodge; he was my chief. Once when I was on an air force base in Alaska, I had a patient with an ear infection. I gave him tetracycline for it, but he came down with papilledema (optic nerve edema), and I didn't know why. So I called down here and Phil Dodge said there was some evidence that tetracycline could cause that. He told me not to worry, to take him off tetracycline, and he'd be better in two days. He was teaching me from 4,000 miles away.

Dr. Simons: There was a window of time when this was not a very good facility. Phil Dodge arrived just as I left after medical school for training. When I came back to Dodge's department, the change was like night and day. All of a sudden he had a phenomenal faculty, had attracted really good house officers. Phil was the reason why this became a first-class facility again, then Harvey [Colten] expanded on that.

Dr. Wool: When you talk to people, they can't believe how nice everyone is here. We have a word for that in Jewish-Yiddish: 'hamish,' which means a down-to-earth personality.

Dr. Simons: You mention Jim Keating. You could always pick up the phone and call him with questions. If you had been one of his residents, you might be a little scared for the first five years of practice. But after that...

Dr. Kahn: It is not so much a difference between this Children's and other children's hospitals; it's the difference between Children's Hospital and other hospitals in St. Louis. I think there is an extraordinary difference in the feeling of caring for patients; I don't think that happens to the same degree in many other places.

Dr. Kieffer: Just walking into the building, you realize this is a children's hospital. At the front door, you are greeted by a hot-air balloon going up and down, pictures of children on the wall, a train going around. How can you not think about children getting better when you see that?

You have talked about the smells, tastes, sights, and tactile sensations of the hospital. What about sounds?

Dr. Kahn: In the old hospital, the wind would blow and the gratings on the windows rattled. It was one of the things that convinced people that if we didn't build another hospital, we would have to condemn the other one anyway.

Dr. Wolff: I remember very few kids crying; there were more kids crying in my office than here.

Dr. Putnam: When I was an intern, I was on 12W, trying to get some sleep, when I was awakened by a helicopter, part of the transport service, landing just above me. At the same time, I recall trying to convince a kid who'd just lost a tooth on that floor that it was the tooth fairy coming by helicopter.

Dr. Nash: There has been constant improvement. They didn't fix it all at the same time, but bit by bit it all got fixed. At one time, there was nothing, and gradually it all evolved into a big something, and at every phase it has been sort of spectacular to me, to watch it grow, since my first contact in 1952. Now, 54 years later, I wonder what they will do in the next 50 years? It will be a hard act to follow.

Peter B. Kieffer. His family's connection with Washington University goes back a century to his great-grandfather, Alonzo Kieffer, a surgical and anatomy professor at the medical school. Peter Kieffer graduated from the School of Medicine in 1990, and then did his residency training at Children's Hospital from 1990-1993. Afterwards, he went into private practice in Overland, where he remains today.

Peter Putnam. A 1997 graduate of Dartmouth Medical School, he came to St. Louis in 1997 and did his pediatric residency at Children's Hospital for three years, followed by one year as chief resident. He entered private practice with Esse Health in 2001.

Gerald Wool. In 1960, while a medical student at Washington University, he rounded at Children's Hospital — and decided to become a pediatrician. He graduated from medical school in 1962, then was a resident at Children's Hospital and chief resident for the following year. After serving in the military during the Vietnam War, he came back to private practice with The Children's Clinic in St. Louis, retiring in 2002.

Maurice Lonsway, Jr. A 1950 School of Medicine graduate and resident from 1951-1953 at Children's Hospital, he did a fellowship at Children's Hospital in Boston, then returned to St. Louis in 1954 to open The Children's Clinic, retiring in 1993. He received the Distinguished Service Award in 1994. His father, Maurice Lonsway, Sr., had been a resident in the old Maternity Hospital on Jefferson Avenue, located across from a dairy, where "the smell was unbelievable. He was very glad to leave it and come to the new environs of Children's Hospital." Lonsway, Jr., used to round with his father, enticed by "a wonderful drug store in the nurse's building, where they had chocolate sundaes with cherries on top."

Patricia B. Wolff. A 1972 graduate of the University of Minnesota Medical School, who did her pediatric internship at the University of Colorado, she came to Children's Hospital in 1975 as a second-year resident and, in 1976-1977, continued on to do a pediatric fellowship in endocrinology/metabolism. She is a pediatrician in private practice with Forest Park Pediatrics.

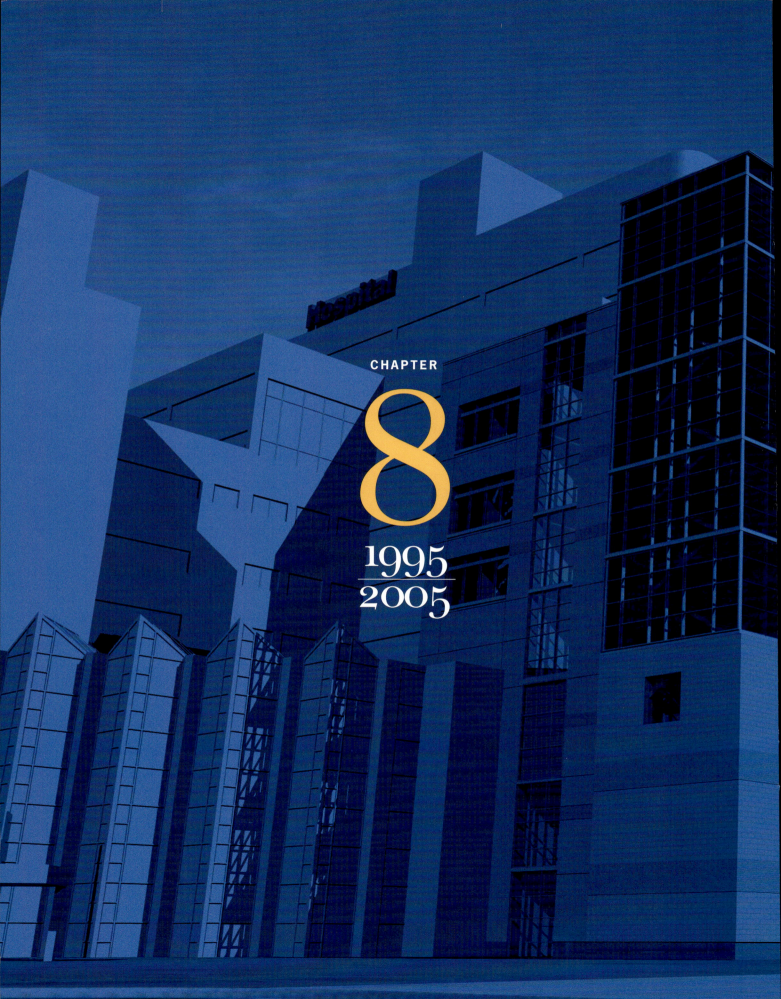

CHAPTER

8

1995
/
2005

New Millennium: Synergy, Progress, and the Promise of Discovery

CHAPTER EIGHT NEW MILLENNIUM: SYNERGY, PROGRESS, AND THE PROMISE OF DISCOVERY

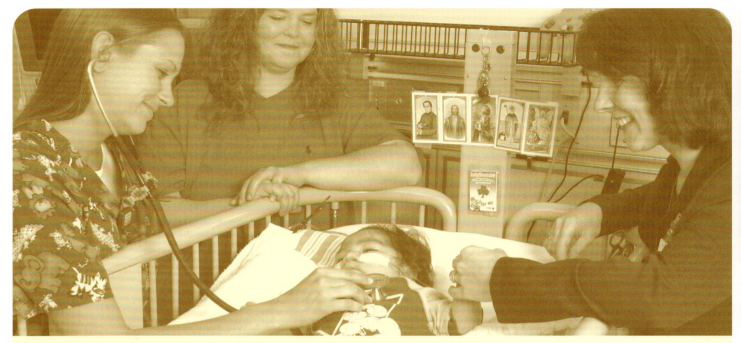

BELOW **Ted W. Frey.** In 1971, Frey joined Children's Hospital as director of fiscal services, became chief operating officer in 1986, and president of the hospital and the hospital's foundation in 1995. "Ted's dedication to doing what's right for kids has been a guiding force at Children's Hospital," said Louis J. Fusz, Jr., hospital board chairman. "That standard motivates him to go the extra mile in serving patients and their families but also has influenced the hospital's increased emphasis on community outreach efforts." Becker Medical Library

Family-Centered Care. Karen Crow (right), family-centered care coordinator, visits with Rebecca Briagas, whose son Agustin received a double-lung transplant at the hospital in 2004. In the mid-90s, Children's Hospital adopted family-centered care concepts that more fully engage parents as active participants in their child's care. Becker Medical Library. Photo by Kimberly Keefe

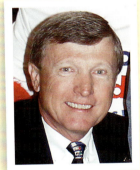

It was a year of seismic administrative change.

In 1995, both of the top pediatric positions in the medical center — the presidency of Children's Hospital and the chairmanship of the Department of Pediatrics — needed to be filled. In addition, the Children's Hospital Board of Trustees announced a new slate of officers, including Martin K. Sneider as chairman and a cohort of first-time members, among them Fred L. Brown, president and chief executive officer of the organization that had recently merged with Children's Hospital: the BJC Health System. In still another move, infectious disease specialist Penelope G. Shackelford became medical staff president.

PREVIOUS PAGE **A computer rendering shows the hospital's east expansion, scheduled to open during winter 2006.** Becker Medical Library
INSET ***Child* magazine named St. Louis Children's Hospital one of the top 10 U.S. Pediatric Hospitals in 2003.** Becker Medical Library

1995
Penelope Shackelford becomes Medical Staff president.

1995
Ted W. Frey is named the new president and senior executive officer of the hospital.

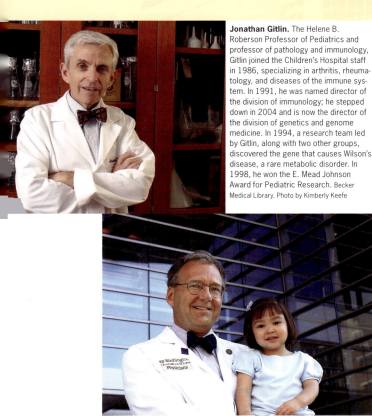

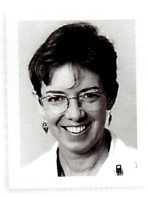

Jonathan Gitlin. The Helene B. Roberson Professor of Pediatrics and professor of pathology and immunology, Gitlin joined the Children's Hospital staff in 1986, specializing in arthritis, rheumatology, and diseases of the immune system. In 1991, he was named director of the division of immunology; he stepped down in 2004 and is now the director of the division of genetics and genome medicine. In 1994, a research team led by Gitlin, along with two other groups, discovered the gene that causes Wilson's disease, a rare metabolic disorder. In 1998, he won the E. Mead Johnson Award for Pediatric Research. Becker Medical Library. Photo by Kimberly Keefe

Penelope G. Shackleford. A 1968 School of Medicine graduate, she joined the faculty in 1972 and was director of the division of pediatric infectious diseases. In 1998, she was named director of the new division of pediatric ambulatory medicine. Her research interests include the development of the immune system. Becker Medical Library

LEFT **Alan L. Schwartz**. A graduate of Case-Western Reserve University in 1974 and its medical school in 1976, Schwartz did his residency at Children's Hospital Medical Center in Boston. He served on the faculty of Harvard University from 1979 to 1986 before joining the pediatric faculty at Washington University School of Medicine, where he became head of pediatrics in 1995. His research focuses on receptor cell biology, intracellular trafficking of molecules, protein turnover, and the regulation of blood coagulation. Becker Medical Library. Photo by Kimberly Keefe

Yet despite this upheaval, it was also a year in which everyone was eager to maintain continuity. Both Children's Hospital and the Department of Pediatrics — set on successful trajectories — were aiming to move forward, but not with revolutionary plans. At Children's Hospital, the main hurdle was adjusting to the BJC merger. And the pediatrics department, after Harvey Colten stepped down, "had a good set of division directors, was in sound financial condition, had a good relationship with its cognate Children's Hospital, and had a good reputation within the University. Many of the things that most pediatric departments around the country lack within their medical centers were already in place," said neonatologist F. Sessions Cole later.

In choosing a successor for Alan Brass, the Children's Hospital board turned to an internal candidate who was well known to them. Ted W. Frey — a 25-year veteran of the hospital administration, who had joined the staff in 1971 as director of fiscal services and was later executive vice president and chief operating officer — became the new president and senior executive officer. One goal, he said, was building an even closer relationship with the Children's Hospital medical staff. "I plan to fully involve physicians in all major decisions affecting our future direction in our shared concern for the health and well-being of the children and families we serve," he said then.

After an international search that included some external as well as two other internal candidates — Cole and cardiology director Arnold Strauss — Alan L. Schwartz, who had spent nearly a decade directing pediatric hematology/oncology, was selected as the new chairman, replacing Harvey Colten. "Dr. Schwartz brings to this most important position outstanding talents as a researcher, clinician, educator and administrator," said William Peck, medical school dean. As for Schwartz himself, he accepted this new position, he said later, because it was "the most exciting pediatric chair in American medicine. The pediatric head sits as a member of the Executive Faculty — and there is no other place in the country where pediatrics has an equal seat at the table with medicine, surgery, and other departments. Here, pediatrics has a voice in every major activity of the School of Medicine, one of the great medical schools in the United States."

1995

STOP (Steps to Prevent Violence) is launched with the American Academy of Pediatrics and the Center to Prevent Handgun Violence.

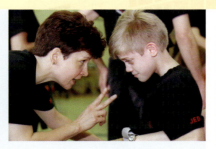

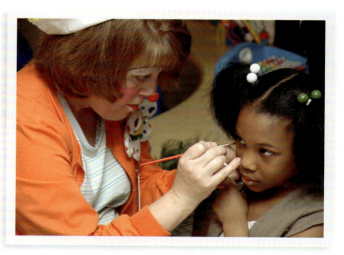

Clown Docs. The Clown Docs program, supported by individual donations, began at Children's Hospital in 1999 at the instigation of School of Medicine cardiology faculty member Dana R. Abendschein and his wife Jane. Here, "Nurse Sniggles" paints the face of Jayla Turner at the hospital's annual "Celebrate Spring" party in child life services. Becker Medical Library. Photo by John Twombly

In 1998, pediatric neurologist Janice E. Brunstrom, who had joined the Department of Neurology in 1995 as a postdoctoral research fellow, founded the Pediatric Neurology Cerebral Palsy Center at Children's Hospital and became its director. Her goal was to create a focal point for research and clinical care, where physicians could devise new therapies that would help cerebral palsy (CP) patients achieve maximum mobility and independence.

Today, this Center serves more than 400 patients with its dedicated staff, also consisting of Michael Noetzel, director of clinical and diagnostic neuroscience; neurology nurse coordinator Sandy Arrick; pediatric nurse practitioner Helen Race; and several occupational and physical therapists. The work of other colleagues also benefits the children at the Center, such as seizure specialist K. Liu Lin Thio, pediatric neurologist Bradley Schlaggar, and orthopaedic surgeon Scott Luhmann. Among their activities is a martial arts program for CP patients, the first of its kind in the U.S.

Through the Carol and Paul Hatfield Cerebral Palsy Sports and Rehabilitation Center, children with CP can participate in camps, swimming, basketball and other physical activities designed to promote increased strength and better body control.

Brunstrom, who has received numerous awards for her work, including the highest honor of the United Cerebral Palsy Women's Board in 2001, is a role model for her patients, since she herself was born with CP. "I tell [my patients] up front," she said in 2001, "that I expect them to do their very best and give something back to the world."

Cerebral Palsy Center. Jan Brunstrom, director of the hospital's Cerebral Palsy Center, talks to 10-year-old Jedediah Farmer at a 2001 martial arts class sponsored by the Center. Becker Medical Library. Photo by Tim Parker

EARLY ADVANCES

As a condition of his hiring, Schwartz had asked for a giant financial commitment that would make possible the construction of a pediatric research building, planned along unconventional lines. Instead of research space organized by division, this new facility would place investigators exploring similar research themes alongside one another, regardless of divisional affiliation, in laboratories built without walls between them. An important spur to this project was the growth in pediatric research over the previous decade, with research grants now totaling more than $11 million annually. Most came from the National Institutes of Health (NIH), which named the Department of Pediatrics a Child Health Research Center of Excellence in 1995. "I did not feel that pediatrics had ever taken full advantage of the depth and breadth of the research environment at the School of Medicine — not even within its own talent pool in pediatrics — and I wanted to help to catalyze that," said Schwartz later.

In 1998 came the official announcement that this 10-story, 226,000-square-foot building, designed by architect Ralph Johnson with major input from Schwartz, would go up, with six of its floors dedicated to pediatric research laboratories. Scientists previously housed in five different sites around campus would now be located in one place, thus freeing up space on the tenth and eleventh floors of Children's Hospital for expansion. In this new building, scientists would devote their work to projects within four broad research themes: developmental biology; molecular and cellular biology; immunity, infection, and inflammation; and patient-oriented research. The financial underpinning of this project was a monumental $20 million gift from James S. McDonnell III, John F. McDonnell, and the JSM Charitable Trust.

In the midst of sweeping facilities changes across the entire medical center, other building projects were also proceeding. In November 1995, a ground-breaking ceremony took place

1995
U.S. Rep. Richard Gephardt visits the hospital to discuss the impact of new Medicaid legislation, which reduced the number of insured patients in most hospitals, including Children's.

1995
Alan L. Schwartz becomes the new head of pediatrics, replacing Harvey Colten.

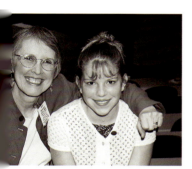

Barbara Cole. Pictured here with patient Shannon Mattie, Cole was a member of the hospital's medical staff for 30 years, and was director of the division of nephrology from 1988 until her retirement in 2001. The hospital's annual Quality Award is named in her honor. Becker Medical Library

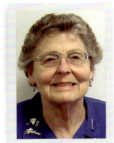

Dorothy Hanpeter. A volunteer at Children's Hospital for 28 years, retired teacher Dorothy Hanpeter focuses on reassuring parents of surgical patients in the same-day surgery waiting room. Becker Medical Library

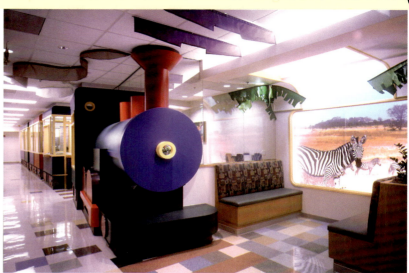

Dana Brown Emergency Unit. A Pediatric Level 1 Trauma Center, this facility was renovated to appeal to children, with its zoo-themed waiting area and registration space that looks like a train. It is named for businessman and philanthropist Dana Brown, who died in 1994. Becker Medical Library

on South Newstead for an expanded Child Development Center, with room for 235 employee children. In that same month, the hospital also announced a $21.5 million expansion plan — some 31,475 square feet in all — that would accomplish several things: more than double space in the emergency room, re-named the Dana Brown Emergency Unit; develop the Hale Irwin Center for Pediatric Hematology/Oncology; create space for a future expansion of the Pediatric Intensive Care Unit; and expand the ambulatory surgery area. The hospital also launched a major re-engineering effort, planned by 15 teams of staff members and community physicians who worked together to create efficient new systems while also reducing costs.

SCHWARTZ-FREY ERA ACCOMPLISHMENTS

Together, Schwartz and Frey began actively moving to fill key positions both from the existing medical staff and from outside it. From within, Schwartz appointed Cole as the first vice chairman of the pediatrics department, taking charge of such external affairs as government relations; in another internal move, David B. Wilson, a 1986 M.D./Ph.D. graduate of the School of Medicine, became the new director of the pediatric hematology/oncology division. From outside, Schwartz recruited others to expand this division, including Robert J. Hayashi. Charles B. Huddleston was named director of the division of cardiothoracic surgery, while Richard Todd was appointed psychiatrist-in-chief. In 1998, Joseph St. Geme III became director of the division of infectious diseases succeeding Penelope G. Shackelford, who moved over to head the new division of pediatric ambulatory medicine. George S. Bassett became the first full-time chief of pediatric orthopaedics, Steven D. Shapiro the director of the division of allergy and pulmonary medicine, and Neil White the director of endocrinology and metabolism.

Thanks to an initiative called the "Joint Chairs Program," involving cooperation between Children's Hospital and the School of Medicine, four new named professorships were added in 1998 as F. Sessions Cole became the Park J. White, MD, Professor of Pediatrics; James P. Keating, the W. McKim Marriott, MD, St. Louis Children's Hospital Professor of Pediatrics; Jeffrey L. Marsh, the Apolline Blair St. Louis Children's Hospital Professor of Surgery; and Arnold W. Strauss, the Alumni Professor of Pediatrics, succeeding Schwartz, now the Harriet B. Spoehrer Professor. Two more were established in 2000. One, the Helene B. Roberson professorship of pediatrics, was awarded to immunologist Jonathan Gitlin, while the Dana Brown/St. Louis

NOVEMBER 1995

1995 — The National Institutes of Health (NIH) names the Department of Pediatrics a Child Health Research Center of Excellence.

1995 — Ground is broken for an expanded Child Development Center.

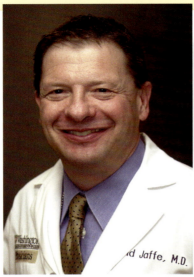

David Jaffe. First chair of the Division of Pediatric Emergency Medicine and the Dana Brown/St. Louis Children's Hospital Professor of Pediatrics, Jaffe oversees the Emergency Department — third-largest in Missouri — which treats 50,000 children each year. Jaffe is widely known as a founder of the field of pediatric emergency medicine. Becker Medical Library

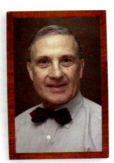

Gordon R. Bloomberg. A resident at Children's Hospital, Bloomberg went on to spend 39 years in private practice, with a subspecialty in pediatric allergy. He then joined the full-time faculty of the department of pediatrics, pursuing his interest in asthma research, especially among inner-city children. He served as medical staff president from 1998 to 2000. Becker Medical Library

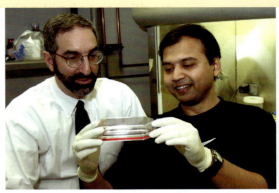

David H. Gutmann. A neurologist who joined the hospital staff in 1994, Gutmann became director of a new, multi-disciplinary center specializing in research and clinical care for neurofibromatosis, a complex genetic disorder that causes tumors to grow on nerves in the brain and body. Gutmann, the Donald O. Schnuck Family Professor of Neurology and professor of genetics and pediatrics, is a national expert on this disorder. He is shown here with postdoctoral researcher Biplab Gasgupta in the lab. Washington University School of Medicine

Children's Hospital professorship was given to emergency medicine head David Jaffe, the first such chair in the country.

The new administration kept a sharp focus on residency selection and training, which by the 1990s involved a considerable winnowing effort. In 1996, the program had nearly 700 applicants; from this pool, some 200 were interviewed and 22 selected from an array of medical schools that included Michigan, Rochester, Duke, Vanderbilt, Baylor, the University of Chicago, and Washington University. One attraction for these students was the highly successful COPE program, in which 67 community pediatricians now participated. It received the Outstanding Teaching Award for 1996 from the Ambulatory Pediatric Association.

With the help of the Medical Staff, now under the leadership of pediatrician Gordon R. Bloomberg, and with the participation of the full-time medical faculty, Children's Hospital increased its emphasis on quality with the founding of the Quality Improvement Council in 1997, followed the next year by the Office of Pediatric Quality Management (OPQM), directed by Barbara R. Cole and Gary LaBlance. In 1999, the OPQM established the Family Advisory Council,

memories *Kathleen Long*

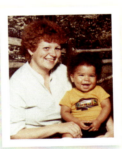

Photo courtesy of Kathleen Long

Kathleen Long, RRT, NPS, day shift coordinator of respiratory therapy, came to Children's Hospital in 1979 from Jewish Hospital, where she worked in pathology. She did on-the-job training in respiratory therapy, concurrently obtaining an associate's degree in that field. At first, she was a certified respiratory therapy technician, then passed an exam to become a registered respiratory therapist (RRT). In 2000, she passed the pediatric neonatal specialty exam (NPS). She was a staff therapist until 10 years ago, when she was promoted to coordinator.

"When my son, Kameron Harper, was born in March 1979, I was a smoker, so he had a few respiratory issues as a baby — frequent colds, pneumonia, wheezing — and I didn't know why. He even ended up at Children's a couple of times, and one of the therapists, Alice Hemphill, taught me how to do postural drainage to clear his lungs. I realized that maybe he had those problems because I smoked. It took me until 1984 to quit but finally I did and now he is 27, completely well.

"Between Kameron being admitted and Alice teaching me, it sparked my interest, so one day I went over and talked to Children's Hospital about a job. Alice happened to be there the day I applied, and she told my boss, Mike Gruzeski, 'She knows postural drainage, hire her!' Children's was paying 20 cents an hour more than Jewish: $4.48 hour. That was appealing to me because I was a single mom and needed the money — I thought 'maybe I'll work there for a while.'

"I have been here ever since. Children's can still be hard if kids are really sick or don't make it, but there are so many success stories that I can't imagine working anywhere else."

1996

The Health Insurance Portability and Accountability Act of 1996 (HIPAA) is enacted with government-mandated privacy rules.

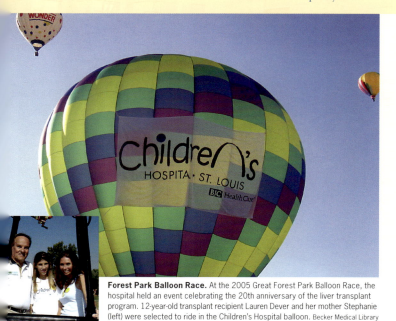

Forest Park Balloon Race. At the 2005 Great Forest Park Balloon Race, the hospital held an event celebrating the 20th anniversary of the liver transplant program. 12-year-old transplant recipient Lauren Dever and her mother Stephanie (left) were selected to ride in the Children's Hospital balloon. Becker Medical Library

which sought advice from parents whose children required frequent hospital care, and a year later Children's Hospital launched the successful "Waste and Waits" quality improvement program. In 1994, the hospital also began offering "CARES," an after-hour, referral-only emergency care service, headed by Brian Skrainka and later by pediatrician Douglas Carlson.

Meanwhile, Children's Hospital physicians — full-time faculty and part-time clinical faculty alike — benefited from the Washington University Physician Network (WUPN), which negotiated equitable payer contracts. Complicating the work of all these physicians, however, was a new federal policy: government-mandated privacy rules in the Health Insurance Portability and Accountability Act of 1996 (HIPAA) program.

CLINICAL AND RESEARCH ADVANCES

Research grants helped bolster the critical work done by physician-scientists. In 1997, pathologist Carl H. Smith, director of the clinical laboratories, received a $1.1 million grant to study cellular mechanisms of the transfer of nutrients from a mother to her unborn baby; in the same year, Alan L. Schwartz received a $1.1 million grant to investigate a cell surface receptor molecule, LRP, that his group had discovered in 1990, as well as

memories T.S. Park

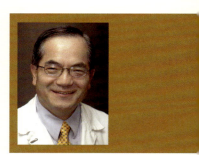

Today, T.S. Park is the Shi H. Huang Professor of Neurological Surgery, professor of pediatrics and of anatomy and neurobiology, and neurosurgeon-in-chief at St. Louis Children's Hospital. In 1971, he earned his medical degree from Yonsei University in Seoul, Korea, then did his neurosurgery residency at the University of Virginia, followed by a pediatric neurosurgery fellowship at the University of Toronto. In 1990, he came to St. Louis from the University of Virginia, where he was an associate professor of neurological surgery and pediatrics. He has earned international acclaim for advancing the selective dorsal rhizotomy procedure in children with spastic cerebral palsy.

"When I came here in 1990, pediatric neurosurgery was not a full-fledged service; at first, I did not even have a chair or a desk, and my telephone was on the floor. I had no clinic, no operating room, and no equipment either, so I saw the patients in my office. I'm sorry I didn't take a picture of the scene.

"Actually, I hadn't expected to have these things ready when I arrived. When I was recruited from the University of Virginia, I said we would build it all together. So I gave Ralph Dacey, the chief of neurosurgery, a wish list when I came — and that was all I needed. The hospital administrators — Alan Brass, Ted Frey — and I never wrote any letters back and forth: We just talked and solved any problems that way. I have the highest admiration for those people; they were really dedicated to this institution.

"Basically, we built a whole new program together, including a clinic, office space, and an operating room. Today, we are one of premier pediatric neurosurgery programs in the world, with patients from some 34 countries. But I have great memories of building the program here, and I always felt that I had wonderful support."

1996

The heart and lung transplant programs at the hospital each mark a milestone: their 100th transplant.

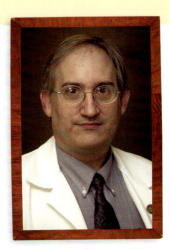

Aaron Hamvas. A 1981 School of Medicine graduate and resident from 1981 to 1984, Hamvas did a fellowship in newborn medicine at Children's Hospital from 1987 to 1990 and is today medical director of the Neonatal Intensive Care Unit. Becker Medical Library

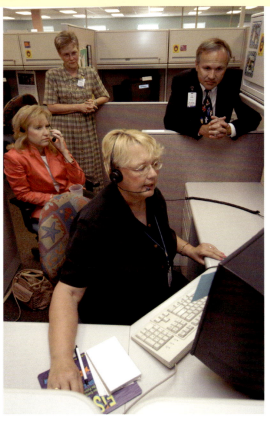

another $1.1 million grant to continue studying molecular mechanisms for the regulation of protein degradation within the cell. Neurosurgeon-in-chief T.S. Park — among a handful of pediatric neurosurgeons nationwide to receive such funding — won a $1.2 million grant from the NIH to study the inflammatory response that can damage blood vessels in newborn brains. A Specialized Center Research grant in cardiology, awarded to Arnold Strauss and colleagues from the National Heart, Lung and Blood Institute in 1999, funded research into the basic molecular mechanisms responsible for heart formation, while David Perlmutter won an important program project grant from the NIH to investigate the cellular pathogenesis of pediatric liver disease.

Surgery also advanced with new procedures. In 1995, orthopaedic surgeon Keith H. Bridwell did a ground-breaking spinal fusion procedure on a 14-year-old scoliosis patient, who had earlier undergone a heart and double-lung transplant performed by cardiothoracic surgeon Eric N. Mendeloff. The heart and lung transplant programs each marked their 100th transplant in the following year; by 1997, more than 60 percent of all pediatric lung transplants in the nation were taking place at Children's Hospital. The transplant programs also pioneered procedures such as a combined lung and liver transplant, as well as a living donor lung transplant and later a living donor liver transplant, performed by surgeon Jeffrey Lowell.

Other areas made significant progress. Under Rodney P. Lusk, the otolaryngology program remained a pioneer in sinus surgery for children, while the Cleft Palate and Craniofacial Deformities Institute led in the treatment of facial deformities. Jonathan Gitlin continued his ground-breaking work on the role of copper and iron in human biology, T.S. Park performed his 500th selective dorsal rhizotomy procedure on a five-year-old patient in 1997, and the cochlear implant program celebrated its 100th procedure. The Cystic Fibrosis Center, under the direction of pulmonologist George B. Mallory, Jr., had grown to one of the 10 largest in the United States; the Childhood Asthma Management Program (CAMP) published new research on inhaled steroids. Children's Hospital also launched a new Adolescent Center, under the direction of pediatrician Lynn White, and a hospitalist program under physicians Douglas Carlson and Jeffrey Dawson. In 1996, the pediatric dentistry program began the only hospital-based program in the region for special-needs children. The outpatient pain management

1996
The COPE program receives the Outstanding Teaching Award from the Ambulatory Pediatric Association.

1997
A collaborative ambulatory services program is begun with Missouri Baptist Medical Center.

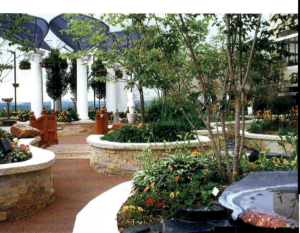

Olson Family Garden. This 8,000-square-foot garden, located on the eighth floor, is a rooftop space — home to more than 7,000 plants and flowers — designed for children and families who need a place for quiet reflection. It is named for donors Bruce and Kim Olson. Becker Medical Library

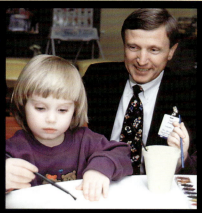

Ted Frey. Hospital president Ted Frey enjoys the company of three-year-old patient Laura Jenkins as she gets creative in the Child Life Services playroom. Becker Medical Library

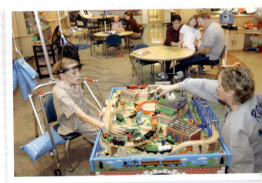

BELOW **Child Life Services.** In 1963, Marian Alexander lost her daughter to leukemia, and afterwards became a dedicated volunteer at Children's Hospital. Altogether, she contributed some 25,000 hours of time, particularly in the Child Life Services activity room. That room, which offers arts and crafts, board games, a teen lounge, and a school room, has been renamed in her honor. Becker Medical Library

program, begun in 1992 as one of only a handful in the United States, continued to expand under director M. Barry Jones.

And Children's Hospital worked with other hospitals in the region on cooperative ventures to help children. Under the umbrella of Project ARK (AIDS/HIV Resources for Kids), established in 1995, hospitals throughout the area that treated HIV-positive children combined their medical, psychosocial, and educational services. Children's Hospital and SSM Cardinal Glennon Children's Hospital also began coordinating their government relations efforts.

THE BJC MERGER

Under the aegis of the BJC Health System, Children's Hospital and its staff began working toward effective consolidation. As BJC's new head of regional pediatrics, F. Sessions Cole was charged with creating a regional, integrated healthcare delivery system. In 1997, the St. Louis Metropolitan Pediatric Council — made up of medical staff members and administrators from throughout the system — met to formulate a coordinated vision of which pediatric goals and strategies to pursue for the immediate future. They established a list of seven on which to focus: clinical and service quality, health status and child advocacy, service delivery coordination, service development and accessibility, organizational effectiveness and internal relationship development, cost management, and marketing and external relationship development.

Other partnerships also began to develop, such as the collaborative ambulatory services program with Missouri Baptist Medical Center in 1997. New services, including a new pediatric hospice program — the first in the area — became available to patients from throughout the system. Building on the experience of the Missouri Baptist alliance, Children's Hospital also forged a partnership with Christian Hospital Northwest Hospital.

But the merger with BJC hit some rough spots in the early years. Suddenly, Children's Hospital administrators were no longer the last word in decision-making for the hospital. One of the disputed areas was legislative lobbying, which had previously been done for Children's Hospital by a dedicated lobbyist, familiar with children's special health care needs. Now BJC consolidated that job with advocacy for the medical center's adult-focused hospitals — and thus, in the view of Children's Hospital administrators, diluted the message. With time, Children's acquired its own lobbyist again, as BJC recognized the need to separate the two functions.

Another issue was BJC's implementation of a

1997
The cochlear implant program celebrates its 100th procedure.

1997
The Adolescent Center is launched.

memories *Velma Hunt*

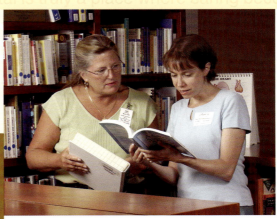

Family Resource Center. Laura Noce, left, health information nurse in the hospital's Family Resource Center and Georgiana Ladas Grant, FRC librarian, help parents access information from the Center's library of child health and disease materials. Becker Medical Library

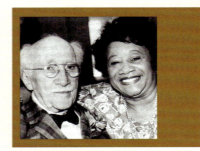

Velma Hunt and Park J. White in 1987.

Velma Hunt, who has worked at Children's Hospital since 1957, has been called "an angel" by grateful families. She has held various jobs over the years: aide, wardmaster, the first African-American evening intake supervisor, patient welcoming coordinator, and since her retirement from full-time work in 1995, a patient liaison in the Emergency Room. All the while, she has shown exemplary devotion to the hospital. As physician Neil Middelkamp puts it, "Mrs. Hunt can resolve virtually any situation with her knowledge of the hospital and her endowed calm and compassion. She is always very helpful to the parents and patients even when they are agitated, concerned, lost, or whatever." Velma Hunt's son, Ken Hunt, has worked as a unit secretary in the neonatal intensive care unit for 26 years.

"Some of us live many years and never know what our calling is — but I know mine. I had never had any thought of working in a hospital, but Dr. Park White, who was a member at Pilgrim Congregational Church UCC when I joined, was responsible for my being here. Now everything I do, I do in his memory.

"It has been a joy and a privilege to work here, and in 1960 when I lost my oldest son, Albert Hunt III, who drowned at age 12 on a Boy Scout trip, I wouldn't have been able to cope if it hadn't been for Children's Hospital.

"Today, I try to be useful, that's all I can say. When parents are waiting in the emergency room with their children, we need everyone's eyes and ears open. For example, I have learned to look at the child who is covered up. One time we had a family with twins, and the mother indicated that one of the babies was ill. When I pulled the blanket back, the baby was smiling. I had a strange feeling and asked to see the other one — and he was turning blue! By following my intuition, we were able to avoid a tragedy.

"It bothers me that some people in the community are not aware of what a great gem they have sitting here in the middle of St. Louis. The founders of Children's Hospital had a vision. We as stewards must preserve that vision and continue to carry on this sanctuary for all of God's children."

new approach to Medicaid patients. Even before the merger, the University had begun working with the medical center hospitals to establish their own Medicaid-affiliated health plan, CarePartners HMO. Now BJC decided to limit its managed care coverage to only two Medicaid-affiliated plans — CarePartners and Health Care USA, a privately sponsored program — omitting two other large plans. That meant Children's Hospital had access to only 65 percent of the Medicaid population. In part as a result of this change, the number of Medicaid patients seen in the Emergency Room dropped by some 20 percent within a year; inpatient volume also fell off. The access problem for Children's Hospital was alleviated early in 2004, when BJC expanded its coverage to a third Medicaid-managed plan.

CHILD AND FAMILY ADVOCACY

Advocacy efforts — legislative, educational, medical, and community — continued to gain importance. One example was the STOP (Steps to Prevent Violence) campaign, launched in 1995 with the American Academy of Pediatrics and the Center to Prevent Handgun Violence; another was the Children's Hospital Injury Prevention Coalition, a safety education program coordinated by emergency unit charge nurse Angie Klocke. Some physicians also moved into an advocacy role, such as F. Sessions Cole, a supporter of prenatal care. In addition, the hospital began giving advocacy awards to

1997

The Quality Improvement Council is founded.

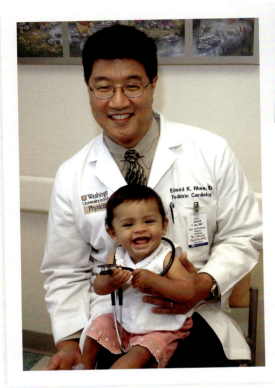

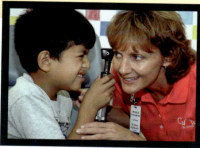

Putting patients first. Jesus Portillo playfully checks the ear of Michelle Radomski of the Healthy Kids Express mobile health van team. The reverse role-playing puts children at ease before their health screening. Becker Medical Library

LEFT **Edward Rhee with Damaris Ochoa.** In 2004, five-month-old baby Damaris Ochoa of Kansas City, treated at Children's Hospital by Edward Rhee, director of electrophysiology and arrhythmia services, became the youngest child ever to receive a pacemaker for heart failure therapy. Becker Medical Library. Photo by John Twombly

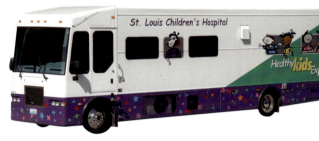

Healthy Kids Express. The hospital's mobile health van outreach program, launched in 2000, was the first of its kind in the area. The van staff serves at-risk children who need routine check-ups and preventive care. Initial funding for the program was provided by the Friends of St. Louis Children's Hospital. Becker Medical Library

people who had improved the lives of children; in 1995, the recipients were Alan Brass for his community advocacy and Gary J. Stangler, director of the Missouri Department of Social Services, for his statewide efforts.

A major thrust of advocacy efforts, both nationally and at the state level, was the expansion of Medicaid benefits, so crucial for uninsured children — and particularly those with chronic illnesses who require frequent hospital care. These were tumultuous times for Medicaid funding, as governments and hospitals often squared off as adversaries, with the governments pressing for greater economy and hospitals for broader coverage. The issue was particularly urgent at Children's Hospital, where nearly half of all patients in 1995 were enrolled in Medicaid.

During the 1990s, the pendulum swung in both directions as new legislation took effect. In 1995, U.S. Rep. Richard Gephardt visited the hospital to discuss the impact of new Medicaid legislation, which reduced the number of insured patients in most hospitals, including Children's Hospital. Then two years later,

Congress enacted the State Children's Health Insurance Program (SCHIP), which helped bridge the gap for low-income working families who earned too much to qualify for Medicaid but also lacked employer-sponsored insurance. In 1998, Gov. Mel Carnahan visited Children's Hospital to sign Senate Bill 632 — the Children's Health Initiative Program — which expanded Medicaid coverage to 90,000 Missouri children previously without insurance, 25,000 of them in the St. Louis area. He received Children's Hospital's Missouri Advocate of the Year award for supporting this legislation.

Several years later, Alan Schwartz said in his annual address, "the ability of providers to reimburse us for our work and commitment is where the challenge lies. In 2002, we saw additional increases to the 45 percent of the state-supported patients for whom we care." The Washington University Physicians and Faculty Practice Plan, led by physician James Crane — the second-largest academic faculty practice in the country — had proved extraordinarily helpful in meeting this challenge, he said.

1997
The Development Board celebrates its 25th anniversary.

1998
The Office of Pediatric Quality Management (OPQM) is established.

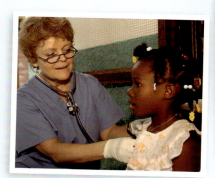

Patricia Wolff with a patient in Haiti.
Courtesy of Patricia Wolff

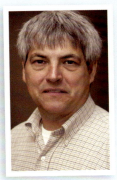

Mark Manary.
Becker Medical Library

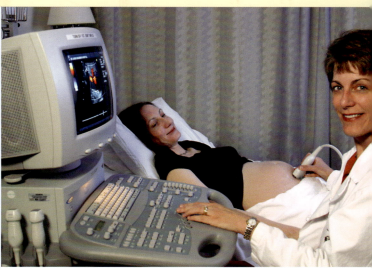

Angela Sharkey. As the director of the hospital's Fetal Heart Center, Sharkey heads a team that specializes in the prenatal screening, diagnosis, and care of fetuses with suspected heart disorders. Becker Medical Library. Photo by Kimberly Keefe

Two Washington University faculty members have been working in distant countries to reduce the devastating problem of childhood malnutrition.

Mark Manary, professor of pediatrics, began a research program in 2001, supported by the St. Louis Children's Hospital Foundation, aimed at saving the lives of starving children in Malawi, one of Africa's poorest countries, where one in eight children die of malnutrition. To help these children, especially toddlers who are most at risk, he uses a novel ready-to-use food — a mixture of peanut butter, sugar, milk powder, oil, and micronutrients — that has had dramatic results. Recovery rates for children who take this mixture for six weeks have soared to 95 percent, as opposed to 25 percent with standard milk-based therapy. Manary is a 1982 graduate of the School of Medicine, who did his residency at Children's Hospital from 1982 to 1985.

In 2004, Patricia B. Wolff, associate professor of clinical pediatrics who also did her residency at Children's Hospital, established a new program: Meds & Food for Kids (MFK). Its aim is to save the lives of dangerously malnourished children in Haiti and other developing countries through medical services, nutrition education, prescription drugs, and the same fortified peanut butter mixture that Manary pioneered. As it is in Malawi, malnutrition is a severe problem in Haiti, where 80 percent of the people live below the poverty line and 129 of every 1,000 children will die before their fifth birthday.

COMMUNITY HEALTH OUTREACH

Just as Children's Hospital expanded its advocacy efforts, it did the same with community outreach, in part through the successful nurse-staffed Answer Line (454-KIDS). To meet the needs of high-risk mothers and infants, the hospital's Maternal Child Program expanded, providing a continuum of care after discharge. A new Mobile Intensive Care Unit — streamlined and enlarged — was introduced in 1998, and in 2000 Children's Hospital launched the first mobile health van of its kind in the area, Healthy Kids Express™, that would bring medical attention to urban elementary and middle schools.

To help inner-city children avoid injury, Children's Hospital used a grant from the Robert Wood Johnson Foundation to build safe playgrounds at area schools; other programs targeted bike helmets, car seat installation, immunization, smoking, and infectious disease prevention. The Safe Kids campaign also stressed the importance of avoiding accidents, while a new coalition of pediatricians, including Alison Nash, worked on such issues as lead poisoning, teen sexuality, mental health, and maternal postpartum education. Through a new partnership with Grace Hill Neighborhood Services health centers, three nurse practitioners helped the Grace Hill staff perform health exams on north St. Louis children.

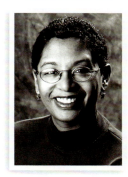

Alison Nash. A St. Louis pediatrician, Alison Nash entered practice in 1989 with her father, pediatrician Homer E. Nash, Jr. She received Children's Hospital's 1998 Community Advocate of the Year award for her tireless work in improving the health of children. She has also been a preceptor in the COPE program. Becker Medical Library

1998
A new Mobile Intensive Care Unit is introduced.

1998
Governor Mel Carnahan signs Senate Bill 632, the Children's Health Initiative Program, at the hospital.

> *"In 1998, U.S. News & World Report's annual guide to "America's Best Hospitals" ranked Children's Hospital as one of the best in the United States."*

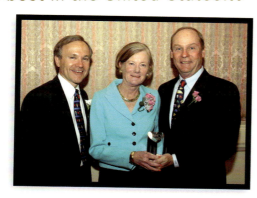

Louis J. Fusz, Jr. Lou Fusz (right) has been an active supporter of the hospital for over 20 years. He is past chairman of the Board of Trustees and served as chairman of the Foundation board from 2005-2006. He and his wife Corie received the hospital's 2004 Heart of Gold award, presented here by Lee Fetter, in recognition of their philanthropic gifts and commitment to child health. Becker Medical Library. Photo by Steve Dolan.

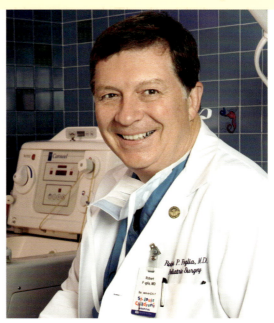

Robert P. Foglia. In 1990, Foglia, formerly on the Harvard Medical School staff and then UCLA, was appointed surgeon-in-chief and director of pediatric general surgery by Children's Hospital and the School of Medicine. Becker Medical Library. Photo by Kimberly Keefe.

Some physicians even extended their help internationally, such as cardiothoracic surgeon Eric Mendeloff and lung transplant coordinator Grace McBride, who volunteered in Trinidad during 2001 as part of a team to repair children's congenital heart defects. Pediatrician Mark Manary began important nutritional work in Malawi; later, clinical faculty member Patricia B. Wolff adapted Manary's findings to save the lives of malnourished toddlers in Haiti.

FUND-RAISING PROGRESS

As they had from the beginning, donors continued to play a critical role in funding the hospital's efforts. In 1995, the NADAH Women's Organization continued their nearly two-decade old tradition when they donated $14,000 to the Cleft Palate and Craniofacial Deformities Institute. In 1997, 26 Children's Circle of Care members — recognized for their gifts of at least $10,000 per year — donated more than $1.4 million to Children's Hospital; and in that same year, a trust left by Louis and Daisy Gutman helped fund bone marrow transplants for children, regardless of their financial circumstances. The Development Board, founded in 1972, celebrated its 25th anniversary in 1997 — having raised a total of $12.8 million.

Annual fund-raising events took place, many of them backed by key sponsor Enterprise Rent-A-Car and the Enterprise Rent-A-Car Foundation: Children's Under the Big Top, the Boone Valley Classic, CAROUSEL, the Children's Hospital Day at Six Flags, the Ladies' Golf Classic, and the Hale Irwin/St. Louis Children's Hospital Golf Benefit, which by 2000 would raise some $8 million for Children's Hospital. Soon another annual golf tournament, the Joe Buck Classic, would raise money to support community outreach and advocacy programs.

At the same time, volunteers remained a key part of the effort to make patients feel comfortable. From Jan Achuff and her goose puppet, "Waddles," to Marian Alexander who tirelessly helped in Child Life Services, some 350 volunteers per day in 1996 — who spent a total of 38,000 hours a year — helped out at Children's Hospital. Each year, the Friends of St. Louis Children's Hospital organization awards scholarships, named for long-time volunteer Jane Spoehrer, to outstanding high school volunteers.

1998

U.S. News & World Report ranks Children's Hospital as one of the best in the United States.

memories *Dwayne Ingram*

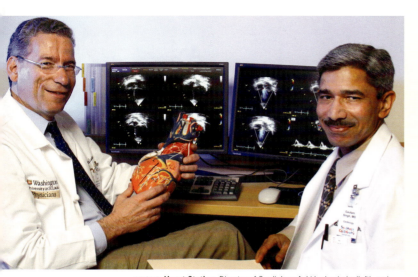

ABOVE **Heart Station.** Director of Cardiology Achi Ludomirsky (left), and cardiologist Gautam Sngh review digital images at the St. Louis Children's Hospital Heart Station Becker Medical Library. Photo by Kimberly Keefe

MOVING FORWARD

By the late 1990s, Children's Hospital was doing extraordinarily well: setting records in overall admissions, same-day surgeries, and total surgical cases. In 1998, *U.S. News & World Report's* annual guide to "America's Best Hospitals" ranked Children's Hospital as one of the best in the United States. During the next year, the hospital had some 12,532 admissions and 61,070 patient days overall.

Its mission, condensed to a single, fundamental purpose by Ted Frey, read simply: "to do what's right for kids." The vision statement, now meshed with the role of the BJC Health System, was related: "Children's Hospital will be the hallmark for quality pediatric care within our region, as well as nationally and internationally. As the flagship for a growing, integrated pediatric health care network, we will lead the development of innovative cost-effective approaches in prevention, primary care and specialty services, with the ultimate goal of improving the health of all children."

In 1999, Louis J. Fusz, Jr., a long-time supporter of Children's Hospital and member of the Board of Trustees since 1988, took over as board chairman, while Barbara Cole became Medical Staff president. A new 700-car garage was underway at the corner of Children's Place and Kingshighway, with a pedestrian bridge planned to allow access to the hospital; in 2000, demolition of the venerable Spoehrer Tower began to make way for this addition. In 2001, a new Diagnostic and Interventional Catheterization Laboratory opened. Along with the transplant service, the newborn medicine program

Dwayne I. Ingram came to Children's Hospital in 1980 as a porter in the cafeteria. Through the years, he has worked in the linen department and central supply; as a clerk in central processing; as a scheduling secretary for the operating rooms; and, since 1990, as patient advocacy coordinator, helping children and their parents.

"My experience here has been shaped by patients I have met over the years. Tia, who came from Hawaii, had a brain tumor; we became buddies. She spent a lot of time here, and I would bring in toys for her to play with. When the doctors had to shave her beautiful, long black hair on one side, she had her mother color the other side green with red streaks. With all she was going through, she still wanted to be a kid and have things to laugh about. She died on October 31, 1991, and her mother always calls me on the anniversary of her death.

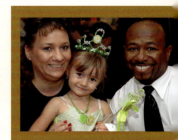

"Around 16 years ago, I bought another little girl, Adina, a baby Big Bird doll before she had open-heart surgery. She and her mother, Rabbi Susan Talve, were back in March 2005 and I happened to run into them. Rabbi Talve said: 'Remember Big Bird?' Adina pulled it out of her backpack; not only had she taken it with her when she had procedures over the years, but she had shared it with other families whose children were having surgery.

"What an honor, what a privilege, to be here and serve these families in whatever way I can. These kids are champions; they are my heroes."

1999
The OPQM creates the Family Advisory Council to obtain advice from parents whose children require frequent hospital care.

1999
Congress passes the Children's Hospital Graduate Medical Education (CHGME) legislation, which provides major funding for residency programs.

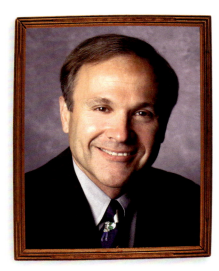

Lee F. Fetter. When Lee Fetter became president of Children's Hospital and senior executive officer of BJC HealthCare in 2002, Steve Lipstein, president and CEO of BJC HealthCare, said this: "We are highly impressed with Lee's credentials for this key leadership role at St. Louis Children's Hospital. He has the right combination of intellect, personality, and values — and he is committed to 'doing what's right for kids.'" Becker Medical Library

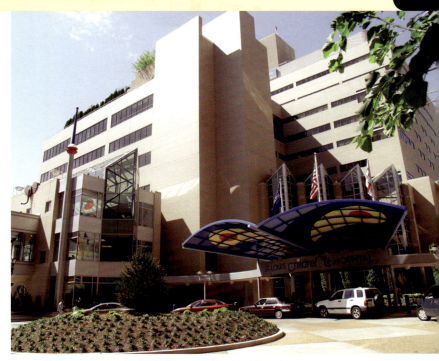

Making patients and families feel welcome. This view of the southeast corner of the hospital shows the ground level entrance and patient drop-off area. This feature opened in 2001, along with the new visitor garage, expanded lobbies, and second-floor pedestrian bridge. Becker Medical Library

remained particularly active, with 97 percent occupancy in 1999 — a steep increase from the 73 percent occupancy in 1995.

Also in 2000, a nine-month planning process, under the leadership of Todd Sklamberg, vice president of pediatric services development, culminated in a five-year strategic plan that would serve as a roadmap for future development. The plan established four key strategic areas: increase the hospital's share of the pediatric market, locally and nationally; continue to strengthen relationships with full- and part-time medical staff; improve relations with the School of Medicine, government bodies, and the community; and, finally, continue to offer strong clinical programs.

New community initiatives also began, such as the Healthy Kids at Play partnership, funded in part by the Danforth Foundation, which provided various St. Louis communities with outreach programs tailored to the children in those areas. A $1 million gift from The Saigh Foundation secured the future of Healthy Kids Express, helping pay salaries of nurses and staff members on the two mobile vans.

These changes took place in the context of sweeping change across the medical center as a "Campus Integration Plan" consolidated ambulatory services at the north end of the campus and inpatient care at the south end. New buildings went up, while familiar buildings were razed. In 2002, long-time medical dean and executive vice chancellor for medical affairs William Peck stepped down, replaced by pediatrician Larry Shapiro, who had graduated from the School of Medicine and once been a resident at Children's Hospital. By now, the medical school was a leader in national rankings, tied for the number two spot in 2004 in the prestigious *U.S. News & World Report* list.

NEW LEADERSHIP OF LEE F. FETTER

In 2002, after 31 years of service to Children's Hospital, Ted Frey retired. After a national search, Children's Hospital announced his successor: Lee F. Fetter, who had been at the School of Medicine since 1983, serving most recently as associate vice chancellor for administration and finance and chief operating officer of the Faculty Practice Plan. From 1993 to 2000, he had

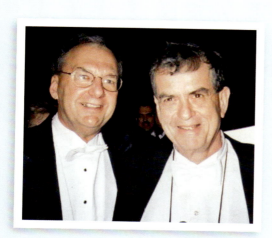

Aaron Ciechanover and Alan Schwartz.

A visiting professor of pediatrics at Washington University School of Medicine since 1987, Aaron Ciechanover won the 2004 Nobel Prize in Chemistry. He was the 22nd Nobel Laureate associated with Washington University. His award, which he shared with two colleagues, honored his work in discovering a process that cells use to eliminate unwanted proteins.

Ciechanover began his work at Washington University with research on cellular biology, conducted during a two-year sabbatical with pediatric department head Alan L. Schwartz. Afterwards, he spent a part of every year at Children's Hospital; otherwise, he was Research Distinguished Professor of Biochemistry at Technion-Israel Institute of Technology in Haifa, Israel.

As he said at the time: "My association with Washington University, which I consider to be my second home, has contributed greatly to my research."

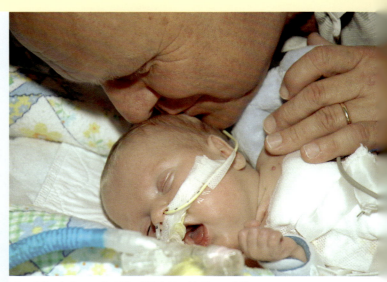

In safe hands. Four-month-old Evan Wells is kissed by his grandfather during his stay at St. Louis Children's Hospital in October, 2004. Evan was the first patient at the hospital to receive a heart transplant from a donor with a different blood type. Becker Medical Library

also been chief financial officer for the School of Medicine, responsible for all business affairs involving the affiliated hospitals, including Children's Hospital. In his year-end address, Alan Schwartz commended the choice. "In my opinion," he said, "the hospital's new president, Lee Fetter, is now and in the future will be the best president of any children's hospital in the United States. There is a fantastic relationship between the department of pediatrics and Children's, and I believe Lee...is going to take the hospital on to the next level."

In turn, Fetter was pleased by what he found. "The hospital was in very good shape when I got here," said Fetter later. "Ted Frey had recruited well, and the fact that there was a strong management team in place — including Velinda Block, Gary LaBlance, and Todd Sklamberg — has helped immensely. While I knew the dynamics of the medical center intimately, I did not at that time know how to run a hospital, so it was important to have that support here. I also felt that our single greatest asset was our affiliation with the medical school — and leveraging that relationship was the way to become even more of a national presence and one of the top 10 children's hospitals in the nation."

A year after he had begun, Fetter assessed his specific priorities. The first was cutting-edge healthcare, its quality assured by several things: intensive reviews of current practice; an educational campaign, sponsored by BJC HealthCare, called "A Pact and our Promise"; and a renewed patient safety culture. Another was continued lobbying efforts on the state and national levels to protect pediatric health care programs from cuts. Others included preserving special relationships with the community pediatricians and gathering information for a new strategic planning effort.

He also underscored the importance of a new building project initiated under Ted Frey's leadership, that was set to begin in 2004. With patient volume up by 15 percent over the previous five years and 275,000 patient visits each year, Children's Hospital would undertake a major expansion and renovation: a $76.5 million project to construct seven floors on the east side of

1999 Barbara Cole becomes Medical Staff president.

2000 Children's Hospital launches Healthy Kids Express, the first mobile health van of its kind in the area.

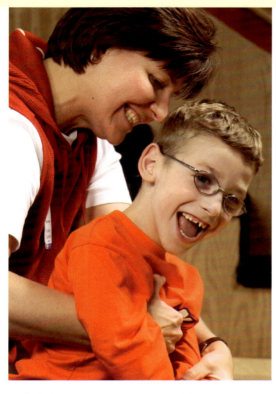

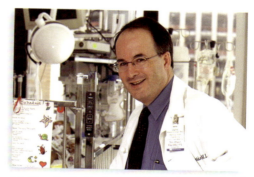

The best medicine. Physical therapist Deann Koyn shares a laugh with patient Aric Christian Wagner during a therapy session. Becker Medical Library

Julio Pérez-Fontán. Director of pediatric intensive care services at Children's Hospital, Pérez-Fontán was also a researcher who studied the effect of denervation on the function of airways in the lungs. He had joined the faculty in 1992, and in 2001 he was named the Alumni Endowed Professor of Pediatrics at the medical school. Becker Medical Library

its building. This new space would add 95,000 square feet to the existing 550,000 square-foot structure, while another 120,000 square feet would be renovated. With this addition, the number of single-occupancy rooms would be substantially increased, so that some 80 percent of patients would have private rooms, the PICU and NICU would both expand, the number of operating rooms would grow, a larger therapy gym would be built, and same-day surgery would increase in size by more than 50 percent. Overall, the number of hospital beds would climb from 235 to 250.

But a key goal was also fund-raising — and Fetter announced the beginning of "the largest fund-raising campaign in the hospital's history." In general, he said later, "I believe that Children's Hospital should be among the top two or three recipients of philanthropy in this area. It has an incredible legacy in St. Louis, this is a very generous community, and our relationship with Washington University makes us outstanding." With no capital campaign mounted since the 1980s, he added, "we had fallen off the radar of generous prospective donors in this community." One of his critical long-term goals,

he said, was to increase annual giving, hold a series of successful capital campaigns, and — working closely with the Children's Hospital Foundation, under Executive Vice President Jim Miller — to build up the endowment.

Almost immediately, this new fundraising had great success. With the Foundation's leadership, backed by the Development and Friends boards, the endowment grew substantially — to $175 million by 2005. Behind the scenes, Children's Hospital began collecting contributions in the silent phase of a $125 million campaign that would be launched officially early in 2006.

CHANGES COMING

After 32 years as the revered director of the residency program, pediatrician James Keating stepped down, turning the leadership over to rheumatologist Andrew White. The residency program was changing, with opportunities in such areas as advocacy and adolescent medicine, as well as an accelerated option into the growing fellowship program. In 1999, Congress passed new legislation, Children's Hospital Graduate Medical Education (CHGME), providing major funding for residency programs, including the

2001

A new Diagnostic and Interventional Catheterization Laboratory opens at the hospital.

SEPTEMBER 2001

A new visitor parking garage opens, with a second floor pedestrian bridge connecting it to the hospital.

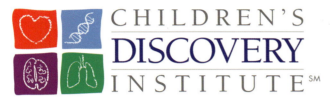

ST. LOUIS CHILDREN'S HOSPITAL
WASHINGTON UNIVERSITY SCHOOL OF MEDICINE

Children's Discovery Institute. In January 2006, Children's Hospital and Washington University School of Medicine launched the Children's Discovery Institute. The collaborative venture will focus extensive research efforts on the most life-threatening diseases of childhood.

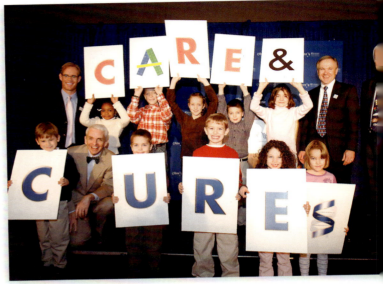

Building for Care, Searching for Cures. A group of energetic youngsters helped Children's Hospital officially launch the Care and Cures comprehensive campaign on January 25, 2006, at the Chase Park Plaza hotel. Joining them are (top row left to right) Joe Buck, Lee Fetter, and Larry Shapiro; and (bottom row, kneeling) Jonathan Gitlin. Becker Medical Library

training program at Children's Hospital. During the first five years after this policy change, Children's Hospital received some $30 million in federal funds to support the cost of physician training. A key voice in maintaining this federal support into the future was the hospital's Children's Advocacy Network (CAN), established in 2004 as an organization of pediatric providers and other supporters willing to contact lawmakers on behalf of children's health.

New division directors took the place of others: Gregory Storch succeeded Carl Smith as director of the division of laboratory medicine, and Louis Muglia taking over from Neil White as division director of endocrinology and metabolism. And faculty members succeeded others in named professorships, as Julio Pérez Fontán became the Alumni Endowed Professor of Pediatrics, succeeding Arnold Strauss; and Robert Strunk replaced the departing David Perlmutter in the pediatric professorship honoring the late pediatrician Donald Strominger.

Relations with community physicians remained strong, as a new effort began — organized in 2003 by physicians Jane Garbutt, Elliot Gellman, and James Keating — involving 66 physicians doing clinical research in their offices. The program, called the Washington University Pediatric and Adolescent Ambulatory Research Consortium (WUPAARC), embarked on community-based studies in such areas as feeding, asthma, gastrointestinal symptoms, and antibiotic resistance. Such efforts as the "Early Bird Rounds" on Friday mornings kept part-time faculty informed as to the full-time faculty's research projects, with broadcasts to 22 sites around the metropolitan area.

CHILDREN'S DISCOVERY INSTITUTE BEGINS

Meanwhile, the total of research grants won by department members continued to rise: to some $16 million in 2001, $17 million in 2002, and nearly $20 million in 2004. By 2005, the pediatrics department would rank fourth nationally in NIH research funding. Full-time faculty continued to publish papers in biomedical journals, some 300 of them in 2001. Among the major grants received was a record-setting $18.5 million grant from the NIH awarded to Michael DeBaun and colleagues to study the effectiveness of blood transfusion therapy as a way to prevent silent strokes in children with sickle cell disease. Others included Jonathan Gitlin's program project grant titled "Mechanisms of Growth and the Overgrowth Syndrome," and a $1.1 million grant from the National Institute of Neurological Disorders and Stroke awarded to R. Mark Grady for his study of muscle-nerve

2002 — Larry Shapiro replaces William Peck as medical dean and executive vice chancellor for medical affairs.

2002 — Ted Frey retires and is replaced as president of the hospital by Lee F. Fetter.

memories *James S. McDonnell*

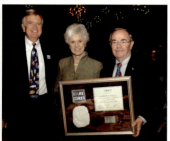

Jim and Libby McDonnell. Jim McDonnell (right) and wife Libby stand with Board of Trustees president Chuck Mueller at the January 2006 launch of the Building for Care, Searching for Cures campaign. McDonnell, the James S. McDonnell Charitable Trust, and the James S. McDonnell Family Foundation provided a $20 million lead gift for the campaign, the largest single gift in the hospital's history. *Becker Medical Library*

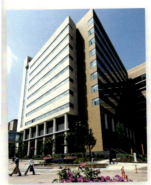

McDonnell Pediatric Research Building.

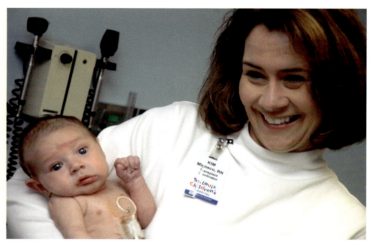

Tiny transplant survivor. Kim Migneco, liver transplant coordinator, holds three-month-old Jacob Gibbs in April 2006. Jacob received a transplanted liver at St. Louis Children's Hospital when he was only 10 days old. *Becker Medical Library*

James S. McDonnell III retired as corporate vice president from McDonnell Douglas in 1991, continuing as a director until the merger with The Boeing Co. Over the past 30 years, he has served numerous terms on the board of Children's Hospital, and was chairman in 1980 and 1981. He is currently back on the board and is also a member of the Washington University School of Medicine National Council. Like his father, aviation pioneer James S. McDonnell, he has also been extraordinarily generous. The McDonnell Pediatric Research Building, dedicated in September 2000, was made possible by a $20 million gift from McDonnell, his brother John F. McDonnell, and the James S. McDonnell Charitable Trust. In 2004, James S. McDonnell III, the James S. McDonnell Charitable Trust, and the James S. McDonnell Family Foundation made a second transformational gift, also of $20 million, to help establish the Children's Discovery Institute, dedicated to finding cures for childhood diseases.

"One day in 1996, Ted Frey, Alan Schwartz, and William Peck came to see me. I was impressed that they came together, representing Children's Hospital, the Department of Pediatrics, and the School of Medicine. They proposed a new Pediatric Research Building — one without interior walls. Heretofore, each department had had its own area for research, which meant that people from one department worked alongside people from the same department. In this new building, researchers from different departments would be intermingled. I thought that was an excellent idea: someone working nearby might think of something you had not, and that might lead you in a new research direction.

"The term 'pediatric research' also struck a chord with me, and eventually led to our gift to construct this building. If you read the plaque on the building, you will see that my family gave it in memory of our daughter, Elizabeth Finney McDonnell, whom we called 'Peggy'; she died of cancer at age two. If a cure for that could be found through work performed in this building, that would be our ultimate reward."

interactions. Facilitating the research of Gitlin and Matthew Goldsmith was a major aquatic addition: a large zebra fish aquarium, installed in the McDonnell Pediatric Research Building. A new Mouse Genetics Core Laboratory developed mouse models of human disease for investigators throughout the medical school.

Nationally, there was a burgeoning of genetic, cellular, and molecular biological research — sparked in part by the work of the Genome Sequencing Center at Washington University — that opened new areas of scientific inquiry. Genomic mapping, said one Children's Hospital prospectus, "provides an unprecedented opportunity to understand the fundamental basis of all human disease. Based on this opportunity, we have a bold vision to cure several childhood diseases....The result: accelerated progress toward cures."

In close cooperation with the School of Medicine, Children's Hospital announced a remarkable new venture, the Children's Discovery Institute. The Institute would focus research, diagnostic, and treatment resources on four deadly illnesses traceable to a genetic

2003
A new program, the Washington University Pediatric and Adolescent Ambulatory Research Consortium (WUPAARC), is organized to conduct community-based pediatric studies.

2004
The hospital's Children's Advocacy Network (CAN) is established.

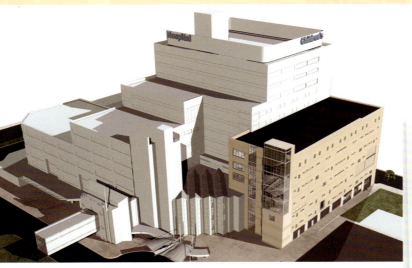

East Expansion. The hospital's seven-story east expansion (shown in tan, lower right) is scheduled for completion in late 2006. When finished, the $76.5 million project will enable the hospital to have 80 percent private rooms, as well as expanded intensive care units, more operating rooms and a larger therapy services gym. Karlsberger Architecture, Inc.

> "As the new millennium began. St. Louis Children's Hospital had much to celebrate."

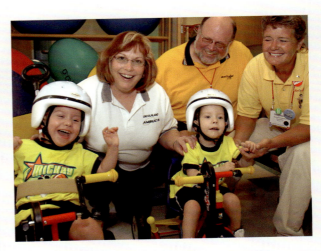

Working hard while having fun. Twins Matt and Zach Sutherland of Florissant, Missouri, get active in the therapy services gym at the hospital. Becker Medical Library

defect: congenital heart disease, malignant brain tumors, musculoskeletal disease, and respiratory disorders, which kill more than 100,000 children nationally each year and 1,000 in the St. Louis area. Interdisciplinary teams of researchers from such areas as physics, bioengineering, epidemiology, cardiology, developmental biology, genetics, computational biology, and nanotechnology would study these diseases. Initial funding for the Institute would be raised as part of the $125 million Building for Care, Searching for Cures comprehensive campaign. In an extraordinary gesture of support, James S. McDonnell III, the James S. McDonnell Charitable Trust, and the James S. McDonnell Family Foundation made a $20 million gift to the fund drive. In recognition of their support, the Children's Hospital Foundation named the pediatric brain tumor component of this effort the McDonnell Children's Cancer Center.

In 2005, the pediatrics department also announced the formation of a new division, Genetics and Genomic Medicine, which would exist within the Department of Pediatrics under the leadership of Jonathan D. Gitlin. Financial support for this division would also come from Children's Hospital as part of the Children's Discovery Institute research collaboration. Six new faculty members, some with interdisciplinary appointments, would be added to this division.

A HISTORY OF PROGRESS

As the new millennium began — and the hospital's 125th anniversary in 2004 began to come in view — St. Louis Children's Hospital had much to celebrate. It continued to receive national accolades for its work. By 2005, for the second time in a row, *Child* magazine had listed it among the 10 best pediatric hospitals in the United States, and *U.S. News & World Report* ranked it as one of the best pediatric hospitals in America, moving it up six slots from 19 to 13. From the American Nurses Credentialing Center (ANCC) it received the Magnet designation, the highest honor in the country for nursing excellence, previously given to only 170 hospitals out of nearly 5,000 nationwide. In another *U.S. News & World Report* listing, the Washington University School of Medicine was ranked third in the nation, with its Department of Pediatrics rated sixth.

Many programs were expanding. By 2005, the lung transplant program — the largest in the world — had performed some 238 transplants,

NOVEMBER 2004

The hospital breaks ground on a $76.5 million expansion and renovation project to construct seven floors on the east side of its building.

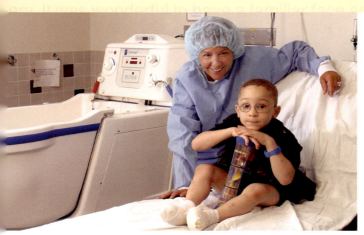

Burn center. Clinical Nurse Specialist Robin Moushey visits with six-year-old Stephen Herron in the hospital's ambulatory burn treatment room. Becker Medical Library. Photo by Kimberly Keefe

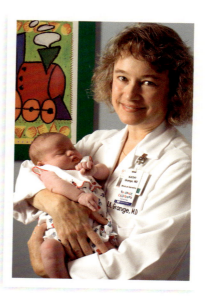

Down Syndrome Clinic. Dr. Kathy Grange, medical director of the Down Syndrome clinic, holds infant Morgan Tremblath. The hospital launched this comprehensive clinic in early 2005 as a place where children with DS can see all their physicians and therapists in a single location. Becker Medical Library

while the cochlear implant program had done more than 200 implants, making it one of the two largest in the nation. In the Cleft Palate and Craniofacial Deformities Institute, physicians had treated more than 2,000 children with cleft lip and palate and 1,500 with other craniofacial problems. By now, Children's Hospital had one of the region's only pediatric sleep clinics, its only dedicated pediatric burn program, a fast-growing minimally invasive surgery program, and nationally recognized programs in asthma, neonatology, sickle cell anemia, and cystic fibrosis. The outlook continued to improve for cancer patients, cared for in the Hale Irwin Pediatric Center for Hematology/Oncology; and for cerebral palsy patients, thanks to the continuing success of selective dorzal rhizotomy surgery, performed by neurosurgeon T.S. Park, and to the work of the Pediatric Neurology Cerebral Palsy Center, headed by neurologist Janice Brunstrom.

More talented physicians joined the staff, including cardiac imaging expert Achi Ludomirsky as the Lewis Larrick Ward Chair of Pediatric Cardiology, and pediatric gastroenterology division head Phillip I. Tarr, an expert on hemolytic uremic syndrome. Others were promoted to leadership positions, such as Edwin Trevathan to chief of the Department of Pediatric and Developmental Neurology and Andrew White as a successor to Jonathan Gitlin as division director of pediatric rheumatology and immunology. Terrie Inder, a New Zealand pediatrician, child neurologist, and expert on newborn brain development, accepted a position in 2005. At the same time, several left to take leadership roles at other medical centers: Arnold Strauss to head pediatrics at Vanderbilt, David Perlmutter to become chairman at Pittsburgh, and Joseph St. Geme to be chairman at Duke.

Relations between Children's Hospital and the Department of Pediatrics have "never been stronger," said Alan Schwartz. "We are intimately interdependent in every one of our key missions, which include patient care, education, scholarship, and community service. I would also use the term 'synergistic.' If you take the talent pool that exists in pediatrics plus the one that exists at SLCH and put them together, you get more than the sum of those two pools. It is a very exciting time, very stimulating."

And the BJC merger had largely turned into an asset for Children's Hospital, bolstering its financial rating to AA status and giving it access to capital as well as lower interest rates. Now the hospital's operating margin had risen to a healthy five percent and above, allowing it to invest in much-needed new technologies. "In my role at the medical school, I was one of the people who negotiated the affiliation agreement

2005

With the Children's Hospital Foundation's efforts, backed by the Development and Friends boards, the hospital's endowment grows to $175 million.

2005

The Department of Pediatrics announces the formation of a new division, Genetics and Genomic Medicine.

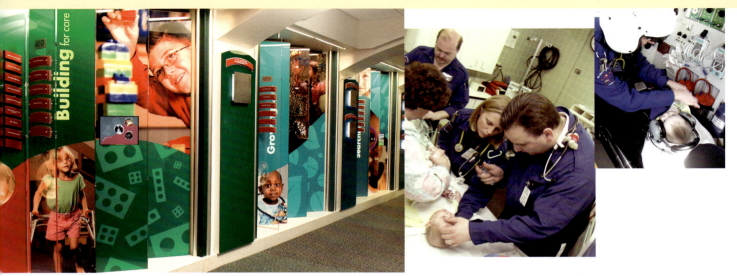

Donor Recognition Hall. On June 26, 2005, Children's Hospital unveiled its new second-floor corridor display, honoring the generosity of significant donors who had made gifts to the hospital since 1980. Becker Medical Library

Transport Team. Children's Hospital Transport Team members check the condition of a seven-month-old girl in the St. Francis Hospital ER before flying back to St. Louis Children's for care (above). In the helicopter, (right) Stacey Eyermann prepares the child for the ride. The headphones protect the baby's ears from the helicopter noise. Becker Medical Library. Photo by John Twombly

> **"Children's Hospital adds luster to BJC because we are so highly regarded in this community."**

with Children's Hospital in 1995, and I saw that the early years were difficult," said Fetter later. "But by 2002, when I joined Children's Hospital, BJC had entered into a new phase of its evolution. I was very comfortable with the senior administrators, I admired the high caliber of professionalism at BJC, and I saw the advantages of having a large entity negotiate both managed care and vendor pricing on our behalf. There also were professional resources in BJC's corporate group — public relations, legal, strategic planning, for example — that we couldn't hire on our own."

On its part, BJC's corporate governance began to change under new president and CEO Steve Lipstein. He viewed each hospital in the BJC system as operating in a unique environment. Thus, the best management model, he said, was a "directed autonomy with congenial controls." Added Lee Fetter: "In the executive staff meetings, Steve Lipstein refers to Children's Hospital as 'that special place' — in part jokingly, but also very admiringly because they know it is a very unique place. Children's Hospital adds luster to BJC because we are so highly regarded in this community.

CHALLENGES FOR THE FUTURE

Still, Children's Hospital, often working in conjunction with the pediatrics department, faced challenges for the future. A key goal remained: the appointment of women pediatricians, so dominant in the profession by 2004, to positions as division directors. Faculty retention and recruitment were, as ever, strongly important, particularly in certain hard-to-fill pediatric subspecialty slots. Despite some additions, the expansion of general pediatric surgery, plastic surgery, cardiothoracic surgery, urology, neurosurgery, and orthopaedic surgery continued to be particular goals. And constant attention to quality remained important, while other kinds of vigilance also came into sharper focus. Since the terrorist events of 2001 in New York and Washington, D.C., disaster preparedness took on a new significance.

Perhaps most critical of all was maintaining — and funding — the original mission of Children's Hospital: finding new ways to provide

Snerdlihc. The hospital's fuzzy mascot, Snerdlihc ("Childrens" spelled backwards) first appeared in 1994 as a hand puppet that visited hospital inpatients. Today, the life-size version of Snerdlihc is worn by hospital volunteers and staff, and makes over 150 community appearances annually. Becker Medical Library

2005
For the second time in a row, *Child* magazine lists the hospital among the 10 best pediatric hospitals in the United States.

2005
Children's Hospital receives the highest honor in the U.S. for nursing excellence: the Magnet designation from the American Nurses Credentialing Center.

January 2006
The hospital announces the largest fundraising endeavor in its history: the $125 million Building for Care, Searching for Cures campaign. The announcement also includes the formal establishment of the Children's Discovery Institute.

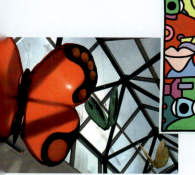

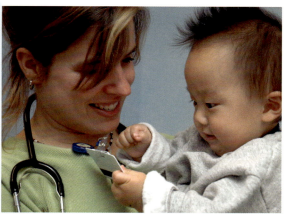

International Adoption Center. Rachel Orscheln, MD, director of the hospital's International Adoption Center, examines nine-month-old Thomas Scholtis from Korea. The hospital launched this comprehensive center in 2005 to meet the health and developmental needs of international adoptees. Becker Medical Library

Both outside and inside, Children's Hospital reflects a child-friendly atmosphere. "You don't feel you're in a hospital when you enter here, and I think the artwork is a big piece of that," says Susan Ebrecht, interior specialist in Facility Services.

Some of the first things that patients see are the animal topiaries out front. Within the circle drive are fiberglass cats, dogs, and fishbowls, created by artist Charlie Houska. In the entrance to the hospital are butterflies and the ever-popular working train.

On the first and third floors are four large acrylic panels specially designed and painted by well-known artist Dale Chihuly. "They are mounted in the windows, and when the sun comes through they just glow," says Ebrecht. A ceramic bench in the rotunda area is made of ceramic pieces that patients designed in workshops.

A large metal rooster, sculpted by Marianist Brother Mel Meyer, is used as a way-finding piece. "People say, 'Go down to the rooster and make a left,'" says Ebrecht. Brother Mel has also done metal wall sculptures and other pieces of art throughout the hospital. Outside the NICU are drawings done by pediatric nurse practitioner Johanna Schloemann.

On the tenth floor are pictures of animals, created by students at Combs School in their music class. They were listening to "Carnival of the Animals" by Saint-Saens, and their teacher asked them to glue pieces of tissue paper onto outlines of the animals. Now the pictures are mounted along the walls on the surgery ward, and patients can press a button under each one to hear the corresponding music.

the best pediatric care available, even when the families of sick children cannot afford it. Advocacy on behalf of Medicaid reimbursement still loomed large, as state and federal governments continued to weigh cuts to the program. "In 10 years, I would like us to be considered one of the top five children's hospitals in the country, have a physical presence beyond the Kingshighway campus, and start an excellent mother's and infant's program," says Fetter.

As it had been from the beginning, the key strength of Children's Hospital remains its dedicated staff. "I've discovered that this is really a remarkable organization, and not just as a hospital but also as an employer," Fetter adds. "As often as I can, I do employee orientations and I tell them that this is a family — a big family and growing, with 2,600 employees — with a very special feeling to it. That is a culture that my predecessors developed over many years. The passion that people feel for this hospital is palpable, and fortunately we've been able to preserve that."

After 125 years of service, St. Louis Children's Hospital had changed in ways that would have astonished the tiny, courageous band of women and homeopaths who had founded it. The small downtown house had turned into a major, state-of-the-art complex on the edge of Forest Park; the women managers had become a professional administrative team, made up of men and women; the volunteer homeopaths had been transformed into a highly skilled medical staff armed with the latest training and technology. As Grace Jones had hoped in 1915, the fledgling hospital had become "an ideal put into life." Yet fundamentally, its mission had changed little. Through the decades, Children's Hospital had continued to offer the same priceless gifts to sick children and their worried families: hope for a healthier future and healing from a host of childhood diseases that could, with the unfolding miracles of medical research, increasingly be vanquished.

Notable Faculty and Staff of St. Louis Children's Hospital and Washington University School of Medicine

AMERICAN PEDIATRIC SOCIETY
Borden S. Veeder: Faculty, 1911; President, 1935
Jean V. Cooke: Faculty, 1918; President, 1949
Hugh McCulloch: Faculty, 1912; President, 1952
Daniel C. Darrow: Faculty, 1925; President, 1957
Henry L. Barnett: WUSM graduate, 1938; House officer, 1938; President, 1982
Ralph D. Feigin: Faculty, 1968; President, 1998
Larry J. Shapiro: WUSM Graduate, 1971; House officer, 1971; President, 2004

JOHN HOWLAND MEDAL RECIPIENTS
Daniel C. Darrow: Faculty, 1925; Medal, 1959
Martha M. Eliot: House officer, 1919; Medal, 1967
Henry L. Barnett: WUSM graduate, 1938; House Officer, 1938; Medal, 1984
Gilbert B. Forbes: House officer, 1941; Medal, 1992

AMERICAN ACADEMY OF PEDIATRICS
Borden S. Veeder: Faculty, 1911; President, 1942
Crawford A. Bost: House officer, 1927; President, 1954
William W. Belford: House officer, 1923; President, 1959
Einor H. Christopherson: WUSM graduate, 1925; House officer, 1926; Executive Director, 1959-67

AMERICAN BOARD OF PEDIATRICS
Borden S. Veeder: Faculty, 1911; President, 1934-41
J. Neal Middelkamp: WUSM graduate, 1948; House officer, 1949; Chairman, 1988
Herbert T. Abelson: WUSM graduate, 1966; House officer, 1966; Chairman 1997

THE SOCIETY FOR PEDIATRIC RESEARCH
Daniel C. Darrow: Faculty, 1925; President, 1940
Mitchell I. Rubin: Faculty, 1928; President, 1947
Henry L. Barnett: WUSM graduate, 1938; House officer, 1938; President, 1960
Gilbert B. Forbes: House officer, 1941; President, 1961
Ralph D. Feigin: Faculty, 1968; President, 1983
Larry J. Shapiro: WUSM graduate, 1971; House officer, 1971; President, 1992
David Perlmutter: Faculty, 1986; President, 1995

CHAIRS OF DEPARTMENTS OF PEDIATRICS
Philip C. Jeans: House officer, 1913; University of Iowa, 1924
Samuel W. Clausen: House officer, 1917; University of Rochester, 1924
Mitchell I. Rubin: House officer, 1928; State University of New York–Buffalo, 1945
Russell J. Blattner: WUSM graduate, 1933; House officer, 1934; Baylor College, 1947
Merl J. Carson: House officer, 1939; University of Southern California, 1950
Milton J. Senn: House officer, 1929; Yale University, 1950
Gilbert B. Forbes: House officer, 1941; University of Texas, Southwestern, 1950; University of Rochester, 1974
William Bradford: WUSM graduate, 1923; House officer, 1923; University of Rochester, 1952
Henry L. Barnett: WUSM graduate, 1938; House officer, 1938; Albert Einstein, 1955
W. Gene Klingberg: WUSM graduate, 1943; House officer, 1943; University of West Virginia, 1960
C. William Daeschner, Jr.: House officer, 1948; University of Texas–Galveston, 1960
Marvin Cornblath: WUSM graduate, 1947; House officer, 1948; University of Maryland, 1968
William W. Cleveland: House officer, 1955; University of Miami, 1969
George N. Donnell: WUSM graduate, 1944; House officer, 1944; University of Southern California, 1971
Ralph D. Feigin: Faculty, 1968; Baylor College, 1977
Barbara Jones: House officer, 1952; University of West Virginia, 1982; University of Kansas, 1985
Herbert T. Abelson: WUSM graduate, 1966; University of Washington, 1983; University of Chicago, 1995
Lynn M. Taussig: WUSM graduate, 1968; House officer, 1968; University of Arizona, 1985
Richard L. Schreiner: WUSM graduate, 1971; House officer, 1971; University of Indiana, 1987
William Crist: House officer and fellow, 1971-2; Mayo Medical School, 1997
Randy A. Kienstra: House officer, 1973; Southern Illinois University, 1988
Larry J. Shapiro: WUSM graduate, 1971; House officer, 1971; University of California–San Francisco, 1991
Alan L. Schwartz: Faculty 1986; Washington University, 1995
Arnold Strauss: WUSM graduate, 1970; House officer, 1970; Faculty 1975; Vanderbilt, 2000
David Perlmutter: Faculty, 1986; University of Pittsburgh, 2001
Joseph St. Geme: Faculty, 1992; Duke University, 2005

CHIEFS OF PEDIATRICS AT HOSPITALS
Montri Mangalasmaya: Chulalongkorn University
Channevat Kashement: House officer, 1955; Mahidal University
M. Remsen Behrer: Fellow, 1949-51; Faculty, 1952; Pittsburgh City Hospital
Horacio Padilla: House officer, 1954-56; Fellow, 1954-56; Guadalajara General Hospital, Mexico
Ihsan Dogramaci: Fellow, 1946-47; Rector, Ankara University, 1963-65; Rector, Hacettepe University, Turkey, 1967-75; president, Bilkent University in Ankara, Turkey, 1985-.
Ernest E. McCoy: House officer, 1951; University of Alberta, Canada, 1970

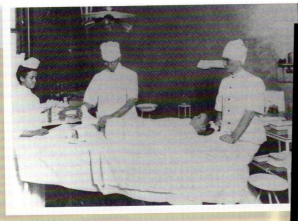
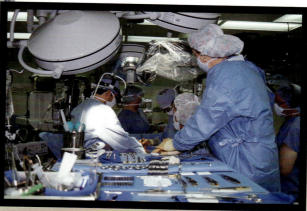

OTHER NOTABLE ACHIEVEMENTS
Katherine Bain: WUSM graduate, 1925; House officer, 1926; Head of Research and Development, U.S. Children's Bureau, 1940
Martha May Eliot: House officer, 1919; Chief U.S. Children's Bureau, 1951
William H. Danforth: House officer, 1955; Faculty, 1957; Vice-Chancellor for Medical Affairs, 1965-71; Washington University chancellor, 1971-95
Ralph D. Feigin: Faculty, 1968; President and Chief Executive Officer, Baylor College of Medicine, 1996
William Crist: House officer and fellow, 1971-72; dean, University of Missouri–Columbia School of Medicine, 2000
Harvey R. Colten: 1986 faculty; Vice-President of Medical Affairs and Dean, Northwestern University School of Medicine, 1997
S. Bruce Dowton: 1986 faculty; Dean, University of New South Wales, Australia, 1998
Larry J. Shapiro: WUSM graduate, 1971; House officer, 1971; Dean, WUSM, 2003
Lynn M. Taussig: WUSM graduate, 1968; House officer, 1968; University of Arizona, 1985; President and CEO of National Jewish Medical and Research Center, 1993

INSTITUTE OF MEDICINE, NATIONAL ACADEMY OF SCIENCES, USA
Dennis Bier: Faculty, 1973
Harvey Colten: Faculty, 1986
William H. Danforth: Faculty, 1971
Ralph Feigin: Faculty, 1968
David L. Rimoin: Faculty, 1967
Alan L. Schwartz: Faculty 1986
Larry J. Shapiro: WUSM graduate, 1971; House officer, 1971; Dean of Washington Unviersity School of Medicine, 2003
Joseph Volpe: Faculty, 1997

BOARD CHAIRS
Apolline Blair 1879-82
Mary McKittrick 1882-1907
Grace Jones 1907-25
Mary Markham 1925-45
Alice Langenberg 1945-50
Roy D. Kercheval 1950-57
James W. Singer, Jr. 1957-60
Hugh M. F. Lewis 1960-62
Edwin M. Johnston 1962-64
Orrin S. Wightman, Jr. 1964-67
Rolla Streett 1967-69
Neal S. Wood 1969-72
Landon Y. Jones 1972-73
Thomas Kenton 1973-76
William Edwards 1976-79
James S. McDonnell III 1979-81
Donald O. Schnuck 1981-84
Andrew E. Newman 1984-86
Neal J. Farrell 1987-89
William E. Cornelius 1990-91
Vincent J. Cannella 1992-94
Martin Sneider 1995-98
Louis J. Fusz, Jr. 1999-2002
Charles W. Mueller 2003-

ADMINISTRATORS
Ruth Riley: Superintendent 1911-12
Claire DeCeu: Superintendent 1912-14
Candice Monfort: Superintendent 1914-17
Louis Burlingham, MD: Administrator 1917-25
Estelle Claiborne: Administrator 1925-54
Lilly D. Hoekstra: Administrator 1954-70
C. Alvin Tolin: President & CEO 1970-84
Linn B. Perkins: President & CEO 1984-85
Ronald G. Evens, MD: President & CEO 1985-88
Alan W. Brass: President & CEO 1988-95
Ted W. Frey: President & SEO 1995-2002
Lee F. Fetter: President & SEO 2002-

HEART OF GOLD RECIPIENTS
The Heart of Gold Award is presented annually to the individual, couple or company who has demonstrated the highest level of philanthropy through gifts of both their time and resources to St. Louis Children's Hospital. The award was first presented in 1997.
Harriet Spoehrer 1997
Doris and Donald Schnuck 1998
Dana Brown 1999
John and Sylvia Londoff 2000
Ollie and Mary Langenberg 2001
Carol and Paul Hatfield 2002
Hale and Sally Irwin 2003
Corie and Lou Fusz 2004
Jim and Libby McDonnell 2005

MEDICAL STAFF DISTINGUISHED SERVICE AWARD
Presented to a member of the St. Louis Children's Hospital Medical Staff who has demonstrated exemplary service and dedication to St. Louis Children's Hospital and its Medical Staff.
James P. Keating 2004
Homer Nash 1998
J. Neal Middelkamp 1996
Maurice Lonsway 1994
David Goldring 1991

ACKNOWLEDGMENTS

This large, exciting project never would have come to fruition without the strong interest and support of Lee Fetter, president of St. Louis Children's Hospital. I am also most grateful for funding that came from three sources: St. Louis Children's Hospital, the St. Louis Children's Hospital Medical Staff, and the Children's Hospital Foundation. Without their generous help, this book would not have been possible.

Others were especially gracious with assistance in fleshing out the narrative. From Washington University School of Medicine, they included three physicians: Alan Schwartz, chairman of the Department of Pediatrics; Lawrence Kahn, who did preliminary research at institutions around the area and was always ready with wise counsel; and Walton Schalick, pediatrician and historian, who was the key advocate for this project and gave outstanding advice on each chapter.

On the hospital side, my particular thanks go to Todd Sklamberg and Steve Kutheis, who provided valuable editorial help, research materials, interview suggestions, and overall guidance for this project. They were in constant contact with the book's production team: Becca Belz, the book's tireless and talented project director; and Scott and Laura Gericke of designlab,inc., its superb designers. Also of great help were public relations manager John Twombly; photographers Tim Mudrovic and Mary Butkus; copy editor Kathy Drury; secretary Patty Rode; and Erin Taylor, who produced the index.

Others were faithful readers of the draft text and helped immeasurably with their comments: Philip Dodge, who met with me several times and provided copies of biographical materials; M. Kenton King, who generously made time for lengthy interviews; J. Neal Middelkamp, who provided invaluable information, critiques, and useful photos. For the nursing interleaf, I appreciate the editorial assistance of Velinda Block and Susan K. Goddard, who both offered comments and reviewed that text.

Underpinning this project was extensive research to find nuggets of information and obscure photos. Librarians from several institutions — archivist Dennis Northcott from the Missouri Historical Society (MHS); photo archivists Ellen Thomasson and Duane Sneddeker, also from MHS; Andrew Harrison and Gerard Shorb of the Alan Mason McChesney Medical Archives at Johns Hopkins University; Shelley Hagen, photo curator at A.G. Edwards; staff from the St. Louis Mercantile Library, Brookings Institution, and St. Louis College of Pharmacy — were of great help. Melinda Frillman of the St. Louis Science Center, Theresa Howard of Creative Services at the School of Medicine, Bob Schmitz and Libby Coleman of BJC HealthCare, Theresa Worley and Susan Starbuck of the Department of Pediatrics, and Kathy Ray from the St. Louis Children's Hospital Library gave us important help with photos, fact-checking, and information. Mary Ellen Benson at Washington University provided crucial help and advice.

But the main source for information and photos was Becker Medical Library. There, photo archivist Philip Skroska was extraordinary, spending untold hours hunting down tiny details, reading the text, and finding elusive photos; we cannot begin to express our gratitude for all that he did to further this project. His archival colleagues Paul Anderson, Martha Riley, Ellen Dubinsky, and Brian McKinney were extremely helpful as well. My sincere thanks also go to my student research assistants Kristin Ehrenberger, Alessandro Medico, and Ezra Mehlman.

Many other people provided documents or photos that were important: Marion Hunt, author of the 1979 history of St. Louis Children's Hospital, kindly sent newspaper clippings from her own files; McKim Marriott, son of one-time pediatric head W. McKim Marriott, generously made available his personal collection of family photos and papers; pediatrician John Martz provided a photo of Alexis Hartmann; the Toverud family of Norway were especially gracious in supplying letters, memories, and photos of their mother and grandmother, Kirsten Toverud. Frank Blair scholar William E. Parrish kindly helped a great deal with information about the Blair children, as did Thomas West Jones and Robert McKittrick Jones III about Grace Richards Jones. Staff members of Children's Hospital also gave time and information to this project, especially Michelle Nelson, Judith Buehler, and Patricia Stolte.

For the nursing interleaf, photos and information came from Doris England, Virginia Hagemann, Shirley Nienhaus, Betty Vallero Reinke, Janice Rumfelt, and Alice Roam; of particular note is Elizabeth O'Connell, who loaned us a treasure trove of materials she had gleaned over the years and spent hours on the phone recalling Children's Hospital history. I would like to thank this group of nurses most cordially for welcoming me to their Washington University School of Nursing reunion in October 2005. Still more thanks go to another attendee, Marie Oetting, who supplied a wonderful story about the hospital and invited me to the reunion.

Let me recognize others who allowed me to speak to them about their memories of Children's Hospital: Helen Aff-Drum, Walter Benoist, Alan Brass, F. Sessions Cole, Harvey Colten, William H. Danforth, Michael DeBaun, Charles Dougherty, Ronald Evens, Lee F. Fetter, Ted Frey, Helen Nash, John Herweg, Velma Hunt, Dwayne Ingram, Lawrence Kahn, James Keating, Kenneth Koerner, Oliver Langenberg, Kathy Long, John Martz, James S. McDonnell III, Ron Morfeld, Hal Morse, Julie Moschenross, T.S. Park, William Peck, Alan Schwartz, Alfred Schwartz, Larry Shapiro, Jessie Ternberg, and Teresa Vietti. The eight community physicians — Lawrence Kahn, Peter Kieffer, Maurice Lonsway, Homer Nash, Peter Putnam, Paul Simons, Patricia B. Wolff, and Gerald Wool — who took part in the roundtable discussion (see the final interleaf in the book) provided delightful reminiscences.

In closing, I would like to dedicate this book to the three wonderful pediatricians who saw my children through the illnesses of childhood: Marsden Fox of Rochester, New York; Kathleen Winters and Patricia B. Wolff of St. Louis. They have my enduring gratitude and respect. Perhaps I could also include someone who brought me through my own diseases and hospitalizations: the late Wilma M. O'Connor, a registered nurse and my mother.

What a privilege it has been to delve into the history of St. Louis Children's Hospital, an institution beloved of so many and for such good reason. It offers a great gift to children and their families: the hope for healing and a brighter future — the very best that medical science, mixed with human compassion, can supply. We are all so fortunate to have this special place in our midst.

SELECTED BIBLIOGRAPHY

The following abbreviations have been used:
SLCH St. Louis Children's Hospital
WUA Washington University Archives
WUBML Washington University Becker Medical Library
WUSM Washington University School of Medicine

Primary Sources

Brookings, Robert. Collection. The Brookings Institution, Washington, D.C.

Dodge, Philip R. "How it Began and Developed: A Brief Autobiographical Sketch." *Journal of Child Neurology*, 14, 8 (August 1999), 537-40.

Goldring, David. Papers. WUBML.

Hartmann, Alexis F., Sr. Papers. WUBML.

Houston, David F. "A University for the Southwest: An Address Delivered Before the Commercial Club of St. Louis." October 31, 1908. WUA.

The Johns Hopkins Medical Institutions, Alan Mason McChesney Medical Archives. Alumnae records.

King, M. Kenton. Interview with Marion Hunt, 1991-92. WUBML.

Lionberger, Isaac. Papers. WUA.

Markham, Mary McKittrick. Journals and diaries. Missouri Historical Society.

Marriott, McKim. Personal family papers and photographs related to W. McKim Marriott. In private possession.

Marriott, Williams McKim. Collected reprints. WUBML.

Martha Parsons Free Hospital for Children. Annual reports. WUBML.

Mauran, Russell & Crowell, Architects; Goldwater, S.S.; and Veeder, Borden Smith. "The St. Louis Children's Hospital: A Hospital Group of a Distinct Character, which Provides for Contagious and Non-contagious Cases, and for Teaching and Research," *The Modern Hospital*, 5, 6 (December 1915), 387-394.

Missouri Republican [newspaper].

Morrow, Ralph. Papers. WUA.

SLCH. Annual reports. WUBML.

SLCH. Brochures, pamphlets, fund-raising publications. WUBML.

SLCH. *Child* [magazines]. SLCH Public Relations Department.

SLCH. Correspondence and memoranda. Miscellaneous Public Relations Files. WUBML.

SLCH. *Doctor's Digest*. WUBML.

SLCH. Elizabeth J. Liggett Memorial, St. Louis Children's Hospital: history of hospital and guide to the building, [1915].

SLCH. Minutes of the Board of Managers. WUBML.

SLCH. *Our Small World*.

SLCH. Records. WUBML.

SLCH. *Small Talk*. WUBML.

SLCH. *Small World*. WUBML.

St. Louis Globe-Democrat [newspaper].

St. Louis Post-Dispatch [newspaper].

St. Louis Star [newspaper].

St. Louis Times [newspaper].

Shaffer, Philip A. Papers. WUBML.

Toverud family. Personal family papers and photographs related to Kirsten Utheim Toverud. In private possession.

Veeder, Borden S. Papers. WUBML.

Washington University, Board of Trustees. Minutes of the Board of Trustees. WUA.

Washington University. *The Dedication of the New Buildings at Washington University Medical School*. St. Louis, April 28, 29 and 30, 1915. St. Louis, [1915].

Washington University Chronicle. WUA.

Washington University Magazine and predecessors. WUA.

Washington University Record. WUA.

WUSM. Annual course bulletins and catalogs. WUBML.

WUSM. Executive Faculty records. WUBML.

WUSM. Office of the Dean, Department of Pediatrics files. WUBML.

WUSM. *Outlook Magazine*. WUBML.

Weekly Bulletin of the St. Louis Medical Society.

White, Park J. Papers. WUBML.

Secondary Sources

Aub, Joseph and Ruth K. Hapgood. *Pioneer in Modern Medicine: David Linn Edsall of Harvard*. Cambridge, MA: Harvard Medical Alumni Association, 1970.

Barclay, Dorothy. "Godmother to the Nation's Youngsters." *New York Times*, April 2, 1952.

Becker Digital Collection, "Beyond TLC: Missouri Women in the Health Science Professions." http://beckerexhibits.wustl.edu/mowihsp/index.htm

Bliss, Michael. *The Discovery of Insulin*. Toronto: McClelland & Stewart, Inc., 1982.

Caal, Carla and Barbara Oliver Korner (eds.). *Hardship and Hope: Missouri Women Writing about their Lives, 1820-1920*. Columbia, MO: University of Missouri Press, 1997.

Cannon, Bradford. "As I Remember: James Barrett Brown," *Annals of Plastic Surgery*, 7(1): July 1981, 79-84.

Cleave, Egbert. *Cleave's Biographical Cyclopedia of Homoeopathic Physicians and Surgeons*. Philadelphia: Galaxy Publishing Co., 1873.

Cone, Thomas E., Jr. *History of American Pediatrics*. Boston: Little, Brown & Co., 1980. WUBML.

Compton, Richard J. and Dry, Camille N. *Pictorial St. Louis: The Great Metropolis of the Mississippi Valley. A Topographical Survey Drawn in Perspective, A.D. 1875*. St. Louis, 1876; Reprinted 1997.

Dictionary of American Biography. New York: Charles Scribner and Sons, 1928-1936 & Supplements. New York: Scribner, c. 1944, Vol. 1-. WUBML.

Crighton, John C. *The History of Health Services in Missouri*. Omaha: Barnhart Press, 1993.

Doisy, Edward. "An Autobiography." *Annual Review Biochemistry*: 45. 1976.

Duncan, T.C. *Diseases of Infants and Children with their Homeopathic Treatment*. Chicago: Duncan Brothers, c. 1878.

Edmonds, William A. *A Treatise on Diseases Peculiar to Infants and Children*. New York: Boericke & Tafel, 1881. SLCH Library.

_____ and S.B. Parsons (eds.). *St. Louis Periscope*. Vol. VII. St. Louis; Fred N. Nixon, 1884.

Faber, Harold K., and Rustin McIntosh. *A History of the American Pediatric Society, 1887-1965*. New York: McGraw-Hill, 1966.

Flexner, Abraham. *Abraham Flexner: An Autobiography*. New York: Simon and Schuster, 1960.

_____ *Medical Education in the United States and Canada : A Report to the Carnegie Foundation for the Advancement of Teaching*. New York: Arno Press, 1972.

Grisham, Marjorie Fox. "History of the Washington University School of Medicine." Unpublished typescript. WUBML.

Hagedorn, Hermann. *Brookings: A Biography*. New York: Macmillan, 1936.

Hall, Corinne Steele. "The Children's Friend: Dr. Aaron J. Steele." Missouri Historical Society Bulletin, 8, 3.

"To honor Alexis F. Hartmann, Sr., M.D.: his students and colleagues have contributed to this issue." *Journal of Pediatrics*, 64, 6, June 1964.

Hunt, Marion. "A Coming of Age with Pediatrics." Washington University School of Medicine, *Outlook Magazine*, spring 1982, 18-24.

_____. "'Extraordinarily Interesting and Happy Years': Martha M. Eliot and Pediatrics at Yale, 1921-1935." *Yale Journal of Biology and Medicine*, 68, 5-6 (Sept.-Dec.1996), 159-170.

_____. "From Childsaving to Pediatrics: A Case Study of Women's Role in the Development of SLCH 1879-1925." Ph.D. thesis, Washington University, 1992. WUBML.

_____. *A Goodly Heritage: St. Louis Children's Hospital"s Centennial History 1879-1979*. St. Louis: SLCH, 1981. WUBML.

_____. "Women and Childsaving: St. Louis Children's Hospital, 1879-1979." Missouri Historical Society *Bulletin*, 36, 2 (January 1980), 65-79.

Hyde, William and Howard Conard (eds.). *Encyclopedia of the History of St. Louis*. New York, Louisville, St. Louis: The Southern History Company, 1899. WUBML.

Jeans, P.C. and W. McKim Marriott. Nutrition: *A Textbook of Infant Feeding for Students and Practitioners of Medicine*. St. Louis: C.V. Mosby, 1947.

King, William Harvey (ed.). *History of Homoeopathy and its Institutions in America: Their founders, benefactors, faculties, officers, hospitals, alumni, etc. with a record of achievement of its representatives in the world of medicine*. New York: Lewis Publishing Company, 1905. WUBML.

Lomax, Elizabeth M.R. *Small and Special: The Development of Hospitals for Children in Victorian Britain*. London: Wellcome Institute for the History of Medicine, 1996.

Marquis, Albert Nelson (ed.), *The Book of Louisans*. 2nd ed., St. Louis: The St. Louis Republic, 1912.

Meckel, Richard A. *Save the Babies: American Public Health Reform and the Prevention of Infant Mortality, 1850-1929*. Baltimore: John Hopkins University Press, 1990.

Memorial Service, Carl V. Moore, M.D.: 1908-1972, Graham Chapel, Washington University, October 29, 1972, three o'clock.

Williams McKim Marriott, 1885-1936: Memorial addresses at a meeting held in the auditorium of the Washington University School of Medicine. Sunday, January 3, 1937. St. Louis: Privately printed, Washington University.

Mosby, C.V. *Little Journeys to the Homes of Great Physicians: William Beaumont-physiologist; Augustus Charles Bernays-surgeon; Williams McKim Marriott-pediatrician*. St. Louis: C.V. Mosby, 1937. WUA.

Morrow, Ralph E. *Washington University in St. Louis: A History*. St. Louis: Missouri Historical Society Press, 1996.

Mueller, C. Barber. *Evarts A. Graham: The Life, Lives, and Times of the Surgical Spirit of St. Louis*. London: BC Decker Inc., 2002.

Nichols, Buford, Angel Ballabriga and Norman Kretchmer (eds). *History of Pediatrics, 1850-1950*. Nestlé Nutrition Workshop Series, Vol. 22. Vevey/New York: Raven Press, c. 1991.

O'Connor, Candace. *Beginning a Great Work: Washington University in St. Louis, 1853-2003*. St. Louis: Washington University, 2004.

Parrish, William E. *Frank Blair: Lincoln's Conservative*. Columbia, MO: University of Missouri Press, 1998.

Pearson, Howard A. *The Centennial History of the American Pediatric Society, 1850-1950*. North Haven, CT: American Pediatric Society, 1988.

Prescott, Heather Munro. *A Doctor of their Own: The History of Adolescent Medicine*. Cambridge, MA: Harvard University Press, 1998. WUBML.

Reps, John William. *Saint Louis Illustrated: Nineteenth-Century Engravings and Lithographs of a Mississippi River Metropolis*. Columbia: University of Missouri Press, 1989.

Risse, Guenter B. *Mending Bodies, Saving Souls*. Oxford: Oxford University Press. 1999.

Robinson, G. Canby. *Adventures in Medical Education*. Cambridge, Massachusetts: Harvard University Press, 1957.

Rosenberg, Charles. *The Care of Strangers: The Rise of America's Hospital System*. New York: Basic Books, 1987.

Stelnicki, Eric, Leroy V. Young, Tom Francel, Peter Randall. "Vilray P. Blair, His Surgical Descendants, and their Roles in Plastic Surgical Development." *Plastic and Reconstructive Surgery*, 103, 7 (June 1999), 1990-2009.

Stevens, Walter B. *St. Louis, The Fourth City 1764-1909*. St. Louis-Chicago: The S.J. Clarke Publishing Co., 1909.

Tolin, C. Alvin. "The Transformation of SLCH into a Complete Hospital." Typescript, April 2, 1984.

Van Ravenswaay, Charles. *St. Louis: An Informal History of the City and Its People, 1764-1865*. St. Louis: Missouri Historical Society Press, 1991.

Veeder, Borden S, "Pediatric Profiles: Williams McKim Marriott, 1885-1936," *Journal of Pediatrics*, 47, 6 (December 1955), 791-801.

White, P.J., Borden S. Veeder, *Journal of Pediatrics*, 56, 2 (February 1960) 139-146.

WUSM Becker Medical Library, "Distinguished Women from Washington University." http://pathbox.wustl.edu/%7Eawn/awntop/distinguished.html

Zahorsky, John. *St. Louis Courier of Medicine*. St. Louis: Courier of Medicine Co., 1904-05.

Zonsius, Patricia M. *Children's Century: Children's Hospital Medical Center, 1890-1990*. Akron: Children's Hospital Medical Center of Akron, 1990.

Author Interviews

Helen Aff-Drum, Alan Brass, F. Sessions Cole, Harvey Colten, William H. Danforth, Michael DeBaun, Philip R. Dodge, Charles Dougherty, Ronald Evens, Lee F. Fetter, Ted Frey, Susan K. Goddard, John Herweg, Velma Hunt, Lawrence Kahn, Dwayne Ingram, James P. Keating, Peter Kieffer, M. Kenton King, Oliver Langenberg, Kenneth Koerner, Kathleen Long, Maurice Lonsway, Jr., McKim Marriott, James S. McDonnell III, J. Neal Middelkamp, Ron Morfeld, Julie Moschenross, Hal Morse, Helen Nash, Homer Nash, Elizabeth O'Connell, Marie Oetting, T.S. Park, William Peck, Peter Putnam, Betty Vallero Reinke, Walton O. Schalick III, Alan Schwartz, Alfred Schwartz, Larry Shapiro, Paul Simons, Jessie Ternberg, Teresa Vietti, Patricia Wolff, and Gerald Wool.

INDEX

Page numbers in *italics* include illustrations.

A

A. Ernest and Jane G. Stein Professorship in Developmental Neurology, 118
Abelson, Herbert, 182
Abendschein, Dana R., 162
Abendschein, Jane, 162
Adams, Raymond D., 107-8
administrators, 183
Adolescent Center, 166
adoption, 20, *181*
advisory committee, 7-8, 37-8, 92
advocacy
  awards for, 168-9, 170
  health care reform, 148-9
  lady board of managers, 70
  legislative lobbying, 167, 168-9, 176
  mission of SLCH and, 145, 172, 180-1
  safety education, 168
Aff-Drum, Helen, *72*, 83, 156
affiliations, 28, 62, 63, 152-3
African-American patients, 26, 46, 51, *65-6*, 88-9
African-American physicians, 87, 90, *92*
Agress, Harry, 131
AIDS epidemic, 149, 167
Alexander, Lamar, 142
Alexander, Marion, 167, 171
Allen, Gerard B., 5, 7, 8, *10*, 13, 26
Allen, Grace, 5, 6
Allen P. and Josephine B. Green Professorship of Pediatric Neurology, 110
Allison, Nathaniel, 43, 45, 71
allopathic medicine and practitioners, 10, 11, 23, 28, 30
Alpha Phi Sorority, *122*
Alumni Endowed Professor of Pediatrics, 163, 176
Ambulatory Care department, 119-20
Ambulatory Pediatric Association, 164
American Academy of Pediatrics (officers), 182
American Board of Pediatrics, 182
American Cancer Society, 120
American Medical Association, 30
American Pediatric Society, 8, 64, 182
American Red Cross, *56*, 57
Ames, Nancy, 121
ANCC Magnet designation, 134-5, 178
Anderson, Charles R., 82
Anderson, Donald C., 119
Anderson, Lori, 152
Anderson, Nathan, 152
anesthesiology division, 152
Answer Line, 146, *166*, 170
antibiotics, 86-7, 88-9
Apolline Blair Professor of Surgery, *111*, 163
appendicitis, 86
"April in Paris," 143
Arness, James, 132
Arrick, Sandy, 162
artwork, *68*, *181*

Aschuff, Jan, 171
Ashcroft, John, 143
asthma management, 146, 166
Atwood, Donna, 97, *98*
Augusta Free Hospital for Children, 23, 24
Auxiliary, 44, 93, *114*, 116, 134, 143
awards given by SLCH
  Community Avocate of the Year award, 170
  George F. Gill Prize in Pediatrics, 67, 71, 73, 81, 111
  Heart of Gold, *170*, 183
  Helen E. Nash Academic Achievement Award, 92
  Keating Outstanding Resident Award, 119
  medical staff distinguished service, 183
  Quality Award, 163
awards received
  for advocacy, 169, 170
  for COPE program, 147
  E. Mead Johnson Award, 144, 145, 161
  Javits Neuroscience Investigator Award, 155
  John Howland Medal, 64, 88, 182
  NIH Child Health Research Center of Excellence, 162
  Nobel Prize winners, 61, 76, *174*
  for nursing excellence, 134-5, 178
  Outstanding Teaching Award, 164
  from United Cerebral Palsy Women's Board, 162

B

Bain, Katherine, 73, 74, 83, 87, 91, 183
Ballew, Debbie, 100, 101
Ballinger, Walter F, II, 110
Banting, Frederick G., 76
Barnes, Robert, 13, 19, 37, *39*
Barnes Hospital, 40-1, 46, 49, *50*, 62, 63, 66, 117
Barnes School of Nursing, 95
Barnett, Henry L., 87, 182
Barr, Dave, 75
Barr, Jessie Wright, 19, 21, 38
Barr, William, 19, 38, 44
Bartlett, Robert, 88
Base Hospital No. 21, *56*, *57*, 130, *131*
Bassett, George S., 163
Bauer, Charles R., 119
Baumgarten, Walter, 43
Beaumont Foundation, 115
Becker, Bernard, 110
Beckman, Mary Elizabeth, *133*, *135*
behavioral problems, services for children with, 70, 85
Behrer, Isbell, *107*
Behrer, M. Remsen, 100, 107, 182
Belford, William W., 182
Bell, James W., 25
Bell, Jane Major, 25

benefits
  "April in Paris," 143
  Auxiliary, 116
  Bob Hope's 100th Birthday Party, *103*, 121, 123
  CAROUSEL, 139, 143
  Children's Miracle Network Telethon, 143
  in early 1900s, *31*
  golf tournaments, 97, 115, 116, *121*, 143, 171
Benoist, Walter, 116
bequests
  Barnes, Robert, 46
  Barnes Hospital, 40-1
  Barr, William, 38, 44
  Butler, James and Margaret, 65
  Russell, Alexander, 38
Best, Charles H., 76
Bielefeld, Paula, *112*
Bier, Dennis, 109, 145, 183
Birth Defects Center, 107
Bisch, Ida, 31
Bishop, Mary McFayden, 82
Bixby, William K., 40
Bixby Professor of Surgery, 66
BJC Health System, 153-4, 160, 161, 167-8, 172, 179-80
Blackfan, Kenneth, 47
Blades, Brian, 88
Blair, Apolline Alexander, *4*, 6, 13, 22, 28, *111*, 163, 183
Blair, Apolline (Mrs. James Blair), 29
Blair, Eveline, 47
Blair, Francis P., Jr., 5
Blair, James, 29
Blair, Montgomery, 5
Blair, Vilray P., 57, *68*, 73, 82
Blattner, Russell J., 82, 87, 88, 91, 96, 182
Blethen, Sandra, 118
Bleyer, Adrien, 83
Block, Velinda, 128, *129*, 174
Bloom, Marshall, 119
Bloomberg, Gordon R., 146, *164*
Blow, Susan, 12
board members.
See also advisory committee
  in 1910, 44
  1989-1993, 152
  admission of men, 92
  Brookings, Robert S., 32-3
  chairmen (listed), 183
  financial recommendations (1970s), 113
  at founding, 6-7, 13
  Fowler, Cora Liggett, 41
  Leighton, George E., *8*
  SLCH expansion 1948-1952, 92
board of lady managers, 59, 69-71
Board of Managers, 93
Board of Trustees, 93, 160, 170
Bob Hope Foundation, 97, 121
Boles, C. Read, 15, 87
Bond, Christopher, 143

Bost, Crawford A., 182
bottle-feeding, 27-8, 67-8, *72*, *133*
Bourgeois, Blaise F.D., 155
Bower, Richard, 127
Bowles, George W., *107*
Boyce, Dr., 26
Boyd, Rev. W.W., 19
Bradford, William, 182
Brass, Alan, 119, *144-5*, 147-8, 151, 152, 154-5, 165, 169, 183
Brazy, Jane E., 119
breast-feeding, 27. *See also* wet nurses
Brewer, Eileen D., 119
Briagas, Austin, *160*
Briagas, Rebecca, *160*
Bricker, Eugene, 82
Bridge, Hudson, 8
Bridwell, Keith H., 166
Brookings, Robert S., 13, 19, 25, *32-3*, 37, 39, 40, 41, 43, 46, 49, 51, 59
Brown, Dana, 143, 163, 183
Brown, Fred L., 154, 160
Brown, James Barrett, *68*, 73, 88
Brunstrom, Janice E., *162*, 179
Buck, Joe, 176
Building for Care, Searching for Cures campaign, 178
Bulkley, Mary E. ("Minnie"), 13, *20*, 21, 27, 51, 70
Burford, Tom, 97, 98, 100, 101
Burlingham, Louis H., *62*, 66, 131, 182, 183
Burlis, Norbert W., 100, 101
burn center, *179*
Butler, James Gay, *65*, 66, 89
Butler, Margaret L., *65*, 66, 89
Byars, Louis T., 82

C

Calvin, Lincoln, 87
Campbell, James, *12*, 13, *27*, 74
Campbell, Robert, 12
Campbell, Virginia Kyle, 12
cancer. *See* oncology
Cannella, Vincent J., 152, 183
Cantor, Eddie, 94, 100
Capen, Frances Pond, 11
Capen, George D., 11
Cardinal Glennon Children's Hospital, 93, 143, 153, 167
cardiology, 100-1, *172*, 179. *See also* transplant program
Care and Cures campaign, *176*
"CARES" service, 165
Carlson, Douglas, 165, 166
Carnahan, Mel, 169
Carnegie, Andrew, 40
CAROUSEL, 139, 143
Carson, Merl J., 82, 98, 182
Catlin, Theron, 74, 82
Catlin Fellowship, 91
"Celebrate Spring" party, *162*
Centennial Gala Committee, 120

Cerebral Palsy Center, *162*, 179
Chalhub, Elias G., 119
Chandler, Warren, 93, *94*
chaplaincy staff, *149*
"Cherry Carnival," 48, 50
Chihuly, Dale, 181
Child Development Center, *139*, 163
Child Guidance Clinic, 71, 75, 85, 97
Child Life Services, 134, *167*, 171
Child magazine, 150, *159*, 178
Child Neurology Society, 88
Childhood Asthma Management Program (CAMP), 146, 166
Children's Advisory Committee, 126
Children's Advocacy Network (CAN), 176
Children's Circle of Care, 171
Children's Discovery Institute, *176*, 177-8
Children's Health Network, 152
Children's Health Services, 152
Children's Hospital Injury Prevention Coalition, 168
Children's Hospital Magazine, 137
Children's Medical Executive Committee (CMEC), 147
Children's Miracle Network Telethon, 143
Children's Research Foundation, 84, 85-6
Children's United Research Effort, 155
Christian Hospital Northwest, 153, 167
Christmastime, *68*, 85, *114*, 149, 155
Christopherson, Elinor H., 182
Ciechanover, Aaron, 174
Claiborne, Estelle, 73, 83, 88, *93*, *94*, *95*, *131*, 182, 183
Clarke, Rev. James W., *94*
Clarke, William C., 119
Clausen, Samuel W., 62, 182
Cleary, Thomas G., 119
Cleft Palate and Craniofacial Deformities Institute, 110, 166, 171, 179
Cleveland, William W., 182
Clopton, Malvern, 43, *57*
Clown Docs program, *162*
cochlear implants, 152, 166, 178
coffee shop, 114
Cole, Barbara, 119, 148, *163*, 164, 172
Cole, Carol Skinner, 64
Cole, F. Sessions, 90, 145, 147, 155, 161, 163, 167, 168
Collins, Francis S., 164
Collisson, William, 6, 7, 8, 30
coloring book developed, 132
Colten, Harvey R., 119, *141*, 144, 145-8, 151, 154, *155*, 157, 161, 183
Combs School, 181
Community Avocate of the Year award, 170
Community Fund, 70
community health outreach, 170-1
community initiatives, 173

Community Outreach Practice Experience (COPE), 147, 155, 164
community physicians, reminisces of, *156-7*
community physicians, ties to, 146-7, 148, 155, 176
Comstock, T. Griswold, *6*, 11, 12, 38
contagious disease ward, 22-3, 25
Conway, James F., 119, *120*, 122, 123
Conzelman, Jimmy, 93
cookbook published, 114
Cooke, Jean Valjean, *60*, 61, 62, 74, 87, 90, 98, 182
Coomer, Sarah, *129*
Cooney, Charlene, 138
Copher, Glover, 66
Cordonnier, Justin, 110
Cori, Carl, 81
Cori, Gerty, 81
Cornblath, Marvin, 182
Cornelius, William, 152, 183
Crist, William, 119, 182, 183
critical care medicine, 146
Crocker, Albert, 87
Crow, Karen, *160*
Cummings, John C., 6, 7, 30
Cupples, Martha S., 21
Cupples, Samuel, 7, *10*, 13, 19, 37, 41
Cystic Fibrosis Center, 166
cystic fibrosis clinic, 127

D

Dacey, Ralph G., Jr., 146, 165
Daeschner, C. William, Jr., 182
Damone, Vic, 121
Dana Brown Emergency Unit, *163*
Dana Brown/St. Louis Children's Hospital professorship, 163-4
Danforth, Donald, Jr., 113, 123
Danforth, John, 143
Danforth, William H., 94, 97, 106, 109, 119, 120, 123, 142, 183
Danforth Chapel, 94
Danforth Foundation, 94, 173
Darling (head of nursing school), 130
Darrow, Daniel C., 73, *88*, 96, 182
Daughaday, William, 118
Davie, Joe, 141
Davis, Edith January, 37, 73, 75
Davis, John T., 38
Dawson, Jeffrey, 166
day care center, 120, *139*
DeBaun, Michael R., *148*, 176
DeCeu, Claire, 182, 183
Dehner, Louis, 145
Dempsey, Edward, 99, *104*, 105
Denny-Brown, Derek, 107
dentistry division, 144, 166
Department of Pediatrics, 161, 178, 179
  SLCH MDs as chairs at other institutions (listed), 182

Department of Pediatrics: heads
  Colten, Harvey R., *141*
  Dodge, Philip R., 107-12
  Goldring, David (acting head), *104*, 106-7
  Hartmann, Alexis F., 75, *80-6*
  Howland, John, 43, *45-7*
  Marriott, Williams McKim, *52-3*, 58, 61-4
  Schwartz, Alan L., *161*
  Veeder, Borden Smith (interim head), 60
Depression era, 74-5, 80
desegregation, 89-90
Deutch, Max, *85*, 87
Development Board, 116, 143, 171
Dever, Lauren, 165
DeVivo, Darryl C., 110, 118, 125
Devoto, Claire, 122
diabetes research, 76-7, 142
Diagnostic Center, 151
dialysis unit, 115, *149*
diarrheal diseases, 27-8, 74
Dickson, Grace Allen, 10
Dietary Department, *112*
diphtheria, 8-9, 61, 67
diseases report (1904), *31*
dispensary, *30*, 45, 73
Dock, George, 44-5, 51, 53
Doctor's Digest, 149
Dodge, Philip R., *106-12*, 108, 113, 119, *120*, 125, 126, 127, 135, 157
Dodson, W. Edwin, 108, 110, 119
Dogramaci, Ihsan, 182
Doisy, Edward A., 76
Dolan, Peggy, 149
Donald O. Schnuck Family Professor of Neurology, 164
Donald Schnuck Professor of Pediatrics, 127
donations. *See also* bequests; endowments; fund-raising; grants; specific donors
  in 1980s, 143
  for building fund (1883), 13
  Children's Research Foundation, 84, 85-6
  from Community Fund Campaign, 74
  for contagious disease pavilion, 33
  from Danforth Foundation, 94
  of iron lung, 75
  for leukemia research, 90, *91*
  for medical school, 40
  for metabolism ward, 73
  from Murphy, Missouri 4-H, 101
  to neurology, 114
  for NICU, 119
  for operating expenses (1907), 37
  for outreach programs, 173
  for pediatrics dept., *106*
  for psychology laboratory, 116
  for research building, 162
  Ridge Farm, *47*, 48
  of rooms/wards (1890s), 25

  for Spoehrer Tower, 115, 116
  for third hospital (1915), 40, 41-2, 45
Donnell, George N., *182*
Donor Recognition Hall, *180*
Dougherty, Charles H., 106, 108, 147
Doval, John H., 87
Down Syndrome clinic, 179
Dowton, S. Bruce, 141, 145, 183
Drewes, Ted, 143
Duncan, T.C., 9, 27
Dyer, Eddie, *98*

E

E. Mead Johnson Award, 144, 145, 161
Ebrecht, Susan, 181
ECMO (extracorporeal membrane oxygenation), 144, *152*
Edison Center Atrium Cafeteria, 153
Edmonds, William A., 7, 14-15, 30
Edsall, David L., 40, 46
education. *See also* interns; nursing education; residency program; Washington University School of Medicine; *specific schools*
  homework, 149
  kindergarten for patients, 24, 26
  in mental health issues, 86
  pediatric instruction begins, 8
  at Ridge Farm, 70
  vocational education for disabled children, 70
Edwards, Diane, 101
Edwards, William L., 120, 183
Eliot, Martha May, *64*, *65*, 88, 182, 183
Eliot, William Greenleaf, 19, 24, 65
Elizabeth J. Liggett Memorial Building, 42, 49
Elman, Robert, 82
Ely & Walker Dry Goods, 26
Emergency Maternal and Child Care Program (EMIC), 88
emergency services, *145-6*, *151*, 156, *163*, 165
encephalitis, 75, 84, 87
endowments. *See also* bequests; grants
  in 1890s, 25, 26
  in 2000s, 175
  Grace Jones Floor, 94
  for infectious disease, 74
  James Gay Butler Endowment Fund, 65
  for obstetrics department, 63-4
  psychiatry chair, 97
England, Doris Asselmeier, *112*, 112-13, *135*
Erganian, Jane, 156
Erlanger, Joseph, *60*, *61*
Escobedo, Marilyn B., 119
Evens, Ronald G., 120, 126, *139*, *140-1*, 142-4, *143*, 144, 183
Executive Faculty, 66, 105, 107, 139, 161
Eyermann, Stacey, *180*

F

Facility Services, 181
Family Advisory Council, 164
Family-Centered Care, *160*
Family Resource Center, 168
Famous-Barr, 93
Farrell, Neal J., 144, 183
Feigin, Ralph D., *109*, 118, 125, 182, 183
fellowships, 74, 82, 91
Ferguson, Tom, 97, 101
Fern Waldman Fund, 90, *91*
Fetal Heart Center, *170*
Fetter, Lee, 139, 140, 153, *170*, *172-3*, *176*, *180*, 181, 183
Fields, Elizabeth, *122*
50th anniversary celebration, 74
Filley, John D., 45
financial structure/conditions. *See also* donations; fund-raising
  in 1880s, 26-7
  in 1907, 37
  in 1970s, 113-14
  in 1980s, 139-40, 143-4, 150
  in 1994, 155
  BJC Health System and, 179-80
  budget (1936-37), *83*
  Evens' strategies, 142
  mergers, 153
  reconstruction (1970s), 117-18
  Tolin on, 127
fires at SLCH, *24*, 116, 147
Fischel, Walter, 57
Fischel, Washington E., 30
Fishman, Marvin A., 110, 125
Flexner, Abraham, 33, *40*, 49, 58, *59*, 60
Flye, M. Wayne, *126*
Foglia, Robert P., 146, 152, *171*
Forbes, Gilbert B., 81, 82, 87, 98, 182
Ford, Richard F., 123
Ford Foundation, 95
Forest Park Balloon Race, 165
Forest Park Preservation Fund, 122
Fowler, Cora Liggett, 41-2, 43-4, 45, 49
Fowler, John, 41
Fowlkes, Erin, *129*
Fraley, Moses, 5
Fraley, Rose Harsh, 5, 74, 92
Frankin, Edward C., 5, 11, 30
Fredbird, *152*
Frey, Ted W., 117, 119, 140, 143, 154, 160, 161, 163-5, *167*, 172, 173, 177, 183
Friends of St. Louis Children's Hospital, 114, 171
fund-raising. *See also* benefits; donations; endowments; grants
  in 1880s, 11-13
  in 1980s, 143
  in 1990s, 171
  Auxiliary activities, 114, 116, 143
  by board of lady managers in 1920s, 69-71

brochure (1950), 80
Building for Care, Searching for Cures campaign, 178
"Canes to Cranes," *155*
"Cherry Carnival," 48, 50
for expansion 1948-1952, 92-5
for expansion 1960s, 98-9
for expansion/renovation plans 2004-06, 174
for heart-lung pump, 100, *101*
in late 1800s, 26-7
for research building in 1960s, 106-7
for residency program, 175-6
for second building (1884), 13, 19-20, 123-4
Stevenson, Virginia on, 12
for third building (1915), 33, 40-1, 45
during WWI, 56
Furlong, Thomas, 19
Furlow, Leonard, 88
Fusz, Corie, *171*, 183
Fusz, Louis J., Jr., 160, *171*, 172, 183

G

Gans, Lawrence, 150
Garbutt, Jane, 176
Gasgupta, Biplab, 164
Gasser, Herbert S., 61
gastroenterology, 119, 144
Gellman, Elliot, 146, 176
General Education Board, 49, 59-60, 63-4, 67, 73-4
Genetics and Genomic Medicine, 178
genetics program, 115, 177
Genome Sequencing Center, 177
George F. Gill Prize in Pediatrics, 67, 71, 73, 81, 111
Gephardt, Richard, 169
Geppert, Leo J., 88
Gibbon, John H., Jr., 100
Gibbon-Mayo Heart-Lung Pump, *101*
Gibbs, Jacob, 177
gift shop, 114
Gill, George F., 67, *71*, 73, 81, 111
Ginther, Bertha, *99*
Girand, Jane, *135*
Gitlin, Jonathan D., 145, 155, *161*, 163, 166, 176, 178, 179
Gleason, Wallace A. ("Skip"), 111-12, 119
Goddard, Susan K., *112*, 113, 132, *135*
Going, Ina, 133
Goldman, Lawrence, 83-4
Goldring, David, 81, 82, 87, 89, 99, *100-1*, *104*, *106-7*, 109, *122*, 157, 183
Goldring, Evelyn, 107
Goldsmith, Matthew, 177
Goldwater, S.S., 46
golf tournaments, 97, 115, 116, *121*, 143, 171
Good Samaritan Hospital, *10-11*, 30

INDEX

Page numbers in *italics* include illustrations.

G (cont.)
Goodman, Charles H., 6, 7, 13, *20*, 21, 22, 37, 38
Grace Hill Neighborhood Services, 170
Grady, R. Mark, 176
Graham, Benjamin B., 5
Graham, Christine Biddle Blair, *5*, 29, 45, 47, 48, 51
Graham, Evarts A., 66, 73, 80, *81*, 86
Grange, Kathy, *179*
Granoff, Dan, 145
Grant, Georgiana Ladas, *168*
Grant, Julia Dent, 25
grants. *See also* endowments
   for air-conditioning, 95
   for community health outreach, 170
   for dialysis unit, 115
   GEB, for medical school, 49, 59-60
   for Neuropsychiatry, 85
   NIH, for research, 96, 114-15, 147, 162, 166, 176
   for research, 99, 148, 165-6, 176-7
Gratz, Anderson, 45
Gratz, Benjamin, 45
Gray, W. Ashley, Jr., 106, *107*
Green, Allan P., 110
Green, John, 67
Green, Josephine B., 110
Green, Sue, 146
Green Foundation, 114
Greenwood, Robert S., 119
Griffin, Kathleen, *139*
Gruzeski, Mike, 164
Gundelach, Charles H., 7
Gutierrez, Fernando, 101
Gutierrez, Rudolfo, *98*
Gutman, Daisy, 171
Gutman, Louis, 171
Gutmann, David H., *164*
Guy, Katherine L., 46
Guze, Samuel, 99, 110, 116

H
Hagedorn, Hermann, 32, 33
Hagemann, Virginia, *132*, 135
Hale Irwin Center for Pediatric Hematology/Oncology, 163, 179
Hale Irwin Golf Tournament, 116, 143
Hall, Corinne Steele, 23
Hall, Frederick Aldin, 51, 74
Hall, John, 87
Hamm, Harry, 116
Hampton, Oscar, 88
Hamvas, Aaron, *166*
Hanpeter, Dorothy, *163*
Hansen, Kyle, *144*
Hanto, Douglas, 150
Harbison, Samuel, 82
Hardaway, W.A., 23, *24*
Harper, Kameron, 164
Harriet B. Spoehrer Professorship, 163
Harrison, Stanley, 87

Hartmann, Alexis F., Jr., 87, 100
Hartmann, Alexis F., Sr., 67, 74, 75, *76-7*, 80-6, 87, 89, 91, *93*, *94*, *98*, 105, *107*
Hatfield, Carol, 182, 183
Hatfield, Paul, 182, 183
Hauff, Marni, 155
Hauff, Warren, 155
Hayashi, Robert J., 163
Haymond, Morey, 118
Health Care for Kids, 153
health care reform, 148
Healthy Kids at Play, 173
Healthy Kids Express, 169, 170, 173
heart disease, 98, 100-1. *See also* cardiology; transplant program
Heart of Gold award, *170*, 183
Heart Station, *172*
Heinbecker, Peter, 82
Helen E. Nash Academic Achievement Award, 92
Helene B. Roberson Professor of Pediatrics, 161, 163
hematology/oncology, 112, 179
Hempelmann, T.C., 67
Hemphill, Alice, 164
Henderson, John B., 5, 7
Henderson, Mary Foote, 5, 6
Hermann E. Spoehrer Children's Research Tower, 115, 116
Hernandez, Antonio "Tony", 97, 100, *122*
Herron, Stephen, *179*
Herweg, Dorothy Glahn, *82*, *135*, 156
Herweg, John, *82*, 86-7, 88, 106
Heys, Florence, 87, 91
Higgins, Ronald, Jr., 87
Hillman, Laura A., 119
Hirshberg, Gary, 152
Hoekstra, Lilly, 95, 113, *131*, 135, 182, 183
Hoffmann and Sauer, 115
Hoffmann Partnership, 123
Holland, Julia Rumsey, 89
Holt, L. Emmett, Sr., 8, 27
home visits, 44-5
Homeopathic Medical College of Missouri, 5, *21*, 30, 42
homeopathic medicine and practitioners, 4-6, 10, 11, 14-15, 21, 25-6, 29-31, 43
Homer G. Phillips Hospital, 83, 87, 89, 90
Hope, Bob, 97, *98*, 99, *104*, *121*, 123, *132*
Hope, Linda, *98*, 121
Hopper, Hedda, 94
Horatio Padilla, 182
hospitals, attitudes towards in early 1900s, 29
housekeeping staff, *99*
Houska, Charlie, 181
Houston, David F., 33, *39*, 41
Houston, Helen, 33, 39, 41
Howland, John, 43, 44, 45, *46-7*, 52, 53, 58, 60, 64, 88, 182

Huang, Shi H., 165
Huddleston, Charles, 150, 163
Humphrey, Harvey, 101
Hunt, Ken, 168
Hunt, Marion, 92
Hunt, Velma, *168*
Hurford, Phelps G., 62

I
immigrants, 9, 26
immunology, 120
incubators, 28, *85*, 96
Inder, Terrie, 179
infectious disease, 22-3, 25, 86-7, 109. *See also* specific diseases
influenza epidemic of 1918, 57
Ingram, Dwayne I., *172*
Institute of Medicine, National Academy of Sciences, 183
insulin research, *76-7*
intensive care, 119, *138*, *146*, *149*, 170
International Adoption Center, 181
interns, 64-5, 88
iron lung, 72, 75, 156
Irvine-Jones, Edith, 73
Irwin, Hale, *115*, 116, 143, 163, *179*, 183
Irwin, Sally, 183
Ittleson Foundation, 96-7

J
Jackes, Margaret, 114
Jackson, Benjamin F., 113
Jacobi, Abraham, 8, 27
Jacobsen, Carlyle, 85
Jaffe, David M., 145-6, *164*
James G. and Margaret L. Butler Ward, 65-6, 89
James Gay Butler Endowment Fund, 66
James S. McDonnell Charitable Trust, 162, 177, 178
James S. McDonnell Family Foundation, 177, 178
January, Julia, 73
Jaudon, Joseph C., 82, 83
Javits Neuroscience Investigator Award, 155
Jeans, Philip C., 48, 57, 67, 68, 96, 182
Jenkins, Laura, *167*
Jennie Mallinckrodt Ward, *60*
Jerrauld, Park, 107
Joe Buck Classic, 171
John Howland Medal, 64, 88, 182
Johnson, Ralph, 162
Johnston, Edwin M., 97, *107*, 183
Johnston, Meredith, 57
Joint Chairs Program, 163-4
Jones, Barbara, 182
Jones, Dorothy J., 82, *111*
Jones, Grace Richards, 19, 22, 31, *32-3*, *36*, 39, 41, 42, 46, 48, 49, 50, 51, 56, 64, 69, 70, 74, 92, 94, 181, 183

Jones, Landon Y., 182, 183
Jones, Laura Gray, 114
Jones, Lorraine, 45
Jones, M. Barry, 167
Jones, Nippy, *98*
Jones, Robert McKittrick, *33*, 38, 39, 40, 41
Jostes, Frederick, 88
Junior Clerkship, 111

K
Kahn, Jane, *107*
Kahn, Lawrence, 89, 100, *107*, 133, 156
Kaufman, Bruce, 146
Keating, James P., 109, 118, *119*, *151*, 157, 163, 175, 176, 183
Keating Outstanding Resident Award, 119
Keenan, William, 116
Keim, Lois, 63, 70
Keinstra, Randy A., 119
Kelly, Benjamin, 12
Kennedy, Walter J., 87
Kenton, Thomas, 182, 183
Kercheval, Royal D., *93*, *94*, 99, 183
Kieffer, Peter B., *157*
Kienstra, William, 182
King, Alexa, *134*
King, M. Kenton, 106, 107, 108, 109, 115, 141, 152
Kingsley, James P., 9-10
Kipnis, David, 118
Kirklin, John, 101
kissing babies, *70*
Kleinberg, Rosalyn, *139*
Klingberg, William Gene, 90, 182
Klingensmith, Georganna J., 119
Klocke, Angie, 168
Knight, Charles F., 154
Koerner, Kenneth, *85*, 91
KPLR-Channel 11, 143
Kreusser, Katherine L., 147

L
LaBeaume, Emma U., 44
LaBlance, Gary, 164, 174
laboratories, 29
Lactate-Ringer's solution developed, 74
Landau, William, 108
Landon, Michael, *109*
Langenberg, Alice M., *89*, 92, *93*, *94*, 183
Langenberg, Mary, 182, 183
Langenberg, Ollie, 182, 183
Langer, Jacob C., 152
Laura Weil Kindergarten, *24-5*, 26
Lee, Elizabeth Blair, 5
leeches, 142
Leighton, George E., 7, *8*
leukemia, 90

Lewis, Hugh, 97, 183
Lewis Larrick Ward Chair of Pediatric Cardiology, 179
library, *168*
Life Seekers, 119
Liggett, Elizabeth J., 41, *42*
Liggett, John E., 41
Lincoln, Edith, 96
Link, Theodore, 41
Linton, M.I., 11
Lionberger, Isaac, 49
Lipstein, Steve, 173, 180
Litzinger, Nancy W., 146
Loeb, Leo, 66, *82*
Loeb, Virgil, 67
Loeffler, Gisella, *68*
Londe, Sol, 82, 87
Londoff, John, 182, 183
Londoff, Sylvia, 182, 183
Long, Christine Graham, 29
Long, Kathleen, *164*
Lonsway, Maurice, Jr., 156, *157*, 183
Lonsway, Maurice, Sr., 62, 83, 156
Lowe, George, 87
Lowell, Jeffrey A., 150, 166
Luckey, Carol, *135*
Ludomirsky, Achi, *172*, 179
Luhmann, Scott, 162
Lusk, Rodney P., 152, 166
Luton, L.S., 29, 37, 38, *42*
Luyties, Carl J., *22*, 26
Luyties, Diedrich R., 7, 11, 22

M
Maas, Edith H., 64, 65
Mackinnon, Susan, 148
Makley, Torrence A., 87
Mallinckrodt, Edward, Sr., 38, 40, 59, *60*
Mallinckrodt, Jennie, 38, 59, *60*
Mallinckrodt Chemical, 93
Mallinckrodt Institute of Radiology, 73, 90, 98, 127
Mallory, George B., Jr., 166
Mallory, Susan, 148
Manary, Mark, *170*, 171
Mangalasmaya, Montri, 182
Manley, Charles, 110
March of Dimes, 107
"Margie Goes to St. Louis Children's Hospital," 132
Markham, George D., 38, 73
Markham, Mary McKittrick, 29, 38, 45, 73, 74, *94*, 183
Marriott, Williams McKim, 33, 49, *52-3*, *55*, *58*, *59*, 60-4, 66, *70*, 71-2, 75, *76-7*, 96, 119, 130, 163
Marsh, Jeffrey L., 110, *111*, 144, 147, 163
Marshall, Dick, 157
Martha Parsons Free Hospital, 23, 24, 25, 31, 43
Martin, Chester, 114

Martin, Frank F., 88
Martz, John C., 91, *96*
Maternal Child Program, 170
Mattie, Shannon, *163*
Mattison, Richard E., 146
Mauran, Russell & Crowell, 45
McAlister, William H., *152*
McBride, Grace, 171
McCall, Mary, 46
McCoy, Ernest E., *182*
McCulloch, Hugh, 57, 67, 69, 72, 73, 89, 96, *182*
McDonnell, Elizabeth Finney, *177*, *183*
McDonnell, James S., III, 119, *120*, 123, 143, 162, *177*, *178*, *183*
McDonnell, James S., Jr., 106, *177*
McDonnell, John F., 162, *177*
McDonnell, Libby, *177*, *182*
McDonnell Children's Cancer Center, 178
McDonnell Pediatric Research Building, *177*
McElwee, Lucien C., 22, *29*
McGann, Kathleen, 149
McKenna, Joseph, 122
McKittrick, Hugh, 6, 13, 19, 25
McKittrick, Mary Weber Cutter, *6*, 7-8, 13, 22, 25, *31*, *183*
McKnight, Robert, 101
McKusick, Victor A., 107
MedAssist Program, 143
Medicaid, 143, 150, 168, 169
medical diagnostics division, 151
medical genetics, 123
medical school. *See* Washington University School of Medicine
Medical Staff. *See also* interns; residency program
  in 1879, *12*
  in 1890s, *21*
  in 1919, *54-5*, *65*
  in 1930s, *81*, 82-3
  in 1942, *86*
  in 1957, *87*
  in 1991, *147*
  in 1994, *155*
  attitude of, 154
  clinical faculty, role of, 156-7
  decision-making, 161
  distinguished service awards, *183*
  faculty, notable (listed), 182-3
  integration of, 87, 90, 92
  international volunteer work, 170
  president (2005), 106
  Quality Improvement Council, 164
  surgical staff (1920), *69*
  women on, 64, 72, 73, 83, 148
  WUPN, 165
  during WWI, *56-7*
  during WWII, *86*, 87-8
Meds & Food for Kids (MFK), 170
Mendeloff, Eric N., 166, 171
meningitis, 86
mental health, 85, 86, 96, 97, 116, 146
Merritt, Dianne F., 148

Merritt, Katherine K., 64, 65
metabolism ward, 73
Meyer, Mel, 181
Middelkamp, J. Neal, *87*, 106, 168, *182*, *183*
Middelkamp, Roberta, 135
Migneco, Kim, *177*
milk. *See under* nutrition
Miller, James, 110, 175
Miller, Trudy, *142*
mission statement, 145, 172, 180-1
Missouri Advocate of the Year, 169
Missouri Baptist Medical Center, 167
Missouri Medical College, 28
Missouri Republican, 18
Mobile Intensive Care Unit, 170
Monfort, Candice, *182*, *183*
Moore, Carl V., 106
Moore, Robert, *93*
Moore, Terry, *98*
Morfeld, Ron, *140*
Morse, Rev. Harold S. ("Hal"), *149*
mortality rates, 8-10, 73, 86, 90
Mosby, C.V., 68
Moschenross, Julie, *125*
motto (of SLCH), 43
Mouse Genetics Core Laboratory, *177*
Moushey, Robin, *179*
Moyer, Carl, 105, *105*
MRI unit, 151
Mueller, C. Barber, 88, 134
Mueller, Charles W. ("Chuck"), *177*, *183*
Muglia, Louis, 176
Munger, Donna B., *33*
Murdock, Howard, 82
Murphy, Fred T., 49, 57, 60, 66
Murphy, John, 57
Musial, Stan, 98, 156

N

NADAH Women's Organization, 171
Naehr, Mary, *135*
Nash, Alison, *170*
Nash, Helen, *87*, 90, *92*
Nash, Homer E., Jr., *87*, *156*, 170, *183*
National Cystic Fibrosis Foundation, 120
National Institutes of Health, 114-15, 162
Needleman, Philip, *141*
neonatal intensive care unit (NICU), 119, *138*
nephrology, 109
neurofibromatosis, 164
neurology
  Child Neurology Society, 88
  donations, 114
  Javits Neuroscience Investigator Award, 155
  Philip Dodge, 108, 109-10
  professorships, 110, 118, 164, 165
  research, 118
neuropsychiatry department, 85

newborn medicine program, 172-3
Newman, Andrew, 140-1, *183*
Niehoff, Lois, *135*
Nienhaus, Shirley, *135*
Nobel Prize winners
  Banting, Frederick G., 76
  Ciechanover, Aaron, *174*
  Doisy, Edward A., 76
  Erlanger, Joseph, *61*
  Gasser, Herbert S., 61
Noble, J.W., 7
Noble, Lizabeth Halsted, 7, 21
Noce, Laura, *168*
Noetzel, Michael J., 149, 162
Nurse Sniggles, *162*
nurses' aides, 133
nursing education
  in 1944, 95
  Marriott on, 130
  rotation process, 131-2
  school established, 37, 129
  students 1908-25, 38, *130*
nursing staff, 128-35
  in 1879, 128-9
  in 1900s, *18*, *19*, 38
  in 1942, 86
  in 1944, 95
  in 1980, 134
  alumnae annual luncheon, 134
  Colten, Harvey R., on, 151
  difficulties, 58
  Goddard, Susan K., *112*, 133
  honors received, 134-5, 178
  importance of, 129-30
  Kahn, Lawrence on, 133
  Moschenross, Julie, *125*
  as parent substitutes, 131
  Red Cross in WWI, *56*
  relationship with patients, 133, 134
  salaries of, 18, 58, 130
  shared governance model, 134
  shortages (1920s, 1930s), 64, 130
  specialty-related wards, 113, 132-3, 135
  Ternberg, Jesse on, 133
  Tolin, C. Alvin on, 118-19
  uniforms, 132
  in WWI, 130, *131*
  in WWII, 88, 130-1
nutrition
  Dietary Department, *112*
  formula for infants, 27-8, 67-8, 72, *133*
  malnutrition, 74-5, 77, 170
  Marriott's infant feeding work, 55, 67-8
  milk, 27-8, *133*
  nutrient transfer *in utero*, 165
  toddler's ward, *133*
  vitamin D and rickets, 68
  wet nurses, 62, 63

O

O'Brien, Margaret, 132
obstetrics department, 63-4
occupational therapy, 63, 70, 90, *95*, 149
Ochoa, Damaris, *169*
O'Connell, Elizabeth, 95, 121, 131, *132*, 133, 135, *135*
Oetting, James, 134
Oetting, Marie, 134
O'Fallon, Caroline Schutz, *25*, 26
Office of Pediatric Quality Management (OPQM), 164
Ohning, Byrd Dell, 121, 133, *135*
Olin, Ann W., 111, 124
Olin, Spencer T., 111, 124
Olson, Bruce, 167
Olson, Kim, 167
Olson Family Garden, *167*
oncology, 82, 90, 112, 154, 178, 179
100th anniversary celebration, 120, 121, 123
Opie, Eugene L., 47, 60, 66
orphanages, affiliation with, 63
Orsheln, Rachel, 181
Osler, William, 30
Osmond Foundation, 143
Osterkamp, Lucille, 114
otoscope and ophthalmoscope, 99
Outpatient Department, 84, *91*, 111, 120
Outstanding Teaching Award, 164
Owens, Frank, *126*

P

Pagliara, Anthony, 110, 118
parents
  as participants in care, 160
  staying with children, 134
  visiting hours, 135
Park, Edwards, 52, 53, 59, 68
Park, T.S., *146*, *165*, 166
Park J. White Professorship in Pediatrics, 90, 147, 163
Parker, Mary, 118
parking garage built, 120
Parsons, Charles, 23
Parsons, Martha Pettus, 23
Parsons, Scott B., *11*, 12, 13, 21, 25-6, 30
Parsons, Scott E., 30, 31, 37, 42
Part-Time Advisory Group (PTAG), 147
pathology department, 29
Patient Care Team, *135*
patients
  African Americans, 26, 46, 51, 65-6, 88-9
  crafts, *37*, *63*
  education, 24, 26, 70, 149
  exercise, benefits of, 61
  number of/census, *31*, 37, 73, 94, 114, 120, 126, 150
  relationships with, 133, 134

Peabody, Francis Weld, 59
Peck, William, 152, 155, 161, 173, 177
Pediatric Clinical Research Center, 109
Pediatric Convulsion Clinic, 98
pediatric hospitals, founding of, 8
pediatric intensive care unit (PICU), *146*, *149*
Pediatric Oncology Group, 112, 154
pediatricians, characterized, 89
pediatricians-in-chief
  Colten, Harvey R., *141*
  Dodge, Philip R., 109, *125*
  Hartmann, Alexis F., Sr., *80-6*
  Marriott, Williams McKim, *52-3*
pediatrics. *See also* Department of Pediatrics
  medical school curriculum, 62
  Veeder on state of (1910), 44
penicillin, 86, 87, 88-9
Pérez-Fontán, Julio, 146, 176
Perkins, Linn B., *113*, 114, 117, 119, *120*, *124*, 125, 126, *183*
Perley, Anne M., 83, 87, 98
Perlmutter, David H., 144, 145, 166, 176, 179, 182
Petross, Teresa, 147
Pettus, Charles Parsons, 43
pharmacy, *142*
physical therapy, 149, *178*
physicians. *See* interns; Medical Staff; residency program
Pickering, Larry, 111, 119
Pierson, Charles E., 101
Plax, Steven I., 147
play therapy, 67
Pluek, Les, *85*
Poelker, John H., 122
poliomyelitis, 75, 89, 96
Pope, Mary, 73
Porter, E.F., Jr., 121
Portillo, Jesus, *169*
poverty
  admission baths, 72
  health care for inner city children, 153
  and mortality rates, 8
Powers, John Ray, 87
premature infant ward, 75, *84-5*, 87
Premature Program, 95
Prensky, Arthur L., *109*-10
presidents, *113*, *141*, *160*, *183*
Private Corridor, 134
professorships, 163-4
  A. Ernest and Jane G. Stein Professorship in Developmental Neurology, 118
  Allen P. and Josephine B. Green Professorship of Pediatric Neurology, 110
  Alumni Endowed Professor of Pediatrics, 163, 176
  Apolline Blair St. Louis Children's Hospital Professor of Surgery, *111*, 163
  Bixby Professor of Surgery, 66

INDEX

Page numbers in *italics* include illustrations.

P (cont.)
Dana Brown/St. Loius Children's Hospital professorship, 163-4
- Donald O. Schnuck Family Professor of Neurology, 164
- Donald Schnuck Professor of Pediatrics, 127
- Harriet B. Spoehrer Professorship, 163
- Helene B. Roberson Professor of Pediatrics, 161, 163
- Park J. White Professor of Pediatrics, 90, 147, 163
- Shi H. Huang Professor of Neurological Surgery, 165
- Spencer T. and Ann W. Olin Distinguished Professor, 111
- W. McKim Marriott Professor of Pediatrics, 119, 163

Project ARK (AIDS/HIV Resources for Kids), 167
psychiatry, 70, 85, 96, 97, 146
psychology laboratory, 116
public relations department, 116, 146
pulmonary division, 145
Putnam, Peter, 156, *157*

Q
Quayle, Kimberly S., 148
Quality Award, 163
Quality Improvement Council, 164
Queeny, Edgar M., 105
Queeny, Edith Schneider, 115
Queeny Tower, 105

R
Race, Helen, 162
radiology, 73, 90, 98. *See also* Mallinckrodt Institute of Radiology
Radomski, Michelle, *169*
Randolph, Jay, *122*
Ranken-Jordan Home for Convalescent Crippled Children, 115
Ratzan, Susan K., 119
Recchia, Kimberlee Coleman, 148
recreational therapy, *138*
Rector, Eleanor Johnson, *83*
rehabilitation services, 149
Reinke, Betty Vallero, 134, 135
Remsen, Ira, 39
research
- in 1920s, 67, 74
- in 1970s, 118
- in 1980s, 144
- in 1990s, 155, 165-6
- on asthma, 146, 166
- cancer, 82, 112
- Children's Research Foundation, 84, 85-6
- by Cole, F. Sessions, *147*
- by Colten, Harvey R., *141*
- C.U.R.E., 155
- on diabetes, 76-7, 142

- E. Mead Johnson Award, 144, 145, 161
- on encephalitis, 84, 87
- federal grants, 99
- funding: Dempsey vs. Hartmann, 99, 105
- GEB grant, 67
- grants, in 2000s, 176-7
- by Hartmann, Alexis F., *76-7*, 81
- on infant nutrition, 67-8, 68, 165, 170
- on insulin and diabetes, *76-7*
- Javits Neuroscience Investigator Award, 155
- on leukemia, 90, *91*
- by Marriott, W. McKim, 53
- McDonnell Pediatric Research Building, *177*
- in neurology, 118
- new building (2006), 162
- NIH Child Health Research Center of Excellence award, 162
- NIH grants, 96, 114-15, 147, 155, 166, 176
- Pediatric Clinical Research Center, 109
- on sickle cell disease, 148, 176
- on SIDS, 145, 155
- Society for Pediatric Research, 182
- on sulfa drugs, 86-7
- Tower Building, 98-9, 106-7, 115, 116
- on Wilson's Disease, 161
- WUPAARC community-based studies, 176
- during WWII, 87

residency program
- in 1949, *93*
- in 1953, *95*
- in 1970s, 111-12
- in 1990s, 164
- in COPE program, 147
- financial support for, 175-6
- food vouchers, 83
- Keating Outstanding Resident Award, 119
- lab work, 154
- women, *83*, 97, 148

resident exchange program, 74, 82, 83
respiratory care, *134*, 164
restructuring in 1993, 152
Rhee, Edward, *169*
Rheumatic Fever Program, 95
rheumatology department, 145
Riddle, Brandon, *126*
Ridge Farm, 47, 48, 57, 66, *67*, 70, 75, *87*, 89
Rieper, Rose, 88
Riley, Ruth, 182, 183
Rimoin, David, 115, 183
Ricoh, David, 85
Roam, Alice, *135*
Robert Wood Johnson Foundation, 170
Roberson, Helene B., 163
Robertson, Rev. C.F., 7, 13
Robertson Tyler, *150*
Robinson, G. Canby, 32, 41, 47
Robson, Alan M., 109, 124, 126-7

Roche, Maurice, 88
Rockefeller Foundation, 85
Rockefeller Institute, 59
Rodgers, Denise, *134*
Rogers, Lucious, 146
Rohlfing, Edwin H., 47
Roper, Charles, 101
Rose, Cora Lee King, *114*
Rosenbaum, Joan, *144*
Rosenberg, Charles E., 25
Rotch, Thomas M., 28
Roth, Hattie, 26
Rothbaum, Robert, 150
Rothman, Steven, *155*
Rubin, Mitchell I., 182
Rumfelt, Janice McKiernan, *129*, *135*
Rupe, Wayne A., 62, 83
Ruprecht, Charles M., 113
Russell, Alexander, 37, 38

S
Sachs, Ernest, 73
Safe Kids campaign, 170
Saigh Foundation, 173
Salmon, George, 88
Sansoucie, Krista, *118*
Santiago, Julio V., 118, *142*, 145, 155
scarlet fever, 9, 74
Schears, Gregory J., 147
Schlaggar, Bradley, 162
Schloemann, Johanna, 181
Schloss, Oscar, 58, 60, 62-3
Schmidt, Irene, *88*
Schmitz, Guy, 106
Schnuck, Donald O., *124*, 127, *139*, 164, 183
Schnuck, Doris, 139, 183
Schoendienst, Red, 156
Schoenecker, Perry, 109
scholarships, 171
Scholtis, Thomas, *181*
schools. *See* education
Schreiner, Richard L., 112, 119, 182
Schwab, Sidney, 57, 67
Schwartz, Alan L., 108, 144, 145, 148, *155*, 161, 162, 163-6, 169, *174*, 177, 179, 182, 183
Schwartz, Alfred, 82
Schwartz, Henry G., 88
Schwartz, Kathleen B., 119
Schwartzman, Bernard, 87
Scott, Wendell, 98
Scoville, Janet, *91*
Second Century Banquet, 108
Seilheimer, Dan K., 119
Senn, Milton J., 182
Senturia, Ben H., 82
Seper, Maureen, *134*
70th anniversary celebration, *93*
Sgarlata, Norine, *135*
Shackelford, Penelope G., 119, 160, *161*, 163

Shaffer, Philip A., 52, *53*, 61, 62, 71-2, *76-7*, 85
Shahan, William E., 66
Shapiro, Larry J., 111, 112, 119, 173, *176*, 182, 183
Shapiro, Steven D., 163
Sharifi, Mustafa, 126
Sharifi, Rafik, 126
Sharkey, Angela, 148, *170*
Shearer, William T., *118*, 119, 120, 125
Sheehan, Michael B., 119
Shenoy, Surenda, 150
Shi H. Huang Professor of Neurological Surgery, 165
Shields, John, 101
Shriners Hospital, 153
sickle cell disease, 148, 176
Simmons, Carrie, 31
Simmons, E.C., 31
Simons, Paul, *156*
Singer, James W. Jr., 97, 101, 183
Singh, Gautam, *172*
6 Westmoreland Place, 33
Skelton, Red, 132
skin grafts, 68
Sklamberg, Todd, 172, 174
Skrainka, Brian, 165
Slaughter, Enos, 98
Sluder, Greenfield, 43
Sly, William S., 115, *123*, 125
Small Talk, 84, 95, 96, 131-2
Smith, Carl H., 165, 176
Smith, Job Lewis, 8, 27
Smith, Margaret G., 75, 83, *105*
Smith, Richard, 107
Smyth, F. Scott, 74
Sneider, Martin K., 160, 183
Snerdlihc, 180
Snyder, Rev. John, 19, 20, 23
So, Samuel S.K., 152
Social Service Department, 44-5, 48, 70-1, 75
social service work, 73, 107, 130
social work department, *139*
Society for Pediatric Research, 182
Somogyi, Michael, 76, *77*
Spahr, Mary, 73
Spalding, Lucille S., 131
Spencer, Selden, 43
Spencer T. and Ann W. Olin Distinguished Professor, 111
Spencer T. and Ann W. Olin Foundation, 124
Spoehrer, Harriet Baur, *115*, 116, 143, 163, 183
Spoehrer, Hermann F., 115, 116
Spoehrer, Jane Baur, *115*, 171
Spoehrer Tower, 107, 115, 116, 123, 151, 172
Spray, Thomas, *150*, 151-2
Springfield Hospital, 153
St. Geme, Joseph, III, 163, 179, 182
St. Jude Children's Research Hospital, *141-2*

St. Louis
- in 1874, 5
- child welfare in, 73
- mortality rates in, 9-10, 73
- pollution in 1800s, *8*, 9
- population in late 1800s, 9

St. Louis Blues, 116
St. Louis Business Journal, 140
St. Louis Cardinals, 98, 116, 132, *152*, 156
St. Louis Children's Hospital
- dedication of staff, 181
- excellence recognized, 149-50, 171, 172, 178 (*See also* awards received)
- faculty/staff notable achievements, 182-3
- first patients, 12
- five-year strategic plan (2000), 173
- founding of, 4-8, 11-12
- future, challenges of, 180-1
- mission statement, 145, 172, 180-1
- motto, 43
- naming of, 8
- rating, 31
- restructuring in 1993, 152

St. Louis Children's Hospital buildings
- first building, *1-2*, 12
- second building (1884), *17-18*, 19, *21*, *22*, 47
- third building (1915), 33, *34-5*, 43-4, 45-6, 49, *49-50*
- expansion in 1920s, *71*, 72
- expansion in 1948-1952, *78-9*, 91-5
- expansion in 1960s, 98-9, *102-3*
- expansion in 1980s, 119, *120-3*, *124*, 126-7, *136-9*
- expansion in 1990s, 151-2, *153*, 162-3
- expansion/renovation plans 2004-06, *158-9*, 173, 174-5, *178*
- wards, *18*, *23*, *26*, *51*, *60*, *66*, *69*, *133*

St. Louis Children's Hospital Foundation, 152, 170, 175, 178
St. Louis Children's Pediatric Physician Hospital Organization (PPHO), 148
St. Louis City Hospital, 83
St. Louis Community Chest, 92
St. Louis Globe-Democrat
- account of visit to children, 74
- on cystic fibrosis clinic, 127
- fund-raising, 69
- on heart-lung pump, 101
- on infant mortality, 9-10
- on NICU nurses, 119
- on proposed expansion (1976-84), 121-2, *123*
- on skin grafts, 68
- on SLCH, 74

St. Louis Maternity Hospital, 63, 116
St. Louis Medical College, 24
St. Louis Medical Society, 11
St. Louis Mercy Hospital, 83
St. Louis Metropolitan Pediatric Council, 167

St. Louis Periscope, 14
St. Louis Post-Dispatch
  on devotion of nursing staff, 135
  on expansion (1976-79), 121-2, 123
  fund-raising after fire, 24
  Marriott on infant care and feeding, 70
  on O'Connell, Elizabeth, 132
  on Park White, 90
  on sulfa drugs, *86*
St. Louis Society for Crippled Children, 95
St. Louis Star, 74
St. Luke's Hospital, 152-3
Stahl, Philip, *139*
Stallings, Minnola, 73
Stangler, Gary J., 169
Stark, Ann R., 119
Stechenberg, Barbara W., 119
Steele, Aaron J., 23, 24
Stein, A. Ernest, 118
Stein, Jane G., 118
sterilizing room (1890s), *21*
Stevenson, Virginia, 6, 7, 8, 12, 51, 74
Stimson, Julia, 44-5, *48*, *56*, *57*, 130, *131*
Stolar, Mary, 122
STOP (Steps to Prevent Violence), 168
Storch, Gregory, 149, 176
Strauss, Arnold W., 100, 101, 111, 119, *145*, 155, 161, 163, 166, 176, 179, 182
Streett, Rolla, 113, 183
Strominger, Donald, *127*
Strunk, Robert C., 127, 145, *146*, 148, 155, 176
Sudden Infant Death Syndrome, 145, 155
sulfa drugs, 86-7
surgery. *See also* transplant program
  in 1890s, 27
  in 1906-07, 37
  in 1911, *36*
  in 1920s, 69, *73*
  in 1984, 127
  Apolline Blair Professor of Surgery, *111*, 163
  Bixby Professor of Surgery, 66
  cochlear implants, 152, 166, 178
  expansion in 1990s, 152
  first woman surgical resident, 97
  for heart disease, 98
  heart-lung pump, *100-1*
  leeches and, 142
  neurosurgery staff, 146, 165
  new procedures in 1990s, 166
  operating rooms, *36*, *68*, *73*, *183*
  Shi H. Huang Professor of Neurological Surgery, 165
  "Short Stay Surgery" program, 127
  skin grafts, 68
  Ternberg, Jessie L., 110
  ward in 1890s, *25*
Sutherland, Matt, *178*
Sutherland, Zach, *178*
Sutton, Howie, 127

Swaine, Richard, 107
Swisher, Charles, 150
syphilis research, 67

T
Talve, Adina, 172
Talve, Rabbi Susan, 172
Tarr, Phillip I., 179
Taussig, Lynn M., 182, 183
technology
  in 1990s, 151
  in early 1900s, 29
  heart-lung pump, *100-1*
  Heart Station, 172
  incubators, *28*, *85*, 96
  iron lungs, 72, 75
  "rapidograph" X-ray technique, 98
  Shapiro, Larry on, 111
Ternberg, Jessie L., *97*, 98, 133, 156
Terry, Robert, 27
tetany, 53
Texauer, Gloria, 87
Thach, Bradley T., *145*
therapy services gym, *178*
Theron Catlin fellowships, 82
Thio, K. Liu Lin, 162
Thomas, Danny, 142
Thornton, Jack, 87-8
Throop, George R., 52, 75, 82
Thurston, Donald L., 97-8, 106, *107*, 142
Thurston, Jean Holowach, 88, 98
Thurston's Cocktail, 142
Tice, Norman J., 143
Tillman, Mary Anne, *141*, 147
Toan, Barrett, 143
Todd, Howard, 150
Todd, Richard, 163
toddler's ward, *133*
Tolin, C. Alvin, 111, *113*, 114, 117, 118-19, *120*, 124, 125, 126, 127, 183
tornado hits SLCH, 97
Toverud, Svein Utheim, 65
Tower Building, 107, 115, 116, 123, 151, 172
transplant program
  bone marrow, 150, 151
  cornea, 150
  enlarged in 1990s, 151-3
  heart, 150, 166, *174*
  international prominence, 150
  intestines, 150
  kidney, 150
  liver, *126*, 150, 165, 166, 176
  lung, 150, 166, 178
thymus, 118
Transport Team, *180*
Treat, Caroline, 8, 12
Treat, Samuel, 8, 12
Tremblath, Morgan, *179*
Trevino, Lee, 116
Turnbaugh, Billy, *107*

Turner, Jayla, *162*
Tuttle, George M., *41*, *42*, 43, 46, 50
Tuttle, Rev. Daniel S., 50
Twain, Mark, 9
21st General Hospital at Fort Benning, 86
"Twigs," 114, 116, 143
Tychsen, Lawrence, 146
Tyrala, Eileen E., 119

U
Uhrig's Cave, 27
Unanue, Emil, 141
United Way, 114
U.S. News & World Report, 149, 171, 172, 173, 178
Utheim, Kirsten, *64*, 65

V
Vallé, Isabel, 32
Vallero, Betty, 134, 135
Van Reken, David V., 119
Veeder, Borden Smith, 36, 44, 47, 49, 52, 53, *56*, *57*, 58, 60, 67, 72, 182
vice chancellor for medical affairs, 106
Victorian Society in America, 122
Vietti, Teresa J., *91*, 106, 129, *154*
visiting hours, 135
Volpe, Joseph J., 110, 118, 144, 155, 183
volunteers. *See also* Auxiliary
  in 1950s, 97
  in 1990s, 171
  Jane Baur Spoehrer, 115
  physicians, international work, 170
  staff members in WWI, 57
  teen-aged, 98, *106*

W
W. McKim Marriott Professor of Pediatrics, 119, 163
Waldman, Meyer, 90
Waldman, Regina, 90, *91*
Walker, George S., 7, 11, 21, 30
Wallace, Harry, *93*
Walton, Franklin, 88
Waltz, Sally, 152
Wannamaker, Lewis, 107
Ward, Lewis Larrick, 179
Washington University
  affiliation of SLCH with, 28
  and Missouri Medical College, 28
  and new SLCH building (1980s), 124
  and SLCH advisory committee, 8
  and St. Louis Medical College, 24
Washington University Family HIV Clinic, 149
Washington University Hospital, 39-40
Washington University Medical Care Group Health Plan, 120

Washington University Medical Center (WUMC), 117
Washington University Pediatric and Adolescent Research Consortium (WUPAARC), 176
Washington University Physician Network (WUPN), 165
Washington University School of Medicine. *See also* Department of Pediatrics
  Children's Discovery Institute, *176*, 177-8
  dedication, 50
  ethics class, 66
  faculty/staff notable achievements, 182-3
  GEB grants, 49, 59-60
  initial funding for, 49
  national ranking, 173
  pediatric curriculum, 62
  planning/vision for, 38-40
  post-graduate courses (1920s), 63
  woman on faculty, 64, 65
  women students, 64, 83
  WU Dean Edward Dempsey, *104*
Washington University School of Nursing, 129, *130*
"Waste and Waits" program, 165
Watkins, John B., 146
Webb, Gabriel, 150
Weeks, Paul, 110
Weil, Laura, 26, 47
Weiner, Meyer, 67
Weiss, Dorothy Wilkes, 74
Welch, William H., 50, 58, 60
Weldon, Virginia B., 110, 118
Wells, Evan, *174*
Wells, Jane, 74
Wells, Sam, 141
wet nurses, 62, 63
Wheeler, Claribel, 71
White, Andrew, *175*, 179
White, Harvey L., 73
White, Lynn, 166
White, Neil, 163, 176
White, Park J., 53, 66, 73, 75, 83, 87, 89, *90*, 92, 99, *141*, 147, 163, *168*
Whitehorn, John, 85
Whitener, Betty, *135*
Whitney, Caroline, 73
whooping cough, 9
Wightman, Orrin S. Jr., *106*, *107*, 183
Wilson, David B., 163
Wilson, Larry, 116
Wilson's Disease, 161
Wolff, Patricia B., 147, 156, *157*, *170*, 171
women
  as division directors, 180
  first woman chief resident, *83*
  first woman surgical resident, 97
  in medical school, 64, 83
  on medical school faculty, 64
  as physicians, 64, 72, 73, 83, 148, 156

Women's Association of Ladue Chapel, 114
Wood, Anna L., 37, 129
Wood, Neal, 113, 114, 183
Wool, Gerald, 156, *157*
World War I, *56-7*, 130, *131*
World War II, *86*, 87-9, 130-1
Worthington, Dorothy, 73
Wright, Mary, *65*
Wuller, Mike, 140
Wultmann, Hulda, 156

Y
Yeatman, James, 6, 7, 8, 19-20, 21
Yesley, Grace, *133*
Young, John, 87

Z
Zahorsky, John, *28*, 43
Zentay, Paul, 82
Zueschel, Cathy, *133*

This book was typeset using New Baskerville and News Gothic types and printed on Lustro Patina text with end sheets on Rainbow Endleaf – Gold. Printed by Garlich Printing Company in St. Louis, Missouri, using a Heidelberg CD 102S+LX 6-color press in an edition of 5,600. Bound by BindTech, Inc. in Nashville, Tennessee. Designed by Scott and Laura Gericke of designlab,inc in Webster Groves, Missouri. SPRING 2006